Complementary and Alternative Medicine

Complementary and Alternative Medicine

Edited by
Pedro Cahill

Larsen & Keller
www.larsen-keller.com

Complementary and Alternative Medicine
Edited by Pedro Cahill
ISBN: 978-1-63549-071-8 (Hardback)

Larsen & Keller

Published by Larsen and Keller Education,
5 Penn Plaza,
19th Floor,
New York, NY 10001, USA

Cataloging-in-Publication Data

Complementary and alternative medicine / edited by Pedro Cahill.
p. cm.
Includes bibliographical references and index.
ISBN 978-1-63549-071-8
1. Alternative medicine. 2. Medicine. 3. Traditional medicine.
4. Integrative medicine.
I. Cahill, Pedro.
R733 .C66 2017
615.5--dc23

The publisher's policy is to use permanent paper from mills that operate a sustainable forestry policy. Furthermore, the publisher ensures that the text paper and cover boards used have met acceptable environmental accreditation standards.

Printed and bound in China.

For more information regarding Larsen and Keller Education and its products, please visit the publisher's website www.larsen-keller.com

Table of Contents

Preface

Alternative medicine comprise of those medicinal and healing practices that do not follow medical diagnosis for intervention and treatment. They are based on local or traditional belief systems and have slow effects. This textbook will explain in detail the diverse methods of treatment that exist in alternate medicine. It will also elaborate on the different types of techniques used under this field. The topics included in this text on complementary and alternative medicine are of utmost significance and are bound to provide incredible insights to readers. Those in search of information to further their knowledge will be greatly assisted by this textbook.

To facilitate a deeper understanding of the contents of this book a short introduction of every chapter is written below:

Chapter 1- Alternative medicine is not science based and has no proven healing effect on patients. In fact, alternative medicines are disapproved of and have at times proven to be very harmful. The chapter on complementary and alternative medicine offers an insightful focus, keeping in mind the subject matter.

Chapter 2- Naturopathy is one of the forms of alternative medicines; it includes homeopathy, ozone therapy and acupuncture. The practice of naturopathy is considered harmful by many, as it not evidence based medicine. The following section will not only provide an overview, it will also delve deep into the topics related to it.

Chapter 3- Anthroposophic medicine includes treatment techniques such as massages, exercises and counseling. It tends to explain health and natural medicine in terms of spirituality and science both. The philosophy behind anthroposophic medicine is known as anthroposophy. This text will provide an integrated understanding of anthroposophic medicine.

Chapter 4- Homeopathy is a form of alternative medicine. They are scientifically not considered effective for treating any condition. Some of the aspects of homeopathy that have been discussed are homeopathic dilutions, electrohomeopathy, arsenicum album and regulation and prevalence of homeopathy. The topics discussed in the section are of great importance to broaden the existing knowledge on homeopathy.

Chapter 5- Ayurveda medicine has its roots in the Indian history. The plants used in Ayurveda are Azadirachta indica, Cedrus deodara, Terminalia arjuna and Phyllanthus emblica. This text has been carefully written to provide an easy understanding of the varied facets of Ayurveda.

Chapter 6- The use of plants for the purpose of medicine is termed as herbalism. It also, at times, includes fungal and bee products. This chapter focuses on the history of herbalism and also lists herbs with known adverse effects. In order to completely understand herbalism, it is necessary to understand the theories and approaches related to herbalism.

Chapter 7- Osteopathy focuses on massages and other physical manipulation of muscle tissues. Craniosacral therapy is a form of alternative therapy that is used in gently manipulating the joints of the cranium. Muscle energy technique, joint manipulation, osteopathic manipulative medicine and osteopathic medicine in the United States have been explained in the following chapter.

Chapter 8- Chiropractic is one of the many forms of alternative medicine. It helps in the curing of the disorders of the musculoskeletal system. This treatment majorly uses manipulation of the spine. The safety of this treatment has been debated as it certainly has adverse effects, and can also cause death in rare cases. The section focuses on the use of the chiropractic treatment and helps the readers in understanding the effects of this treatment.

Chapter 9- The evolution of alternative medicine focuses on the history of alternative medicine and the progress it has made in the last few decades. The users of alternative medicine believe it has healing effects, but these claims have not been proved scientifically. The following chapter carefully analysis the evolution of alternative medicine and provides an extensive understanding of the subject.

I owe the completion of this book to the never-ending support of my family, who supported me throughout the project.

Editor

1

Introduction to Complementary and Alternative Medicine

Alternative medicine is not science based and has no proven healing effect on patients. In fact, alternative medicines are disapproved of and have at times proven to be very harmful. The chapter on complementary and alternative medicine offers an insightful focus, keeping in mind the subject matter.

Alternative Medicine

Alternative medicine or fringe medicine are practices claimed to have the healing effects of medicine but are disproven, unproven, impossible to prove, or only harmful. Alternative therapies or diagnoses are not part of medicine or science-based healthcare systems. Alternative medicine consists of a wide variety of practices, products, and therapies—ranging from those that are biologically plausible but not well tested, to those with known harmful and toxic effects. Contrary to popular belief, significant expense is paid in testing alternative medicine, including over $2.5 billion spent by the United States government, with almost none showing any effect beyond that of false treatment. Perceived effects of alternative medicine are caused by placebo, decreased effects of functional treatment (and therefor also decreased side-effects), and regression toward the mean where improvement that would have occurred anyway is credited to alternative therapies. Alternative medicine is not the same as experimental medicine.

Alternative medicine has grown in popularity and is used by a significant percentage of the population in many countries. While it has extensively rebranded itself: from quackery to complementary or integrative medicine—it promotes essentially the same practices. Newer proponents often suggest alternative medicine be used together with functional medical treatment, in a belief that it "complements" (improves the effect of) the treatment. However, significant drug interactions caused by alternative therapies may instead negatively influence treatments, making them less effective, notably cancer therapy. Despite it being illegal to market alternative therapies for cancer treatment in most of the developed world, many cancer patients use it.

Alternative medical diagnoses and treatments are not included in the science-based curriculum taught in medical schools, and are not used in medical practice where treatments are based on scientific knowledge. Alternative therapies are often based on religion, tradition, superstition, belief in supernatural energies, pseudoscience, errors in reasoning, propaganda, or fraud. Regulation and licensing of alternative medicine and health care providers varies between and within countries.

Alternative medicine has been criticized for being based on misleading statements, quackery, pseudoscience, antiscience, fraud, or poor scientific methodology. Promoting alternative medicine has been called dangerous and unethical. Testing alternative medicine that have no scientific basis has been called a waste of scarce medical research resources. Critics have said "there is really no such thing as alternative medicine, just medicine that works and medicine that doesn't", and the problem is not only that it does not work, but that the "underlying logic is magical, childish or downright absurd". There have also been calls that the concept of any alternative medicine that works is paradoxical, as any treatment proven to work is simply "medicine".

Appeal

Practitioners of complementary medicine usually discuss and advise patients as to available alternative therapies. Patients often express interest in mind-body complementary therapies because they offer a non-drug approach to treating some health conditions.

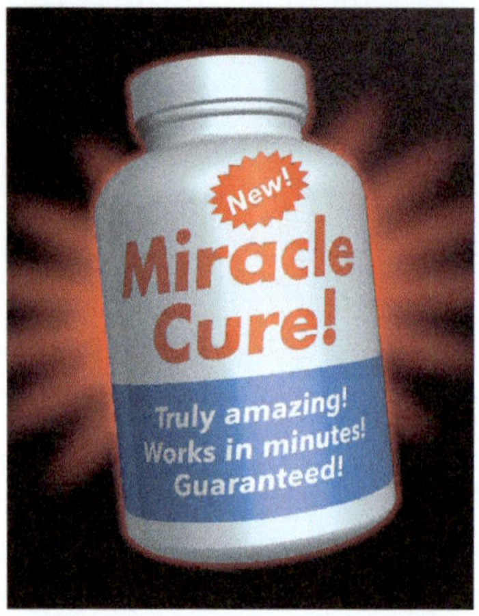

Alternative therapies often make bombastic claims, and frequently include anecdotes from healthy-looking individuals claiming successful treatment.

In addition to the social-cultural underpinnings of the popularity of alternative medicine, there are several psychological issues that are critical to its growth. One of the most critical is the placebo effect—a well-established observation in medicine. Related to it are similar psychological effects, such as the will to believe, cognitive biases that help maintain self-esteem and promote harmonious social functioning, and the *post hoc, ergo propter hoc* fallacy.

Marketing

CAM's popularity may be related to other factors that Edzard Ernst mentioned in an interview in *The Independent*:

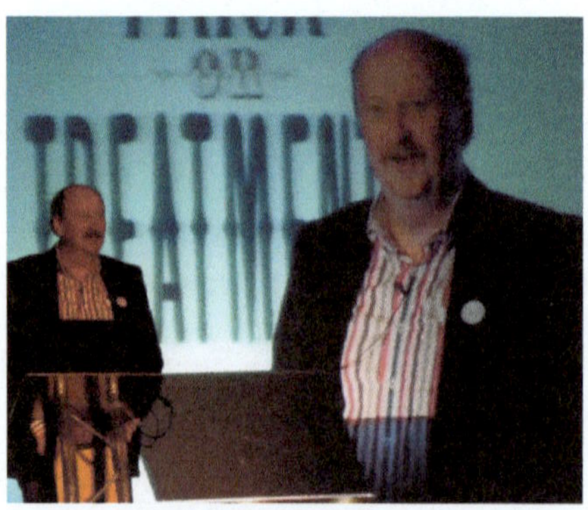

Edzard Ernst in 2012

Why is it so popular, then? Ernst blames the providers, customers and the doctors whose neglect, he says, has created the opening into which alternative therapists have stepped. “People are told lies. There are 40 million websites and 39.9 million tell lies, sometimes outrageous lies. They mislead cancer patients, who are encouraged not only to pay their last penny but to be treated with something that shortens their lives. “At the same time, people are gullible. It needs gullibility for the industry to succeed. It doesn’t make me popular with the public, but it’s the truth.

Paul Offit proposed that “alternative medicine becomes quackery” in four ways: by recommending against conventional therapies that are helpful, promoting potentially harmful therapies without adequate warning, draining patients’ bank accounts, or by promoting “magical thinking.”

A Failure of Mainstream Medicine

In a paper published in October 2010 entitled *The public’s enthusiasm for complementary and alternative medicine amounts to a critique of mainstream medicine*, Ernst described these views in greater detail and concluded:

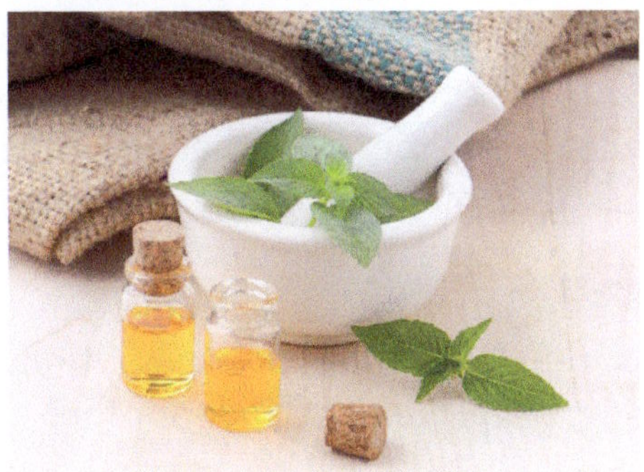

Friendly and colorful images of herbal treatments may look less threatening or dangerous when compared to conventional medicine. This is an intentional marketing strategy.

[CAM] is popular. An analysis of the reasons why this is so points towards the therapeutic relationship as a key factor. Providers of CAM tend to build better therapeutic relationships than mainstream healthcare professionals. In turn, this implies that much of the popularity of CAM is a poignant criticism of the failure of mainstream healthcare. We should consider it seriously with a view of improving our service to patients.

Social Factors

Authors have speculated on the socio-cultural and psychological reasons for the appeal of alternative medicines among the minority using them *in lieu* of conventional medicine. There are several socio-cultural reasons for the interest in these treatments centered on the low level of scientific literacy among the public at large and a concomitant increase in antiscientific attitudes and new age mysticism. Related to this are vigorous marketing of extravagant claims by the alternative medical community combined with inadequate media scrutiny and attacks on critics.

There is also an increase in conspiracy theories toward conventional medicine and pharmaceutical companies, mistrust of traditional authority figures, such as the physician, and a dislike of the current delivery methods of scientific biomedicine, all of which have led patients to seek out alternative medicine to treat a variety of ailments. Many patients lack access to contemporary medicine, due to a lack of private or public health insurance, which leads them to seek out lower-cost alternative medicine. Medical doctors are also aggressively marketing alternative medicine to profit from this market.

Patients can be averse to the painful, unpleasant, and sometimes-dangerous side effects of biomedical treatments. Treatments for severe diseases such as cancer and HIV infection have well-known, significant side-effects. Even low-risk medications such as antibiotics can have potential to cause life-threatening anaphylactic reactions in a very few individuals. Many medications may cause minor but bothersome symptoms such as cough or upset stomach. In all of these cases, patients may be seeking out alternative treatments to avoid the adverse effects of conventional treatments.

Definitions and Terminology

Alternative Medicine

It is loosely as a defined set of products, practices, and theories that are believed or perceived by their users to have the healing effects of medicine, but whose effectiveness has not been clearly established using scientific methods, and whose theory and practice is not part of biomedicine, or whose theories or practices are directly contradicted by scientific evidence or scientific principles used in biomedicine. "Biomedicine" or "medicine" is that part of medical science that applies principles of biology, physiology, molecular biology, biophysics, and other natural sciences to clinical practice, using scientific methods to establish the effectiveness of that practice. Unlike medicine, an alternative product or practice does not originate from using scientific methodology, but may instead be based on testimonials, religion, tradition, superstition, belief in supernatural energies, pseudoscience, errors in reasoning, propaganda, fraud, or other unscientific sources.

In *General Guidelines for Methodologies on Research and Evaluation of Traditional Medicine*, published in 2000 by the World Health Organization (WHO), complementary and alternative medicine were defined as a broad set of health care practices that are not part of that country's own tradition and are not integrated into the dominant health care system.

The expression also refers to a diverse range of related and unrelated products, practices, and theories ranging from biologically plausible practices and products and practices with some evidence, to practices and theories that are directly contradicted by basic science or clear evidence, and products that have been conclusively proven to be ineffective or even toxic and harmful.

The terms-*Alternative medicine, complementary medicine, integrative medicine, holistic medicine, natural medicine, unorthodox medicine, fringe medicine, unconventional medicine,* and *new age medicine* are used interchangeably as having the same meaning and are almost synonymous in some contexts, but may have different meanings in some rare cases.

The meaning of the term "alternative" in the expression "alternative medicine", is not that it is an effective alternative to medical science, although some alternative medicine promoters may use the loose terminology to give the appearance of effectiveness. Loose terminology may also be used to suggest meaning that a dichotomy exists when it does not, e.g., the use of the expressions "western medicine" and "eastern medicine" to suggest that the difference is a cultural difference between the Asiatic east and the European west, rather than that the difference is between evidence-based medicine and treatments that don't work.

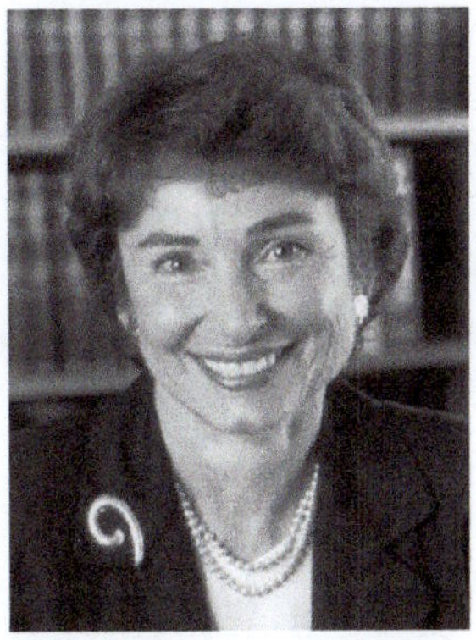

Marcia Angell: "There cannot be two kinds of medicine — conventional and alternative".

Complementary/Integrative Medicine

Complementary medicine (CM) or integrative medicine (IM) is when alternative medicine is used together with functional medical treatment, in a belief that it improves the effect of treatments. However, significant drug interactions caused by alternative therapies may instead negatively influence treatment, making treatments less effective, notably cancer therapy. Both terms refer to use of alternative medical treatments alongside conventional medicine, an example of which is use of acupuncture (sticking needles in the body to influence the flow of a supernatural energy), along with using science-based medicine, in the belief that the acupuncture increases the effectiveness or "complements" the science-based medicine.

Allopathic Medicine

Allopathic medicine or allopathy is an expression commonly used by homeopaths and proponents of other forms of alternative medicine to refer to mainstream medicine. Specifically it refers to the use of pharmacologically active agents or physical interventions to treat or suppress symptoms or pathophysiologic processes of diseases or conditions. The expression was coined in 1810 by the creator of homeopathy, Samuel Hahnemann (1755–1843). In such circles, the expression "allopathic medicine" is still used to refer to "the broad category of medical practice that is sometimes called Western medicine, biomedicine, evidence-based medicine, or modern medicine".

Use of the term remains common among homeopaths and has spread to other alternative medicine practices. The meaning implied by the label has never been accepted by conventional medicine and is considered pejorative. More recently, some sources have used the term "allopathic", particularly American sources wishing to distinguish between Doctors of Medicine (MD) and Doctors of Osteopathic Medicine (DO) in the United States. William Jarvis, an expert on alternative medicine and public health, states that "although many modern therapies can be construed to conform to an allopathic rationale (e.g., using a laxative to relieve constipation), standard medicine has never paid allegiance to an allopathic principle" and that the label "allopath" was from the start "considered highly derisive by regular medicine".

Many conventional medical treatments clearly do not fit the nominal definition of allopathy, as they seek to prevent illness, or remove the cause of an illness by acting on the etiology of disease.

CAM

CAM is an abbreviation of complementary and alternative medicine. It has also been called sCAM or SCAM with the addition of "so-called" or "supplements". The words balance and holism are often used, claiming to take into account a "whole" person, in contrast to the supposed reductionism of medicine. Due to its many names the field has been criticized for intense rebranding of what are essentially the same practices: as soon as one name is declared synonymous with quackery, a new name is chosen.

Traditional Medicine

It refers to the pre-scientific practices of a culture, contrary to what is traditionally practiced in cultures where medical science dominates.

"Eastern medicine" typically refers to the traditional medicines of Asia where conventional bio-medicine penetrated much later.

Problems with Definition

Prominent members of the science and biomedical science community assert that it is not meaningful to define an alternative medicine that is separate from a conventional medicine, that the expressions "conventional medicine", "alternative medicine", "complementary medicine", "integrative medicine", and "holistic medicine" do not refer to any medicine at all.

Others in both the biomedical and CAM communities point out that CAM *cannot* be precisely defined because of the diversity of theories and practices it includes, and because the boundaries between CAM and biomedicine overlap, are porous, and change. The expression "complementary and alternative medicine" (CAM) resists easy definition because the health systems and practices it refers to are diffuse, and its boundaries poorly defined. Healthcare practices categorized as alternative may differ in their historical origin, theoretical basis, diagnostic technique, therapeutic practice and in their relationship to the medical mainstream. Some alternative therapies, including traditional Chinese medicine (TCM) and Ayurveda, have antique origins in East or South Asia and are entirely alternative medical systems; others, such as homeopathy and chiropractic, have origins in Europe or the United States and emerged in the eighteenth and nineteenth centuries. Some, such as osteopathy and chiropractic, employ manipulative physical methods of treatment; others, such as meditation and prayer, are based on mind-body interventions. Treatments considered alternative in one location may be considered conventional in another. Thus, chiropractic is not considered alternative in Denmark and likewise osteopathic medicine is no longer thought of as an alternative therapy in the United States.

Critics say the expression is deceptive because it implies there is an effective alternative to science-based medicine, and that *complementary* is deceptive because it implies that the treatment increases the effectiveness of (complements) science-based medicine, while alternative medicines that have been tested nearly always have no measurable positive effect compared to a placebo.

Different Types of Definitions

One common feature of all definitions of alternative medicine is its designation as "other than" conventional medicine. For example, the widely referenced descriptive definition of complementary and alternative medicine devised by the US National Center for Complementary and Integrative Health (NCCIH) of the National Institutes of Health (NIH), states that it is "a group of diverse medical and health care systems, practices, and products that are not generally considered part of conventional medicine." For conventional medical practitioners, it does not necessarily follow that either it or its practitioners would no longer be considered alternative.

Some definitions seek to specify alternative medicine in terms of its social and political marginality to mainstream healthcare. This can refer to the lack of support that alternative therapies receive from the medical establishment and related bodies regarding access to research funding, sympathetic coverage in the medical press, or inclusion in the standard medical curriculum. In 1993, the British Medical Association (BMA), one among many professional organizations who have attempted to define alternative medicine, stated that it referred to "...those forms of treatment which are not widely used by the conventional healthcare professions, and the skills of which are not taught as part of the undergraduate curriculum of conventional medical and paramedical healthcare courses." In a US context, an influential definition coined in 1993 by the Harvard-based physician, David M. Eisenberg, characterized alternative medicine "as interventions neither taught widely in medical schools nor generally available in US hospitals". These descriptive definitions are inadequate in the present-day when some conventional doctors offer alternative medical treatments and CAM introductory courses or modules can be offered as part of standard undergraduate medical training; alternative medicine is taught in more than 50 per cent of US medical schools and increasingly US health insurers are willing to provide reimbursement for CAM therapies. In 1999, 7.7% of US hospitals reported using some form of CAM therapy; this proportion had risen to 37.7% by 2008.

An expert panel at a conference hosted in 1995 by the US Office for Alternative Medicine (OAM), devised a theoretical definition of alternative medicine as "a broad domain of healing resources ... other than those intrinsic to the politically dominant health system of a particular society or culture in a given historical period." This definition has been widely adopted by CAM researchers, cited by official government bodies such as the UK Department of Health, attributed as the definition used by the Cochrane Collaboration, and, with some modification, was preferred in the 2005 consensus report of the US Institute of Medicine, *Complementary and Alternative Medicine in the United States.*

The 1995 OAM conference definition, an expansion of Eisenberg's 1993 formulation, is silent regarding questions of the medical effectiveness of alternative therapies. Its proponents hold that it thus avoids relativism about differing forms of medical knowledge and, while it is an essentially political definition, this should not imply that the dominance of mainstream biomedicine is solely due to political forces. According to this definition, alternative and mainstream medicine can only be differentiated with reference to what is "intrinsic to the politically dominant health system of a particular society of culture". However, there is neither a reliable method to distinguish between cultures and subcultures, nor to attribute them as dominant or subordinate, nor any accepted criteria to determine the dominance of a cultural entity. If the culture of a politically dominant healthcare system is held to be equivalent to the perspectives of those charged with the medical management of leading healthcare institutions and programs, the definition fails to recognize the potential for division either within such an elite or between a healthcare elite and the wider population.

Normative definitions distinguish alternative medicine from the biomedical mainstream in its provision of therapies that are unproven, unvalidated, or ineffective and support of theories with no recognized scientific basis. These definitions characterize practices as constituting alternative medicine when, used independently or in place of evidence-based medicine, they are put forward as having the healing effects of medicine, but are not based on evidence gathered with the scientific method. Exemplifying this perspective, a 1998 editorial co-authored by Marcia Angell, a former editor of the *New England Journal of Medicine*, argued that:

> "It is time for the scientific community to stop giving alternative medicine a free ride. There cannot be two kinds of medicine – conventional and alternative. There is only medicine that has been adequately tested and medicine that has not, medicine that works and medicine that may or may not work. Once a treatment has been tested rigorously, it no longer matters whether it was considered alternative at the outset. If it is found to be reasonably safe and effective, it will be accepted. But assertions, speculation, and testimonials do not substitute for evidence. Alternative treatments should be subjected to scientific testing no less rigorous than that required for conventional treatments."

This line of division has been subject to criticism, however, as not all forms of standard medical practice have adequately demonstrated evidence of benefit, and it is also unlikely in most instances that conventional therapies, if proven to be ineffective, would ever be classified as CAM.

Similarly, the public information website maintained by the National Health and Medical Research Council (NHMRC) of the Commonwealth of Australia uses the acronym "CAM" for a wide range of health care practices, therapies, procedures and devices not within the domain of conventional medicine. In the Australian context this is stated to include acupuncture; aromatherapy; chiropractic; homeopathy; massage; meditation and relaxation therapies; naturopathy; osteopathy; reflexology, traditional Chinese medicine; and the use of vitamin supplements.

The Danish National Board of Health's "Council for Alternative Medicine" (Sundhedsstyrelsens Råd for Alternativ Behandling (SRAB)), an independent institution under the National Board of Health (Danish: *Sundhedsstyrelsen*), uses the term "alternative medicine" for:

- Treatments performed by therapists that are not authorized healthcare professionals.
- Treatments performed by authorized healthcare professionals, but those based on methods otherwise used mainly outside the healthcare system. People without a healthcare authorisation are [also] allowed to perform the treatments.

Proponents of an evidence-base for medicine such as the Cochrane Collaboration (founded in 1993 and from 2011 providing input for WHO resolutions) take a position that *all* systematic reviews of treatments, whether "mainstream" or "alternative", ought to be held to the current standards of scientific method. In a study titled *Development and classification of an operational definition of complementary and alternative medicine for the Cochrane Collaboration* (2011) it was proposed that indicators that a therapy is accepted include government licensing of practitioners, coverage by health insurance, statements of approval by government agencies, and recommendation as part of a practice guideline; and that if something is currently a standard, accepted therapy, then it is not likely to be widely considered as CAM.

NCCIH Classification

A United States government agency, the National Center on Complementary and Integrative Health (NCCIH), created its own classification system for branches of complementary and alternative medicine that divides them into five major groups. These groups have some overlap, and distinguish two types of energy medicine: *veritable* which involves scientifically observable energy (including magnet therapy, colorpuncture and light therapy) and *putative*, which invokes physically undetectable or unverifiable energy.

The NCCIH classification system is -

1. Whole medical systems: Cut across more than one of the other groups; examples include traditional Chinese medicine, naturopathy, homeopathy, and ayurveda
2. Mind-body interventions: Explore the interconnection between the mind, body, and spirit, under the premise that the mind can affect "bodily functions and symptoms"
3. "Biology"-based practices: Use substances found in nature such as herbs, foods, vitamins, and other natural substances. (Note that as used here, "biology" does *not* refer to the science of biology, but is a usage newly coined by NCCIH in the primary source used for this article. "Biology-based" as coined by NCCIH may refer to chemicals from a nonbiological source, such as use of the poison lead in traditional Chinese medicine, and to other nonbiological substances.)
4. Manipulative and body-based practices: feature manipulation or movement of body parts, such as is done in chiropractic and osteopathic manipulation
5. Energy medicine: is a domain that deals with putative and verifiable energy fields:
    - Biofield therapies are intended to influence energy fields that, it is purported, surround and penetrate the body. No empirical evidence has been found to support the existence of the putative energy fields on which these therapies are predicated.
    - Bioelectromagnetic-based therapies use verifiable electromagnetic fields, such as pulsed fields, alternating-current, or direct-current fields in an unconventional manner.

Types

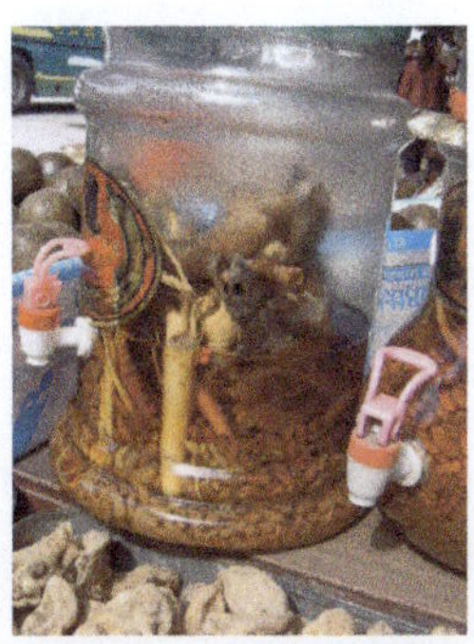

Ready-to-drink traditional Chinese medicine mixture

Alternative medicine consists of a wide range of health care practices, products, and therapies. The shared feature is a claim to heal that is not based on the scientific method. Alternative medicine practices are diverse in their foundations and methodologies. Alternative medicine practices may be classified by their cultural origins or by the types of beliefs upon which they are based. Methods may incorporate or be based on traditional medicinal practices of a particular culture, folk knowledge, supersition, spiritual beliefs, belief in supernatural energies (antiscience), pseudoscience, errors in reasoning, propaganda, fraud, new or different concepts of health and disease, and any bases other than being proven by scientific methods. Different cultures may have their own unique traditional or belief based practices developed recently or over thousands of years, and specific practices or entire systems of practices.

Unscientific Belief Systems

Alternative medicine, such as using naturopathy or homeopathy in place of conventional medicine, is based on belief systems not grounded in science.

	Proposed mechanism	Issues
Naturopathy	Naturopathic medicine is based on a belief that the body heals itself using a supernatural vital energy that guides bodily processes.	In conflict with the paradigm of evidence-based medicine. Many naturopaths have opposed vaccination, and "scientific evidence does not support claims that naturopathic medicine can cure cancer or any other disease".
Homeopathy	A belief that a substance that causes the symptoms of a disease in healthy people cures similar symptoms in sick people.	Developed before knowledge of atoms and molecules, or of basic chemistry, which shows that repeated dilution as practiced in homeopathy produces only water, and that homeopathy is not scientifically valid.

Traditional Ethnic Systems

Alternative medical systems may be based on traditional medicine practices, such as traditional Chinese medicine (TCM), Ayurveda in India, or practices of other cultures around the world. Some useful applications of traditional medicines have been researched and accepted within ordinary medicine, however the underlying belief systems are seldom scientific and are not accepted.

	Claims	Issues
Traditional Chinese medicine	Traditional practices and beliefs from China, together with modifications made by the Communist party make up TCM. Common practices include herbal medicine, acupuncture (insertion of needles in the body at specified points), massage (Tui na), exercise (qigong), and dietary therapy.	The practices are based on belief in a supernatural energy called qi, considerations of Chinese Astrology and Chinese numerology, traditional use of herbs and other substances found in China—a belief that the tongue contains a map of the body that reflects changes in the body, and an incorrect model of the anatomy and physiology of internal organs.
Ayurveda	Traditional medicine of India. Ayurveda believes in the existence of three elemental substances, the doshas (called Vata, Pitta and Kapha), and states that a balance of the doshas results in health, while imbalance results in disease. Such disease-inducing imbalances can be adjusted and balanced using traditional herbs, minerals and heavy metals. Ayurveda stresses the use of plant-based medicines and treatments, with some animal products, and added minerals, including sulfur, arsenic, lead, copper sulfate.	Safety concerns have been raised about Ayurveda, with two U.S. studies finding about 20 percent of Ayurvedic Indian-manufactured patent medicines contained toxic levels of heavy metals such as lead, mercury and arsenic. Other concerns include the use of herbs containing toxic compounds and the lack of quality control in Ayurvedic facilities. Incidents of heavy metal poisoning have been attributed to the use of these compounds in the United States.

Supernatural Energies

Bases of belief may include belief in existence of supernatural energies undetected by the science of physics, as in biofields, or in belief in properties of the energies of physics that are inconsistent with the laws of physics, as in energy medicine.

	Claims	Issues
Biofield therapy	Intended to influence energy fields that, it is purported, surround and penetrate the body.	Writers such as noted astrophysicist and advocate of skeptical thinking (Scientific skepticism) Carl Sagan (1934-1996) have described the lack of empirical evidence to support the existence of the putative energy fields on which these therapies are predicated.
Bioelectromagnetic therapy	Use verifiable electromagnetic fields, such as pulsed fields, alternating-current, or direct-current fields in an unconventional manner.	Asserts that magnets can be used to defy the laws of physics to influence health and disease.
Chiropractic	Spinal manipulation aims to treat "vertebral subluxations" which are claimed to put pressure on nerves.	Chiropractic was developed in the belief that manipulating the spine affects the flow of a supernatural vital energy and thereby affects health and disease. Vertebral subluxation is a pseudoscientific concept and has not been proven to exist.
Reiki	Practitioners place their palms on the patient near Chakras that they believe are centers of supernatural energies in the belief that these supernatural energies can transfer from the practitioner's palms to heal the patient.	

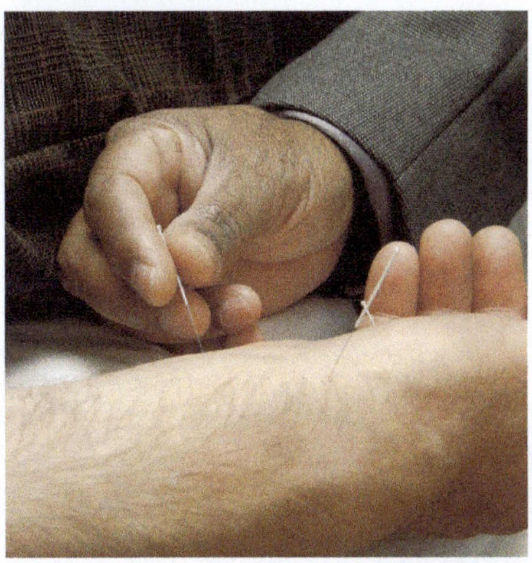

Acupuncture involves insertion of needles in the body.

Holistic Therapy

	Claims
Mind-body medicine	The mind can affect "bodily functions and symptoms" and there is an interconnection between the mind, body, and spirit.

Herbal Remedies and Other Substances Used

Substance based practices use substances found in nature such as herbs, foods, non-vitamin supplements and megavitamins, animal and fungal products, and minerals, including use of these products in traditional medical practices that may also incorporate other methods. Examples include healing claims for nonvitamin supplements, fish oil, Omega-3 fatty acid, glucosamine, echinacea, flaxseed oil, and ginseng. Herbal medicine, or phytotherapy, includes not just the use of plant products, but may also include the use of animal and mineral products. It is among the most commercially successful branches of alternative medicine, and includes the tablets, powders and elixirs that are sold as "nutritional supplements". Only a very small percentage of these have been shown to have any efficacy, and there is little regulation as to standards and safety of their contents. This may include use of known toxic substances, such as use of the poison lead in traditional Chinese medicine.

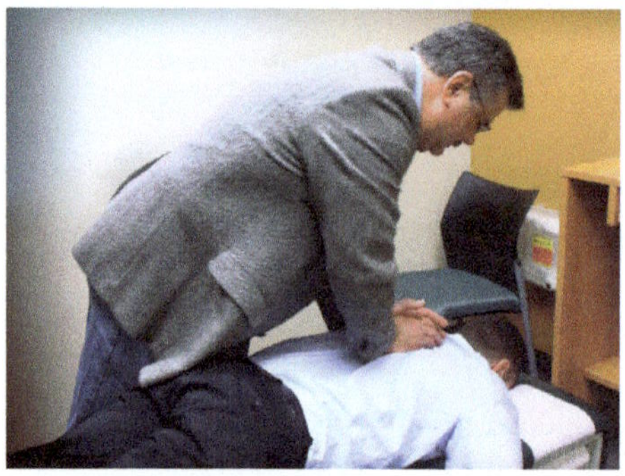

A chiropractor "adjusting" the spine.

Religion, Faith Healing, and Prayer

	Claims
Christian faith healing	There is a divine or spiritual intervention in healing.
Shamanism	A practitioner can reach an altered states of consciousness in order to encounter and interact with the spirit world or channel supernatural energies in the belief that they can heal.

History

The history of alternative medicine may refer to the history of a group of diverse medical practices that were collectively promoted as "alternative medicine" beginning in the 1970s, to the collection of individual histories of members of that group, or to the history of western medical practices that were labeled "irregular practices" by the western medical establishment. It includes the histories of complementary medicine and of integrative medicine. Before the 1970s, western practitioners that were not part of the increasingly science-based medical establishment were referred to "irregular practitioners", and were dismissed by the medical establishment as unscientific and as practicing quackery. Until the 1970's, irregular practice became increasingly marginalized as quackery and fraud, as western medicine increasingly incorporated scientific methods and discoveries, and had a corresponding increase in success of its treatments. In the 1970s, irregular practices were grouped with traditional practices of nonwestern cultures and with other unproven or disproven practices that were not part of biomedicine, with the entire group collectively marketed and promoted under the single expression "alternative medicine".

Use of alternative medicine in the west began to rise following the counterculture movement of the 1960s, as part of the rising new age movement of the 1970s. This was due to misleading mass marketing of "alternative medicine" being an effective "alternative" to biomedicine, changing social attitudes about not using chemicals and challenging the establishment and authority of any kind, sensitivity to giving equal measure to beliefs and practices of other cultures (cultural relativism), and growing frustration and desperation by patients about limitations and side effects of science-based medicine. At the same time, in 1975, the American Medical Association, which played the central role in fighting quackery in the United States, abolished its quackery committee and closed down its Department of Investigation. By the early to mid 1970s the expression "alternative medicine" came into widespread use, and the expression became mass marketed as a collection of "natural" and effective treatment "alternatives" to science-based biomedicine. By 1983, mass marketing of "alternative medicine" was so pervasive that the British Medical Journal (BMJ) pointed to "an apparently endless stream of books, articles, and radio and television programmes urge on the public the virtues of (alternative medicine) treatments ranging from meditation to drilling a hole in the skull to let in more oxygen". In this 1983 article, the BMJ wrote, "one of the few growth industries in contemporary Britain is alternative medicine", noting that by 1983, "33% of patients with rheumatoid arthritis and 39% of those with backache admitted to having consulted an alternative practitioner".

By about 1990, the American alternative medicine industry had grown to a $27 billion per year, with polls showing 30% of Americans were using it. Moreover, polls showed that Americans made more visits for alternative therapies than the total number of visits to primary care doctors, and American out-of-pocket spending (non-insurance spending) on alternative medicine was about equal to spending on biomedical doctors. In 1991, Time magazine ran a cover story, "The New Age of Alternative Medicine: Why New Age Medicine Is Catching On". In 1993, the New England Journal of Medicine reported one in three Americans as using alternative medicine. In 1993, the Public Broadcasting System ran a Bill Moyers special, Healing and the Mind, with Moyers commenting that "...people by the tens of millions are using alternative medicine. If established medicine does not understand that, they are going to lose their clients."

Another explosive growth began in the 1990s, when senior level political figures began promoting alternative medicine, investing large sums of government medical research funds into testing alternative medicine, including testing of scientifically implausible treatments, and relaxing government regulation of alternative medicine products as compared to biomedical products. Beginning with a 1991 appropriation of $2 million for funding research of alternative medicine research, federal spending grew to a cumulative total of about $2.5 billion by 2009, with 50% of Americans using alternative medicine by 2013.

In 1993, Britain's Prince Charles, who claimed that homeopathy and other alternative medicine was an effective alternative to biomedicine, established The Prince's Foundation for Integrated Health (FIH), as a charity to explore "how safe, proven complementary therapies can work in conjunction with mainstream medicine". The FIH received government funding through grants from Britain's Department of Health. In 2008, London's *The Times* published a letter from Edzard Ernst that asked the FIH to recall two guides promoting alternative medicine, saying: "the majority of alternative therapies appear to be clinically ineffective, and many are downright dangerous." In 2010, Brittan's FIH closed after allegations of fraud and money laundering led to arrests of its officials.

In 2004, modifications of the European Parliament's 2001 Directive 2001/83/EC, regulating all medicine products, were made with the expectation of influencing development of the European market for alternative medicine products. Regulation of alternative medicine in Europe was loosened with "a simplified registration procedure" for traditional herbal medicinal products. Plausible "efficacy" for traditional medicine was redefined to be based on long term popularity and testimonials ("the pharmacological effects or efficacy of the medicinal product are plausible on the basis of long-standing use and experience."), without scientific testing. The Committee on Herbal Medicinal Products (HMPC) was created within the European Medicines Agency in London (EMEA). A special working group was established for homeopathic remedies under the Heads of Medicines Agencies.

Through 2004, alternative medicine that was traditional to Germany continued to be a regular part of the health care system, including homeopathy and anthroposophic medicine. The German Medicines Act mandated that science-based medical authorities consider the "particular characteristics" of complementary and alternative medicines. By 2004, homeopathy had grown to be the most used alternative therapy in France, growing from 16% of the population using homeopathic medicine in 1982, to 29% by 1987, 36% percent by 1992, and 62% of French mothers using homeopathic medicines by 2004, with 94.5% of French pharmacists advising pregnant women to use homeopathic remedies. As of 2004, 100 million people in India depended solely on traditional German homeopathic remedies for their medical care. As of 2010, homeopathic remedies continued to be the leading alternative treatment used by European physicians. By 2005, sales of homeopathic remedies and anthroposophical medicine had grown to $930 million Euros, a 60% increase from 1995.

Since 2009, according to Art. 118a of the Swiss Federal Constitution, the Swiss Confederation and the Cantons of Switzerland shall within the scope of their powers ensure that consideration is given to complementary medicine.

By 2013, 50% of Americans were using CAM. As of 2013, CAM medicinal products in Europe continued to be exempted from documented efficacy standards required of other medicinal products.

Individual Systems and Practices

Much of what is now categorized as alternative medicine was developed as independent, complete medical systems. These were developed long before biomedicine and use of scientific methods. Each system was developed in relatively isolated regions of the world where there was little or no medical contact with pre-scientific western medicine, or with each other's systems. Examples are traditional Chinese medicine and the Ayurvedic medicine of India.

Other alternative medicine practices, such as homeopathy, were developed in western Europe and in opposition to western medicine, at a time when western medicine was based on unscientific theories that were dogmatically imposed by western religious authorities. Homeopathy was developed prior to discovery of the basic principles of chemistry, which proved homeopathic remedies contained nothing but water. But homeopathy, with its remedies made of water, was harmless compared to the unscientific and dangerous orthodox western medicine practiced at that time, which included use of toxins and draining of blood, often resulting in permanent disfigurement or death.

Other alternative practices such as chiropractic and osteopathic manipulative medicine were developed in the United States at a time that western medicine was beginning to incorporate scientific methods and theories, but the biomedical model was not yet totally dominant. Practices such as chiropractic and osteopathic, each considered to be irregular practices by the western medical establishment, also opposed each other, both rhetorically and politically with licensing legislation. Osteopathic practitioners added the courses and training of biomedicine to their licensing, and licensed Doctor of Osteopathic Medicine holders began diminishing use of the unscientific origins of the field. Without the original nonscientific practices and theories, osteopathic medicine is now considered the same as biomedicine.

"Irregular Practitioners"

Until the 1970s, western practitioners that were not part of the medical establishment were referred to "irregular practitioners", and were dismissed by the medical establishment as unscientific, as practicing quackery. Irregular practice became increasingly marginalized as quackery and fraud, as western medicine increasingly incorporated scientific methods and discoveries, and had a corresponding increase in success of its treatments.

Dating from the 1970s, medical professionals, sociologists, anthropologists and other commentators noted the increasing visibility of a wide variety of health practices that had neither derived directly from nor been verified by biomedical science. Since that time, those who have analyzed this trend have deliberated over the most apt language with which to describe this emergent health field. A variety of terms have been used, including heterodox, irregular, fringe and alternative medicine while others, particularly medical commentators, have been satisfied to label them as instances of quackery. The most persistent term has been alternative medicine but its use is problematic as it assumes a value-laden dichotomy between a medical fringe, implicitly of borderline acceptability at best, and a privileged medical orthodoxy, associated with validated medico-scientific norms. The use of the category of alternative medicine has also been criticized as it cannot be studied as an independent entity but must be understood in terms of a regionally and temporally specific medical orthodoxy. Its use can also be misleading as it may erroneously imply that a real medical alternative exists. As with near-synonymous expressions, such as unorthodox, complementary, marginal, or quackery, these linguistic devices have served, in the context of processes of professionalisation and market competition, to establish the authority of official medicine and police the boundary between it and its unconventional rivals.

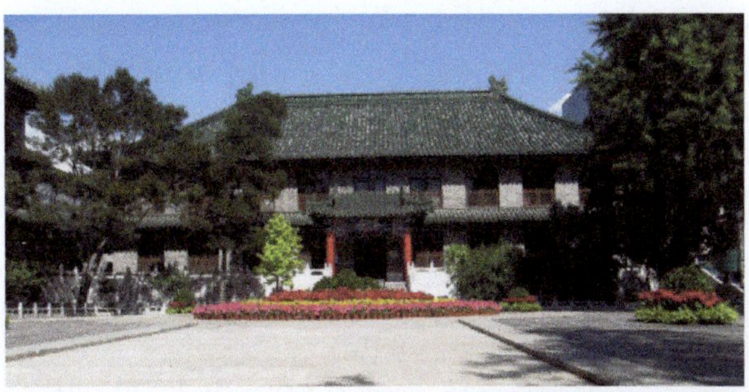

Peking Union Medical College

An early instance of the influence of this modern, or western, scientific medicine outside Europe and North America is Peking Union Medical College.

From a historical perspective, the emergence of alternative medicine, if not the term itself, is typically dated to the 19th century. This is despite the fact that there are variants of Western non-conventional medicine that arose in the late-eighteenth century or earlier and some non-Western medical traditions, currently considered alternative in the West and elsewhere, which boast extended historical pedigrees. Alternative medical systems, however, can only be said to exist when there is an identifiable, regularized and authoritative standard medical practice, such as arose in the West during the nineteenth century, to which they can function as an alternative.

During the late eighteenth and nineteenth centuries regular and irregular medical practitioners became more clearly differentiated throughout much of Europe and, as the nineteenth century progressed, most Western states converged in the creation of legally delimited and semi-protected medical markets. It is at this point that an "official" medicine, created in cooperation with the state and employing a scientific rhetoric of legitimacy, emerges as a recognizable entity and that the concept of alternative medicine as a historical category becomes tenable.

As part of this process, professional adherents of mainstream medicine in countries such as Germany, France, and Britain increasingly invoked the scientific basis of their discipline as a means of engendering internal professional unity and of external differentiation in the face of sustained market competition from homeopaths, naturopaths, mesmerists and other nonconventional medical practitioners, finally achieving a degree of imperfect dominance through alliance with the state and the passage of regulatory legislation. In the US the Johns Hopkins University School of Medicine, based in Baltimore, Maryland, opened in 1893, with William H. Welch and William Osler among the founding physicians, and was the first medical school devoted to teaching "German scientific medicine".

Buttressed by increased authority arising from significant advances in the medical sciences of the late 19th century onwards—including development and application of the germ theory of disease by the chemist Louis Pasteur and the surgeon Joseph Lister, of microbiology co-founded by Robert Koch (in 1885 appointed professor of hygiene at the University of Berlin), and of the use of X-rays (Röntgen rays)—the 1910 Flexner Report called upon American medical schools to follow the model of the Johns Hopkins School of Medicine, and adhere to mainstream science in their teaching and research. This was in a belief, mentioned in the Report's introduction, that the preliminary and professional training then prevailing in medical schools should be reformed, in view of the new means for diagnosing and combating disease made available the sciences on which medicine depended.

Putative medical practices at the time that later became known as "alternative medicine" included homeopathy (founded in Germany in the early 19c.) and chiropractic (founded in North America in the late 19c.). These conflicted in principle with the developments in medical science upon which the Flexner reforms were based, and they have not become compatible with further advances of medical science such as listed in Timeline of medicine and medical technology, 1900–1999 and 2000–present, nor have Ayurveda, acupuncture or other kinds of alternative medicine.

At the same time "Tropical medicine" was being developed as a specialist branch of western medicine in research establishments such as Liverpool School of Tropical Medicine founded in 1898 by

Alfred Lewis Jones, London School of Hygiene & Tropical Medicine, founded in 1899 by Patrick Manson and Tulane University School of Public Health and Tropical Medicine, instituted in 1912. A distinction was being made between western scientific medicine and indigenous systems. An example is given by an official report about indigenous systems of medicine in India, including Ayurveda, submitted by Mohammad Usman of Madras and others in 1923. This stated that the first question the Committee considered was "to decide whether the indigenous systems of medicine were scientific or not".

By the later twentieth century the term 'alternative medicine' entered public discourse, but it was not always being used with the same meaning by all parties. Arnold S. Relman remarked in 1998 that in the best kind of medical practice, all proposed treatments must be tested objectively, and that in the end there will only be treatments that pass and those that do not, those that are proven worthwhile and those that are not. He asked 'Can there be any reasonable "alternative"?' But also in 1998 the then Surgeon General of the United States, David Satcher, issued public information about eight common alternative treatments (including acupuncture, holistic and massage), together with information about common diseases and conditions, on nutrition, diet, and lifestyle changes, and about helping consumers to decipher fraud and quackery, and to find healthcare centers and doctors who practiced alternative medicine.

By 1990, approximately 60 million Americans had used one or more complementary or alternative therapies to address health issues, according to a nationwide survey in the US published in 1993 by David Eisenberg. A study published in the November 11, 1998 issue of the Journal of the American Medical Association reported that 42% of Americans had used complementary and alternative therapies, up from 34% in 1990. However, despite the growth in patient demand for complementary medicine, most of the early alternative/complementary medical centers failed.

Medical Education

Mainly as a result of reforms following the Flexner Report of 1910 medical education in established medical schools in the US has generally not included alternative medicine as a teaching topic. Typically, their teaching is based on current practice and scientific knowledge about: anatomy, physiology, histology, embryology, neuroanatomy, pathology, pharmacology, microbiology and immunology. Medical schools' teaching includes such topics as doctor-patient communication, ethics, the art of medicine, and engaging in complex clinical reasoning (medical decision-making). Writing in 2002, Snyderman and Weil remarked that by the early twentieth century the Flexner model had helped to create the 20th-century academic health center, in which education, research, and practice were inseparable. While this had much improved medical practice by defining with increasing certainty the pathophysiological basis of disease, a single-minded focus on the pathophysiological had diverted much of mainstream American medicine from clinical conditions that were not well understood in mechanistic terms, and were not effectively treated by conventional therapies.

By 2001 some form of CAM training was being offered by at least 75 out of 125 medical schools in the US. Exceptionally, the School of Medicine of the University of Maryland, Baltimore includes a research institute for integrative medicine (a member entity of the Cochrane Collaboration). Medical schools are responsible for conferring medical degrees, but a physician typically may not legally practice medicine until licensed by the local government authority. Licensed physicians in the US who have attended one of the established medical schools there have usually graduated Doctor of Medicine (MD). All states require that applicants for MD licensure be graduates of an approved medical school and complete the United States Medical Licensing Exam (USMLE).

The British Medical Association, in its publication *Complementary Medicine, New Approach to Good Practice* (1993), gave as a working definition of non-conventional therapies (including acupuncture, chiropractic and homeopathy): "...those forms of treatment which are not widely used by the orthodox health-care professions, and the skills of which are not part of the undergraduate curriculum of orthodox medical and paramedical health-care courses." By 2000 some medical schools in the UK were offering CAM familiarisation courses to undergraduate medical students while some were also offering modules specifically on CAM.

United States Government

In 1991, pointing to a need for testing because of the widespread use of alternative medicine without authoritative information on its efficacy, United States Senator Tom Harkin used $2 million of his discretionary funds to create the Office for the Study of Unconventional Medical Practices (OSUMP), later renamed to be the Office of Alternative Medicine (OAM). The OAM was created to be within the National Institute of Health (NIH), the scientifically prestigious primary agency of the United States government responsible for biomedical and health-related research. The mandate was to investigate, evaluate, and validate effective alternative medicine treatments, and alert the public as the results of testing its efficacy.

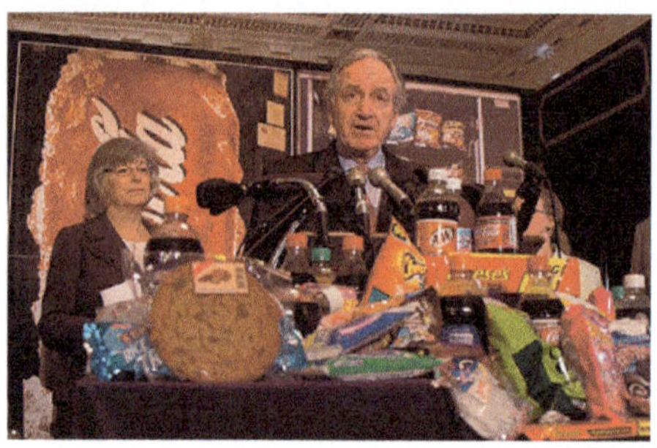

Sen. Tom Harkin at a press conference.

Sen. Harkin had become convinced his allergies were cured by taking bee pollen pills, and was urged to make the spending by two of his influential constituents. Bedell, a longtime friend of Sen. Harkin, was a former member of the United States House of Representatives who believed that alternative medicine had twice cured him of diseases after mainstream medicine had failed, claiming that cow's milk colostrum cured his Lyme disease, and an herbal derivative from camphor had prevented post surgical recurrence of his prostate cancer. Wiewel was a promoter of unproven cancer treatments involving a mixture of blood sera that the Food and Drug Administration had banned from being imported. Both Bedell and Wiewel became members of the advisory panel for the OAM. The company that sold the bee pollen was later fined by the Federal Trade Commission for making false health claims about their bee-pollen products reversing the aging process, curing allergies, and helping with weight loss.

In 1994, Sen. Harkin (D) and Senator Orrin Hatch (R) introduced the Dietary Supplement Health and Education Act (DSHEA). The act reduced authority of the FDA to monitor products sold as "natural" treatments. Labeling standards were reduced to allow health claims for supplements based only on unconfirmed preliminary studies that were not subjected to scientific peer review, and the act made it more difficult for the FDA to promptly seize products or demand proof of safety where there was evidence of a product being dangerous. The Act became known as the "The 1993 Snake Oil Protection Act" following a New York Times editorial under that name.

Senator Harkin complained about the "unbendable rules of randomized clinical trials", citing his use of bee pollen to treat his allergies, which he claimed to be effective even though it was biologically implausible and efficacy was not established using scientific methods. Sen. Harkin asserted that claims for alternative medicine efficacy be allowed not only without conventional scientific testing, even when they are biologically implausible, "It is not necessary for the scientific community to understand the process before the American public can benefit from these therapies." Following passage of the act, sales rose from about $4 billion in 1994, to $20 billion by the end of 2000, at the same time as evidence of their lack of efficacy or harmful effects grew. Senator Harkin came into open public conflict with the first OAM Director Joseph M. Jacobs and OAM board members from the scientific and biomedical community. Jacobs' insistence on rigorous scientific methodology caused friction with Senator Harkin. Increasing political resistance to the use of scientific methodology was publicly criticized by Dr. Jacobs and another OAM board member complained that "nonsense has trickled down to every aspect of this office...It's the only place where opinions are counted as equal to data." In 1994, Senator Harkin appeared on television with cancer patients who blamed Dr. Jacobs for blocking their access to untested cancer treatment, leading Jacobs to resign in frustration.

In 1995, Wayne Jonas, a promoter of homeopathy and political ally of Senator Harkin, became the director of the OAM, and continued in that role until 1999. In 1997, the NCCAM budget was increased from $12 million to $20 million annually. From 1990 to 1997, use of alternative medicine in the US increased by 25%, with a corresponding 50% increase in expenditures. The OAM drew increasing criticism from eminent members of the scientific community with letters to the Senate Appropriations Committee when discussion of renewal of funding OAM came up. Nobel laureate Paul Berg wrote that prestigious NIH should not be degraded to act as a cover for quackery, calling the OAM "an embarrassment to serious scientists." The president of the American Physical Society wrote complaining that the government was spending money on testing products and practices that "violate basic laws of physics and more clearly resemble witchcraft". In 1998, the President of the North Carolina Medical Association publicly called for shutting down the OAM.

In 1998, NIH director and Nobel laureate Harold Varmus came into conflict with Senator Harkin by pushing to have more NIH control of alternative medicine research. The NIH Director placed the OAM under more strict scientific NIH control. Senator Harkin responded by elevating OAM into an independent NIH "center", just short of being its own "institute", and renamed to be the National Center for Complementary and Alternative Medicine (NCCAM). NCCAM had a mandate to promote a more rigorous and scientific approach to the study of alternative medicine, research training and career development, outreach, and "integration". In 1999, the NCCAM budget was increased from $20 million to $50 million. The United States Congress approved the appropriations without dissent. In 2000, the budget was increased to about $68 million, in 2001 to $90 million, in 2002 to $104 million, and in 2003, to $113 million.

In 2009, after a history of 17 years of government testing and spending of nearly $2.5 billion on research had produced almost no clearly proven efficacy of alternative therapies, Senator Harkin complained, “One of the purposes of this center was to investigate and validate alternative approaches. Quite frankly, I must say publicly that it has fallen short. It think quite frankly that in this center and in the office previously before it, most of its focus has been on disproving things rather than seeking out and approving.” Members of the scientific community criticized this comment as showing Senator Harkin did not understand the basics of scientific inquiry, which tests hypotheses, but never intentionally attempts to “validate approaches”. Members of the scientific and biomedical communities complained that after a history of 17 years of being tested, at a cost of over $2.5 Billion on testing scientifically and biologically implausible practices, almost no alternative therapy showed clear efficacy. In 2009, the NCCAM’s budget was increased to about $122 million. Overall NIH funding for CAM research increased to $300 Million by 2009. By 2009, Americans were spending $34 Billion annually on CAM.

In 2012, the Journal of the American Medical Association (JAMA) published a criticism that study after study had been funded by NCCAM, but “failed to prove that complementary or alternative therapies are anything more than placebos”. The JAMA criticism pointed to large wasting of research money on testing scientifically implausible treatments, citing “NCCAM officials spending $374,000 to find that inhaling lemon and lavender scents does not promote wound healing; $750,000 to find that prayer does not cure AIDS or hasten recovery from breast-reconstruction surgery; $390,000 to find that ancient Indian remedies do not control type 2 diabetes; $700,000 to find that magnets do not treat arthritis, carpal tunnel syndrome, or migraine headaches; and $406,000 to find that coffee enemas do not cure pancreatic cancer.” It was pointed out that negative results from testing were generally ignored by the public, that people continue to “believe what they want to believe, arguing that it does not matter what the data show: They know what works for them”. Continued increasing use of CAM products was also blamed on the lack of FDA ability to regulate alternative products, where negative studies do not result in FDA warnings or FDA-mandated changes on labeling, whereby few consumers are aware that many claims of many supplements were found not to have not to be supported.

In 2014 the NCCAM was renamed to the National Center for Complementary and Integrative Health (NCCIH) with a new charter requiring that 12 of the 18 council members shall be selected with a preference to selecting leading representatives of complementary and alternative medicine, 9 of the members must be licensed practitioners of alternative medicine, 6 members must be general public leaders in the fields of public policy, law, health policy, economics, and management, and 3 members must represent the interests of individual consumers of complementary and alternative medicine.

Efficacy

There is a general scientific consensus that Alternative Therapies lack the requisite scientific validation, and their effectiveness is either unproved or disproved. Many of the claims regarding the efficacy of alternative medicines are controversial, since research on them is frequently of low quality and methodologically flawed. Selective publication bias , marked differences in product quality and standardisation, and some companies making unsubstantiated claims, call into question the claims of efficacy of isolated examples where there is evidence for alternative therapies.

The Scientific Review of Alternative Medicine points to confusions in the general population - a person may attribute symptomatic relief to an otherwise-ineffective therapy just because they are taking something (the placebo effect); the natural recovery from or the cyclical nature of an illness (the regression fallacy) gets misattributed to an alternative medicine being taken; a person not diagnosed with science-based medicine may never originally have had a true illness diagnosed as an alternative disease category.

Edzard Ernst characterized the evidence for many alternative techniques as weak, nonexistent, or negative and in 2011 published his estimate that about 7.4% were based on "sound evidence", although he believes that may be an overestimate. Ernst has concluded that 95% of the alternative treatments he and his team studied, including acupuncture, herbal medicine, homeopathy, and reflexology, are "statistically indistinguishable from placebo treatments", but he also believes there is something that conventional doctors can usefully learn from the chiropractors and homeopath: this is the therapeutic value of the placebo effect, one of the strangest phenomena in medicine.

In 2003, a project funded by the CDC identified 208 condition-treatment pairs, of which 58% had been studied by at least one randomized controlled trial (RCT), and 23% had been assessed with a meta-analysis. According to a 2005 book by a US Institute of Medicine panel, the number of RCTs focused on CAM has risen dramatically.

As of 2005, the Cochrane Library had 145 CAM-related Cochrane systematic reviews and 340 non-Cochrane systematic reviews. An analysis of the conclusions of only the 145 Cochrane reviews was done by two readers. In 83% of the cases, the readers agreed. In the 17% in which they disagreed, a third reader agreed with one of the initial readers to set a rating. These studies found that, for CAM, 38.4% concluded positive effect or possibly positive (12.4%), 4.8% concluded no effect, 0.69% concluded harmful effect, and 56.6% concluded insufficient evidence. An assessment of conventional treatments found that 41.3% concluded positive or possibly positive effect, 20% concluded no effect, 8.1% concluded net harmful effects, and 21.3% concluded insufficient evidence. However, the CAM review used the more developed 2004 Cochrane database, while the conventional review used the initial 1998 Cochrane database.

In the same way as for conventional therapies, drugs, and interventions, it can be difficult to test the efficacy of alternative medicine in clinical trials. In instances where an established, effective, treatment for a condition is already available, the Helsinki Declaration states that withholding such treatment is unethical in most circumstances. Use of standard-of-care treatment in addition to an alternative technique being tested may produce confounded or difficult-to-interpret results.

Cancer researcher Andrew J. Vickers has stated:

> "Contrary to much popular and scientific writing, many alternative cancer treatments have been investigated in good-quality clinical trials, and they have been shown to be ineffective. The label 'unproven' is inappropriate for such therapies; it is time to assert that many alternative cancer therapies have been 'disproven'."

Criticism, Legitimacy and Effects

> There is no alternative medicine. There is only scientifically proven, evidence-based medicine supported by solid data or unproven medicine, for which scientific evidence is lacking.
>
> — *P.B. Fontanarosa, Journal of the American Medical Association (1998)*

"CAM", meaning "complementary and alternative medicine", is not as well researched as conventional medicine, which undergoes intense research before release to the public. Funding for research is also sparse making it difficult to do further research for effectiveness of CAM. Most funding for CAM is funded by government agencies. Proposed research for CAM are rejected by most private funding agencies because the results of research are not reliable. The research for CAM has to meet certain standards from research ethics committees, which most CAM researchers find almost impossible to meet. Even with the little research done on it, CAM has not been proven to be effective.

Steven Novella, a neurologist at Yale School of Medicine, wrote that government funded studies of integrating alternative medicine techniques into the mainstream are "used to lend an appearance of legitimacy to treatments that are not legitimate." Marcia Angell considered that critics felt that healthcare practices should be classified based solely on scientific evidence, and if a treatment had been rigorously tested and found safe and effective, science-based medicine will adopt it regardless of whether it was considered "alternative" to begin with. It is possible for a method to change categories (proven vs. unproven), based on increased knowledge of its effectiveness or lack thereof. A prominent supporter of this position is George D. Lundberg, former editor of the Journal of the American Medical Association (JAMA).

Writing in 1999 in *CA: A Cancer Journal for Clinicians* Barrie R. Cassileth mentioned a 1997 letter to the US Senate Subcommittee on Public Health and Safety, which had deplored the lack of critical thinking and scientific rigor in OAM-supported research, had been signed by four Nobel Laureates and other prominent scientists. (This was supported by the National Institutes of Health (NIH).)

In March 2009 a staff writer for *the Washington Post* reported that the impending national discussion about broadening access to health care, improving medical practice and saving money was giving a group of scientists an opening to propose shutting down the National Center for Complementary and Alternative Medicine. They quoted one of these scientists, Steven Salzberg, a genome researcher and computational biologist at the University of Maryland, as saying "One of our concerns is that NIH is funding pseudoscience." They noted that the vast majority of studies were based on fundamental misunderstandings of physiology and disease, and had shown little or no effect.

Writers such as Carl Sagan (1934-1996), a noted astrophysicist, advocate of scientific skepticism and the author of *The demon–haunted world: science as a candle in the dark* (1996), have lambasted the lack of empirical evidence to support the existence of the putative energy fields on which these therapies are predicated.

Sampson has also pointed out that CAM tolerated contradiction without thorough reason and experiment. Barrett has pointed out that there is a policy at the NIH of never saying something doesn't work only that a different version or dose might give different results. Barrett also expressed concern that, just because some "alternatives" have merit, there is the impression that the rest deserve equal consideration and respect even though most are worthless, since they are all classified under the one heading of alternative medicine.

Some critics of alternative medicine are focused upon health fraud, misinformation, and quackery as public health problems, notably Wallace Sampson and Paul Kurtz founders of Scientific Review of Alternative Medicine and Stephen Barrett, co-founder of The National Council Against Health Fraud and webmaster of Quackwatch. Grounds for opposing alternative medicine include that:

- It is usually based on religion, tradition, superstition, belief in supernatural energies, pseudoscience, errors in reasoning, propaganda, or fraud.
- Alternative therapies typically lack any scientific validation, and their effectiveness is either unproved or disproved.
- Treatments are not part of the conventional, science-based healthcare system.
- Research on alternative medicine is frequently of low quality and methodologically flawed.
- Where alternative treatments have replaced conventional science-based medicine, even with the safest alternative medicines, failure to use or delay in using conventional science-based medicine has caused deaths.
- Methods may incorporate or base themselves on traditional medicine, folk knowledge, spiritual beliefs, ignorance or misunderstanding of scientific principles, errors in reasoning, or newly conceived approaches claiming to heal.

Many alternative medical treatments are not patentable,, which may lead to less research funding from the private sector. In addition, in most countries, alternative treatments (in contrast to pharmaceuticals) can be marketed without any proof of efficacy—also a disincentive for manufacturers to fund scientific research.

English evolutionary biologist Richard Dawkins, in his 2003 book *A Devil's Chaplain* , defined alternative medicine as a "set of practices that cannot be tested, refuse to be tested, or consistently fail tests." Dawkins argued that if a technique is demonstrated effective in properly performed trials then it ceases to be alternative and simply becomes medicine.

CAM is also often less regulated than conventional medicine. There are ethical concerns about whether people who perform CAM have the proper knowledge to treat patients. CAM is often done by non-physicians who do not operate with the same medical licensing laws which govern conventional medicine, and it is often described as an issue of non-maleficence.

According to two writers, Wallace Sampson and K. Butler, marketing is part of the training required in alternative medicine, and propaganda methods in alternative medicine have been traced back to those used by Hitler and Goebels in their promotion of pseudoscience in medicine.

In November 2011 Edzard Ernst stated that the "level of misinformation about alternative medicine has now reached the point where it has become dangerous and unethical. So far, alternative medicine has remained an ethics-free zone. It is time to change this."

Placebo Effect

A research methods expert and author of "Snake Oil Science", R. Barker Bausell, has stated that "it's become politically correct to investigate nonsense." There are concerns that just having NIH support is being used to give unfounded "legitimacy to treatments that are not legitimate."

Use of placebos to achieve a placebo effect in integrative medicine has been criticized as, "...diverting research time, money, and other resources from more fruitful lines of investigation in order to pursue a theory that has no basis in biology."

Another critic has argued that academic proponents of integrative medicine sometimes recommend misleading patients by using known placebo treatments to achieve a placebo effect. However, a 2010 survey of family physicians found that 56% of respondents said they had used a placebo in clinical practice as well. Eighty-five percent of respondents believed placebos can have both psychological and physical benefits.

Integrative medicine has been criticized in that its practitioners, trained in science-based medicine, deliberately mislead patients by pretending placebos are not. "quackademic medicine" is a pejorative term used for *integrative medicine*, which medical professionals consider an infiltration of quackery into academic science-based medicine.

An analysis of trends in the criticism of complementary and alternative medicine (CAM) in five prestigious American medical journals during the period of reorganization within medicine (1965–1999) was reported as showing that the medical profession had responded to the growth of CAM in three phases, and that in each phase, changes in the medical marketplace had influenced the type of response in the journals. Changes included relaxed medical licensing, the development of managed care, rising consumerism, and the establishment of the USA Office of Alternative Medicine (now National Center for Complementary and Alternative Medicine). In the "condemnation" phase, from the late 1960s to the early 1970s, authors had ridiculed, exaggerated the risks, and petitioned the state to contain CAM; in the "reassessment" phase (mid-1970s through early 1990s), when increased consumer utilization of CAM was prompting concern, authors had pondered whether patient dissatisfaction and shortcomings in conventional care contributed to the trend; in the "integration" phase of the 1990s physicians began learning to work around or administer CAM, and the subjugation of CAM to scientific scrutiny had become the primary means of control.

Use and Regulation

Prevalence of Use

Complementary and alternative medicine (CAM) has been described as a broad domain of healing resources that encompasses all health systems, modalities, and practices and their accompanying theories and beliefs, other than those intrinsic to the politically dominant health system of a particular society or culture in a given historical period. CAM includes all such practices and ideas self-defined by their users as preventing or treating illness or promoting health and well-being. Boundaries within CAM and between the CAM domain and that of the dominant system are not always sharp or fixed.

According to recent research, the increasing popularity of the CAM needs to be explained by moral convictions or lifestyle choices rather than by economic reasoning.

About 50% of people in developed countries use some kind of complementary and alternative medicine other than prayer for health. A British telephone survey by the BBC of 1209 adults in 1998 shows that around 20% of adults in Britain had used alternative medicine in the past 12 months. About 40% of cancer patients use some form of CAM.

In developing nations, access to essential medicines is severely restricted by lack of resources and poverty. Traditional remedies, often closely resembling or forming the basis for alternative remedies, may comprise primary healthcare or be integrated into the healthcare system. In Africa, traditional medicine is used for 80% of primary healthcare, and in developing nations as a whole over one-third of the population lack access to essential medicines.

Some have proposed adopting a prize system to reward medical research. However, public funding for research exists. Increasing the funding for research on alternative medicine techniques is the purpose of the US National Center for Complementary and Alternative Medicine. NCCIH and its predecessor, the Office of Alternative Medicine, have spent more than $2.5 billion on such research since 1992; this research has largely not demonstrated the efficacy of alternative treatments.

That alternative medicine has been on the rise "in countries where Western science and scientific method generally are accepted as the major foundations for healthcare, and 'evidence-based' practice is the dominant paradigm" was described as an "enigma" in the Medical Journal of Australia.

In the US

In the United States, the 1974 Child Abuse Prevention and Treatment Act (CAPTA) required that for states to receive federal money, they had to grant religious exemptions to child neglect and abuse laws regarding religion-based healing practices. Thirty-one states have child-abuse religious exemptions.

The use of alternative medicine in the US has increased, with a 50 percent increase in expenditures and a 25 percent increase in the use of alternative therapies between 1990 and 1997 in America. Americans spend many billions on the therapies annually. Most Americans used CAM to treat and/or prevent musculoskeletal conditions or other conditions associated with chronic or recurring pain. In America, women were more likely than men to use CAM, with the biggest difference in use of mind-body therapies including prayer specifically for health reasons". In 2008, more than 37% of American hospitals offered alternative therapies, up from 26.5 percent in 2005, and 25% in 2004. More than 70% of the hospitals offering CAM were in urban areas.

A survey of Americans found that 88 percent thought that "there are some good ways of treating sickness that medical science does not recognize". Use of magnets was the most common tool in energy medicine in America, and among users of it, 58 percent described it as at least "sort of scientific", when it is not at all scientific. In 2002, at least 60 percent of US medical schools have at least some class time spent teaching alternative therapies. "Therapeutic touch", was taught at more than 100 colleges and universities in 75 countries before the practice was debunked by a nine-year-old child for a school science project.

Prevalence of Use of Specific Therapies

The most common CAM therapies used in the US in 2002 were prayer (45.2%), herbalism (18.9%), breathing meditation (11.6%), meditation (7.6%), chiropractic medicine (7.5%), yoga (5.1%-6.1%), body work (5.0%), diet-based therapy (3.5%), progressive relaxation (3.0%), mega-vitamin therapy (2.8%) and Visualization (2.1%)

In Britain, the most often used alternative therapies were Alexander technique, Aromatherapy, Bach and other flower remedies, Body work therapies including massage, Counseling stress therapies, hypnotherapy, Meditation, Reflexology, Shiatsu, Ayurvedic medicine, Nutritional medicine, and Yoga. Ayurvedic medicine remedies are mainly plant based with some use of animal materials. Safety concerns include the use of herbs containing toxic compounds and the lack of quality control in Ayurvedic facilities.

According to the National Health Service (England), the most commonly used complementary and alternative medicines (CAM) supported by the NHS in the UK are: acupuncture, aromatherapy, chiropractic, homeopathy, massage, osteopathy and clinical hypnotherapy.

In Palliative Care

Complementary therapies are often used in palliative care or by practitioners attempting to manage chronic pain in patients. Integrative medicine is considered more acceptable in the interdisciplinary approach used in palliative care than in other areas of medicine. “From its early experiences of care for the dying, palliative care took for granted the necessity of placing patient values and lifestyle habits at the core of any design and delivery of quality care at the end of life. If the patient desired complementary therapies, and as long as such treatments provided additional support and did not endanger the patient, they were considered acceptable.” The non-pharmacologic interventions of complementary medicine can employ mind-body interventions designed to “reduce pain and concomitant mood disturbance and increase quality of life.”

Regulation

In Austria and Germany complementary and alternative medicine is mainly in the hands of doctors with MDs, and half or more of the American alternative practitioners are licensed MDs. In Germany herbs are tightly regulated: half are prescribed by doctors and covered by health insurance.

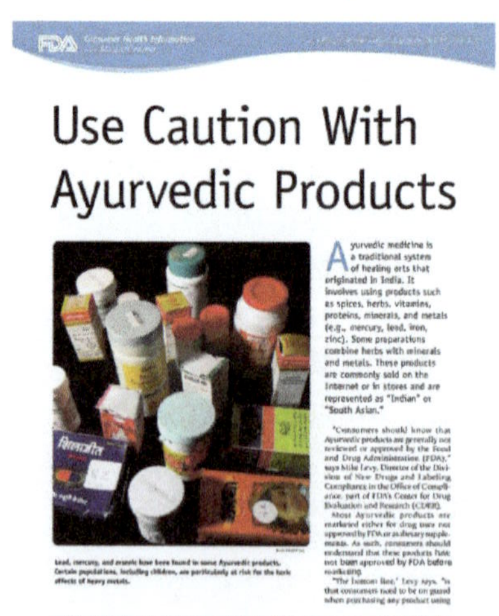

Health campaign flyers, as in this example from the Food and Drug Administration, warn the public about unsafe products.

Some professions of complementary/traditional/alternative medicine, such as chiropractic, have achieved full regulation in North America and other parts of the world and are regulated in a manner similar to that governing science-based medicine. In contrast, other approaches may be partially recognized and others have no regulation at all. Regulation and licensing of alternative medicine ranges widely from country to country, and state to state.

Government bodies in the USA and elsewhere have published information or guidance about alternative medicine. The U.S. Food and Drug Administration (FDA), has issued online warnings for consumers about medication health fraud. This includes a section on Alternative Medicine Fraud, such as a warning that Ayurvedic products generally have not been approved by the FDA before marketing.

Conflicts of Interest

Some commentators have said that special consideration must be given to the issue of conflicts of interest in alternative medicine. Edzard Ernst has said that most researchers into alternative medicine are at risk of "unidirectional bias" because of a generally uncritical belief in their chosen subject. Ernst cites as evidence the phenomenon whereby 100% of a sample of acupuncture trials originating in China had positive conclusions. David Gorski contrasts evidence-based medicine, in which researchers try to disprove hyphotheses, with what he says is the frequent practice in pseudoscience-based research, of striving to confirm pre-existing notions. Harriet A. Hall writes that there is a contrast between the circumstances of alternative medicine practitioners and disinterested scientists: in the case of acupuncture, for example, an acupuncturist would have "a great deal to lose" if acupuncture were rejected by research; but the disinterested skeptic would not lose anything if its effects were confirmed; rather their change of mind would enhance their skeptical credentials.

Risks

Adequacy of Regulation and Cam Safety

Many of the claims regarding the safety and efficacy of alternative medicine are controversial. Some alternative treatments have been associated with unexpected side effects, which can be fatal.

A commonly voiced concerns about complementary alternative medicine (CAM) is the way it's regulated. There have been significant developments in how CAMs should be assessed prior to re-sale in the United Kingdom and the European Union (EU) in the last 2 years. Despite this, it has been suggested that current regulatory bodies have been ineffective in preventing deception of patients as many companies have re-labelled their drugs to avoid the new laws. There is no general consensus about how to balance consumer protection (from false claims, toxicity, and advertising) with freedom to choose remedies.

Advocates of CAM suggest that regulation of the industry will adversely affect patients looking for alternative ways to manage their symptoms, even if many of the benefits may represent the placebo affect. Some contend that alternative medicines should not require any more regulation than over-the-counter medicines that can also be toxic in overdose (such as paracetamol).

Interactions with Conventional Pharmaceuticals

Forms of alternative medicine that are biologically active can be dangerous even when used in conjunction with conventional medicine. Examples include immuno-augmentation therapy, shark cartilage, bioresonance therapy, oxygen and ozone therapies, and insulin potentiation therapy. Some herbal remedies can cause dangerous interactions with chemotherapy drugs, radiation therapy, or anesthetics during surgery, among other problems. An anecdotal example of these dangers was reported by Associate Professor Alastair MacLennan of Adelaide University, Australia regarding a patient who almost bled to death on the operating table after neglecting to mention that she had been taking "natural" potions to "build up her strength" before the operation, including a powerful anticoagulant that nearly caused her death.

To *ABC Online*, MacLennan also gives another possible mechanism:

> And lastly [*sic*] there's the cynicism and disappointment and depression that some patients get from going on from one alternative medicine to the next, and they find after three months the placebo effect wears off, and they're disappointed and they move on to the next one, and they're disappointed and disillusioned, and that can create depression and make the eventual treatment of the patient with anything effective difficult, because you may not get compliance, because they've seen the failure so often in the past.

Potential Side-effects

Conventional treatments are subjected to testing for undesired side-effects, whereas alternative treatments, in general, are not subjected to such testing at all. Any treatment – whether conventional or alternative – that has a biological or psychological effect on a patient may also have potential to possess dangerous biological or psychological side-effects. Attempts to refute this fact with regard to alternative treatments sometimes use the *appeal to nature* fallacy, i.e., "That which is natural cannot be harmful." Specific groups of patients such as patients with impaired hepatic or renal function are more susceptible to side effects of alternative remedies.

An exception to the normal thinking regarding side-effects is Homeopathy. Since 1938, the U.S. Food and Drug Administration (FDA) has regulated homeopathic products in "several significantly different ways from other drugs." Homeopathic preparations, termed "remedies", are extremely dilute, often far beyond the point where a single molecule of the original active (and possibly toxic) ingredient is likely to remain. They are, thus, considered safe on that count, but "their products are exempt from good manufacturing practice requirements related to expiration dating and from finished product testing for identity and strength", and their alcohol concentration may be much higher than allowed in conventional drugs.

Treatment Delay

Those having experienced or perceived success with one alternative therapy for a minor ailment may be convinced of its efficacy and persuaded to extrapolate that success to some other alternative therapy for a more serious, possibly life-threatening illness. For this reason, critics argue that therapies that rely on the placebo effect to define success are very dangerous. According to mental health journalist Scott Lilienfeld in 2002, "unvalidated or scientifically unsupported mental health practices can lead individuals to forgo effective treatments" and refers to this as "opportunity cost". Individuals who spend large amounts of time and money on ineffective treatments may be left with precious little of either, and may forfeit the opportunity to obtain treatments that could be more helpful. In short, even innocuous treatments can indirectly produce negative outcomes. Between 2001 and 2003, four children died in Australia because their parents chose ineffective naturopathic, homeopathic, or other alternative medicines and diets rather than conventional therapies.

Unconventional Cancer "Cures"

There have always been "many therapies offered outside of conventional cancer treatment centers and based on theories not found in biomedicine. These alternative cancer cures have often been described as 'unproven,' suggesting that appropriate clinical trials have not been conducted and that the therapeutic value of the treatment is unknown." However, "many alternative cancer treatments have been investigated in good-quality clinical trials, and they have been shown to be ineffective....The label 'unproven' is inappropriate for such therapies; it is time to assert that many alternative cancer therapies have been 'disproven'."

Edzard Ernst has stated:

> "... any alternative cancer cure is bogus by definition. There will never be an alternative cancer cure. Why? Because if something looked halfway promising, then mainstream oncology would scrutinize it, and if there is anything to it, it would become mainstream almost automatically and very quickly. All curative "alternative cancer cures" are based on false claims, are bogus, and, I would say, even criminal."

References

- Ernst, E. (2008). "Placebo and other Non-specific Effects". In Ernst, E. Healing, Hype, or Harm? A Critical Analysis of Complementary or Alternative Medicine. Imprint Academic, Societas. ISBN 9781845401184.
- Dan Hurley (2006). Natural causes: death, lies, and politics in America's vitamin and herbal supplement industry. New York: Broadway Books. ISBN 978-0-7679-2042-1.
- Pickstone, J. (2006). "Medicine, Society and the State". In Porter, R. The Cambridge History of Medicine. Cambridge University Press. pp. 260–97. ISBN 9780521864268.
- Bivins, R. (2011). "Chapter 32: Histories of Heterodoxy". In Jackson, M. The Oxford Handbook of the History of Medicine. Oxford University Press. pp. 578–97. ISBN 9780199546497.
- Edzard Ernst; Singh, Simon (2008), Trick or Treatment: The Undeniable Facts about Alternative Medicine, New York: W. W. Norton, ISBN 0-393-06661-4
- Lu, Gwei-Djen; Needham, Joseph (1980). Celestial Lancets: a History and Rationale of Acupuncture and Moxa. Cambridge and New York: Cambridge University Press. ISBN 9780521215138.
- Sarris, J.; et al. (2010). Clinical Naturopathy: An Evidence-based Guide to Practice. Elsevier Health Sciences. ISBN 9780729579261.
- Saks, M. (1992). "Introduction". In Saks, M. Alternative Medicine in Britain. Oxford: Clarendon Press. pp. 1–21. ISBN 9780198272786.
- Shapiro, Rose (2010-09-30). Suckers: How Alternative Medicine Makes Fools of Us All. Random House. ISBN 9781409059165.
- Dasgupta, Amitava; Hammett-Stabler, Catherine A (2011). Herbal Supplements: Efficacy, Toxicity, Inter-

actions with Western Drugs, and Effects on Clinical Laboratory Tests. Hoboken NJ: John Wiley and Sons. pp. 202–205. ISBN 9780470433508.

- "The short and irreverant e-dition of The Skeptic's Dictionary - part 1 - sCAM - so-called complementary and alternative medicine - Skepdic.com". skepdic.com. Retrieved 2016-10-15.
- "Naturopathic Medicine". American Cancer Society. 1 Nov 2008. Archived from the original on 3 April 2015. Retrieved 20 Nov 2010.
- "Complementary Medicine — Alternative Medical Systems". WebMD. 2014-01-14. Archived from the original on 2015-06-01. Retrieved 2015-06-04.
- "The Use of Complementary and Alternative Medicine in the United States". National Center for Complementary and Integrative Health. 2015-04-07. Archived from the original on 2015-06-01. Retrieved 2015-06-04.
- Freedman, David H. (July–August 2011). "The Triumph of New-Age Medicine". Archived from the original on 10 May 2015. Retrieved 6 June 2015.
- Kolata, Gina (June 17, 1996), On Fringes of Health Care, Untested Therapies Thrive, The New York Times, retrieved December 22, 2015

2

Naturopathy: A Comprehensive Study

Naturopathy is one of the forms of alternative medicines; it includes homeopathy, ozone therapy and acupuncture. The practice of naturopathy is considered harmful by many, as it not evidence based medicine. The following section will not only provide an overview, it will also delve deep into the topics related to it.

Naturopathy

Naturopathy or naturopathic medicine is a form of alternative medicine employing a wide array of pseudoscientific modalities that are branded as "natural," including homeopathy, herbalism, and acupuncture, in addition to diet and lifestyle counseling. Naturopathic medicine is considered by the medical profession to be ineffective and possibly harmful, raising ethical issues about its practice. Naturopaths and naturopathic doctors have repeatedly been accused of being charlatans and practicing quackery.

The ideology and methods of naturopathy are based on vitalism and self-healing, rather than evidence-based medicine. Naturopathic education contains little of the established clinical training and curriculum completed by primary care doctors, as naturopaths mostly study unscientific notions and learn unproven diagnoses and treatments. Naturopaths generally recommend against modern medicine, including surgery, drugs, and vaccinations, in favor of methods claimed to be holistic and non-invasive. Naturopaths tend to oppose vaccines and teach their students anti- and alternative vaccine practices, resulting in lower vaccination rates. According to the American Cancer Society, "scientific evidence does not support claims that naturopathic medicine can cure cancer or any other disease."

The term "naturopathy" was created from "natura" (Latin root for birth) and "pathos" (the Greek root for suffering) to suggest "natural healing". Modern naturopathy grew out of the Natural Cure movement of Europe. According to the Merriam-Webster Dictionary, the first known use of "naturopathy" in print is from 1901. The term was coined in 1895 by John Scheel and popularized by Benedict Lust, who is considered to be the "father of U.S. naturopathy". Beginning in the 1970s, there was a revival of interest in the United States and Canada, in conjunction with the "holistic health" movement.

History

Naturopaths claim the ancient Greek "Father of Medicine", Hippocrates, as the first advocate of naturopathic medicine, before the term existed. Naturopathy has its roots in the 19th-century Nature Cure movement of Europe. In Scotland, Thomas Allinson started advocating his "Hygienic Medicine" in the 1880s, promoting a natural diet and exercise with avoidance of tobacco and overwork.

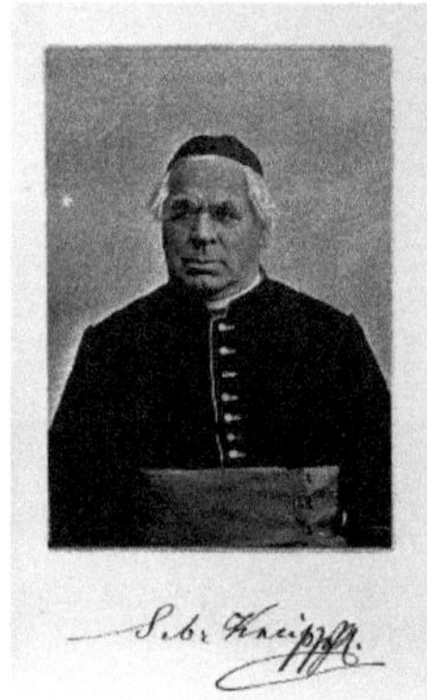

Sebastian Kneipp c. 1898, a Bavarian priest and forefather of naturopathy.

The term *naturopathy* was coined in 1895 by John Scheel, and purchased by Benedict Lust, the "father of U.S. naturopathy". Lust had been schooled in hydrotherapy and other natural health practices in Germany by Father Sebastian Kneipp; Kneipp sent Lust to the United States to spread his drugless methods. Lust defined naturopathy as a broad discipline rather than a particular method, and included such techniques as hydrotherapy, herbal medicine, and homeopathy, as well as eliminating overeating, tea, coffee, and alcohol. He described the body in spiritual and vitalistic terms with "absolute reliance upon the cosmic forces of man's nature".

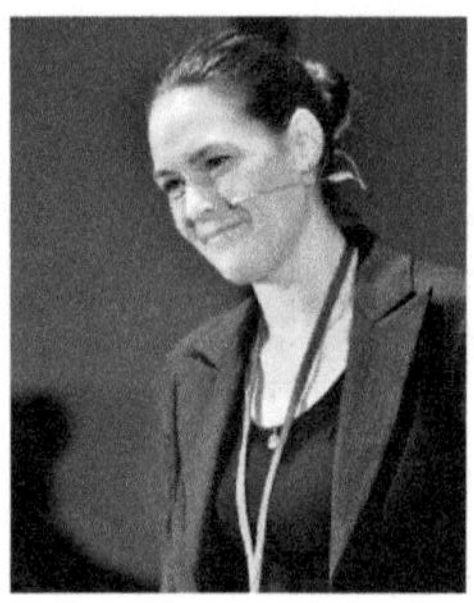

Britt Marie Hermes c. 2016, a former naturopathic doctor and major critic of naturopathic medicine.

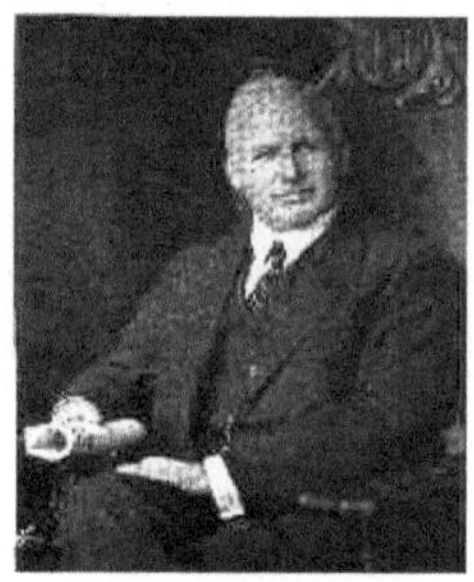

Benedict Lust c. 1902, the founder of naturopathy in the U.S.

In 1901, Lust founded the American School of Naturopathy in New York. In 1902, the original North American Kneipp Societies were discontinued and renamed "Naturopathic Societies". In September 1919, the Naturopathic Society of America was dissolved and Benedict Lust founded the American Naturopathic Association to supplant it. Naturopaths became licensed under naturopathic or drugless practitioner laws in 25 states in the first three decades of the twentieth century. Naturopathy was adopted by many chiropractors, and several schools offered both Doctor of Naturopathy (ND) and Doctor of Chiropractic (DC) degrees. Estimates of the number of naturopathic schools active in the United States during this period vary from about one to two dozen.

After a period of rapid growth, naturopathy went into decline for several decades after the 1930s. In 1910, the Carnegie Foundation for the Advancement of Teaching published the Flexner Report, which criticized many aspects of medical education, especially quality and lack of scientific rigour. The advent of penicillin and other "miracle drugs" and the consequent popularity of modern medicine also contributed to naturopathy's decline. In the 1940s and 1950s, a broadening in scope of practice laws led many chiropractic schools to drop their ND degrees, though many chiropractors continued to practice naturopathy. From 1940 to 1963, the American Medical Association campaigned against heterodox medical systems. By 1958, practice of naturopathy was licensed in only five states. In 1968 the United States Department of Health, Education, and Welfare issued a report on naturopathy concluding that naturopathy was not grounded in medical science and that naturopathic education was inadequate to prepare graduates to make appropriate diagnosis and provide treatment; the report recommends against expanding Medicare coverage to include naturopathic treatments. In 1977 an Australian committee of inquiry reached similar conclusions; it did not recommend licensure for naturopaths.

Beginning in the 1970s, interest waxed in the United States and Canada in conjunction with the holistic health movement. As of 2009, fifteen U.S. states, Puerto Rico, the US Virgin Islands and the District of Columbia licensed naturopathic doctors, and the state of Washington requires insurance companies to offer reimbursement for services provided by naturopathic physicians. South Carolina and Tennessee prohibit the practice of naturopathy.

Naturopathic doctors are actively pushing for more recognition in the U.S. and Canada, but critics argue that naturopathic doctors are misrepresenting their training and exaggerating claims that naturopathic approaches are safe and effective. In 2015, a former naturopathic doctor, Britt Marie Hermes, began writing critically about her experience being trained in and practicing naturopathic medicine.

Practice

A patient undergoing a hydrotherapy session.

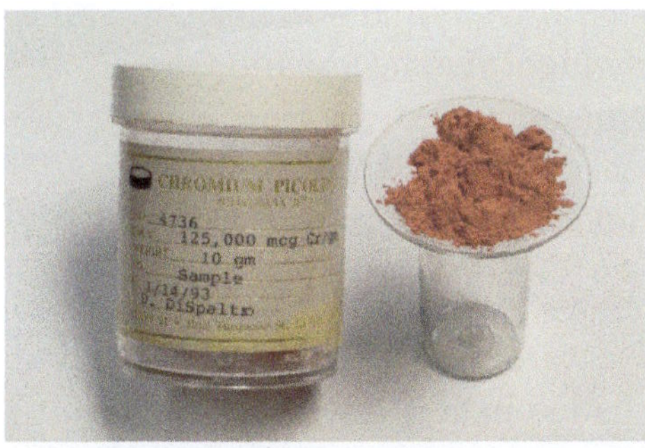

A nutritional supplement of Chromium(III) picolinate, Chromax II.

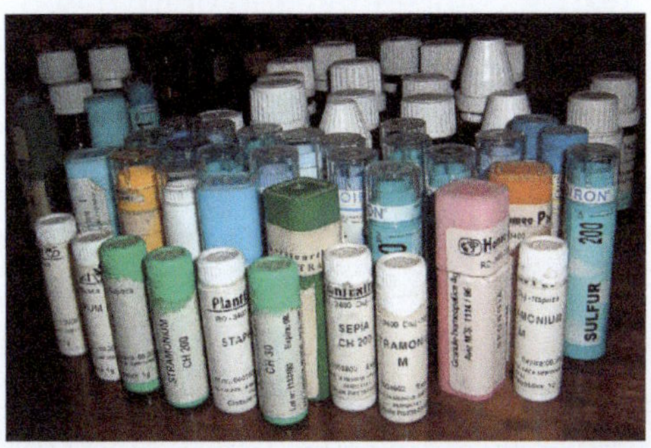

Homeopathic preparations are commonly used by naturopaths. The practice is considered a pseudoscience.

Naturopathic practice is based on a belief in the body's ability to heal itself through a special vital energy or force guiding bodily processes internally. Diagnosis and treatment concern primarily alternative therapies and "natural" methods that naturopaths claim promote the body's natural ability to heal. Naturopaths focus on a holistic approach, often completely avoiding the use of surgery and drugs. Naturopaths aim to prevent illness through stress reduction and changes to diet and lifestyle, often rejecting the methods of evidence-based medicine.

A consultation typically begins with a lengthy patient interview focusing on lifestyle, medical history, emotional tone, and physical features, as well as physical examination. Many naturopaths present themselves as primary care providers, and some naturopathic physicians may prescribe drugs, perform minor surgery, and integrate other conventional medical approaches such as diet and lifestyle counselling with their naturopathic practice. Traditional naturopaths deal exclusively with lifestyle changes, not diagnosing or treating disease. Naturopaths do not generally recommend vaccines and antibiotics, based in part on the early views that shaped the profession, and they may provide alternative remedies even in cases where evidence-based medicine has been shown effective.

Methods

Naturopaths are often opposed to mainstream medicine and take an antivaccinationist stance.

The particular modalities used by a naturopath vary with training and scope of practice. These may include herbalism, homeopathy, acupuncture, nature cures, physical medicine, applied kinesiology, colonic enemas, chelation therapy, color therapy, cranial osteopathy, hair analysis, iridology, live blood analysis, ozone therapy, psychotherapy, public health measures and hygiene, reflexology, rolfing, massage therapy, and traditional Chinese medicine. *Nature cures* include a range of therapies based on exposure to natural elements such as sunshine, fresh air, or heat or cold, as well as nutrition advice such as following a vegetarian and whole food diet, fasting, or abstention from alcohol and sugar. Physical medicine includes naturopathic, osseous, or soft tissue manipulative therapy, sports medicine, exercise, and hydrotherapy. Psychological counseling includes meditation, relaxation, and other methods of stress management.

A 2004 survey determined the most commonly prescribed naturopathic therapeutics in Washington State and Connecticut were botanical medicines, vitamins, minerals, homeopathy, and allergy treatments. A examination published in 2011 of naturopathic clinic websites in Alberta and British Columbia found that the most commonly advertised therapies were homeopathy, botanical medicine, nutrition, acupuncture, lifestyle counseling, and detoxification.

Evidence Basis

Naturopathy lacks an adequate scientific basis, and it is rejected by the medical community. Some methods rely on immaterial "vital energy fields", the existence of which has not been proven, and there is concern that naturopathy as a field tends towards isolation from general scientific discourse. Naturopathy is criticized for its reliance on and its association with unproven, disproven, and other controversial alternative medical treatments, and for its vitalistic underpinnings. Natural substances known as nutraceuticals show little promise in treating diseases, especially cancer, as laboratory experiments have shown limited therapeutic effect on biochemical pathways, while clinical trials demonstrate poor bioavailability. According to the American Cancer Society, "scientific evidence does not support claims that naturopathic medicine can cure cancer or any other disease.

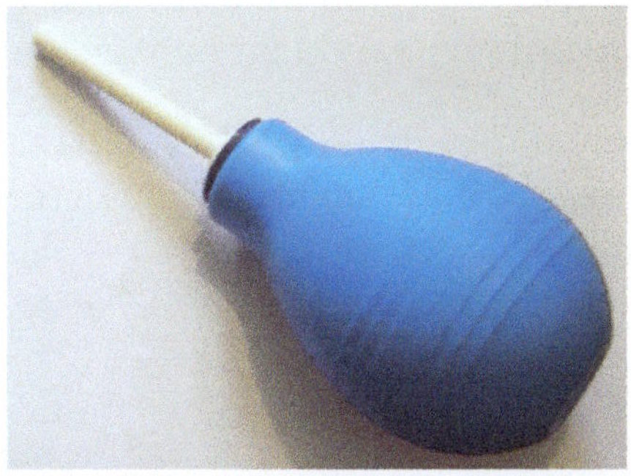

A rectal bulb syringe. Enemas and colonic irrigation are commonly used by naturopaths for a wide range of medical conditions, for which there are no known health benefits.

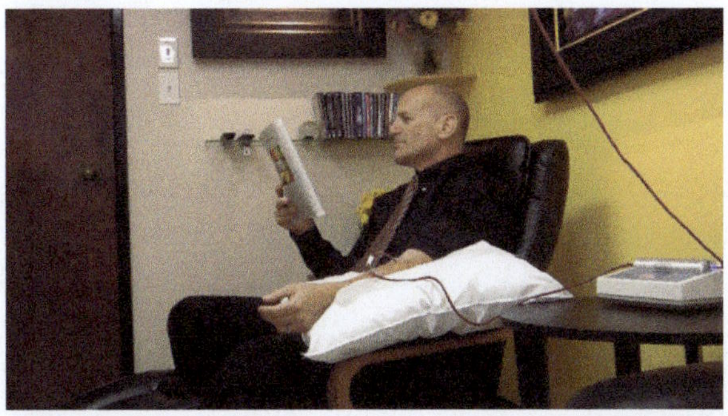

Person undergoing ozone IV therapy with ultraviolet irradiation. The U.S. FDA declares, "Ozone is a toxic gas with no known useful medical application in specific, adjunctive, or preventive therapy.

In 2015, the Australian Government's Department of Health published the results of a review of alternative therapies that sought to determine if any were suitable for being covered by health insurance; Naturopathy was one of 17 therapies evaluated for which no clear evidence of effectiveness was found.

Kimball C. Atwood IV writes, in the journal *Medscape General Medicine*,

Naturopathic physicians now claim to be primary care physicians proficient in the practice of both "conventional" and "natural" medicine. Their training, however, amounts to a small fraction of that of medical doctors who practice primary care. An examination of their literature, moreover, reveals that it is replete with pseudoscientific, ineffective, unethical, and potentially dangerous practices.

Atwood writes that "Physicians who consider naturopaths to be their colleagues thus find themselves in opposition to one of the fundamental ethical precepts of modern medicine. If naturopaths are not to be judged "nonscientific practitioners", the term has no useful meaning".

A retired licensed naturopathic doctor, Britt Marie Hermes, states that "any product that is sold by a naturopath almost guarantees that there is no reliable scientific data to support whatever health claims are made.

According to Arnold S. Relman, the *Textbook of Natural Medicine* is inadequate as a teaching tool, as it omits to mention or treat in detail many common ailments, improperly emphasizes treatments "not likely to be effective" over those that are, and promotes unproven herbal remedies at the expense of pharmaceuticals. He concludes that "the risks to many sick patients seeking care from the average naturopathic practitioner would far outweigh any possible benefits".

The Massachusetts Medical Society states, "Naturopathic practices are unchanged by research and remain a large assortment of erroneous and potentially dangerous claims mixed with a sprinkling of non-controversial dietary and lifestyle advice."

Safety of Natural Treatments

Naturopaths often recommend exposure to naturally occurring substances, such as sunshine, herbs and certain foods, as well as activities they describe as natural, such as exercise, meditation and relaxation. Naturopaths claim that these natural treatments help restore the body's innate ability to heal itself without the adverse effects of conventional medicine. However, "natural" methods and chemicals are not necessarily safer or more effective than "artificial" or "synthetic" ones, and any treatment capable of eliciting an effect may also have deleterious side effects.

Certain naturopathic treatments offered by naturopaths, such as homeopathy, rolfing, and iridology, are widely considered pseudoscience or quackery. Stephen Barrett of QuackWatch and the National Council Against Health Fraud has stated that naturopathy is "simplistic and that its practices are riddled with quackery". "Non-scientific health care practitioners, including naturopaths, use unscientific methods and deception on a public who, lacking in-depth health care knowledge, must rely upon the assurance of providers. Quackery not only harms people, it undermines the ability to conduct scientific research and should be opposed by scientists", says William T. Jarvis.

Vaccination

Naturopathy is based on beliefs opposed to vaccination and have practitioners who voice their opposition. The reasons for this opposition are based, in part, on the early views which shaped the foundation of this profession. A naturopathy textbook, co-authored by Joseph Pizzorno, recalls anti-vaccine beliefs associated with the founding of naturopathy in the United States: "a return to nature in regulating the diet, breathing, exercising, bathing and the employment of various forces" *in lieu* of the smallpox vaccine.

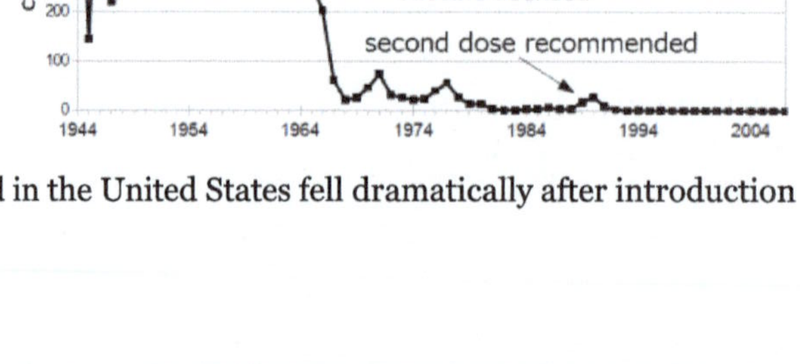

Measles cases reported in the United States fell dramatically after introduction of the measles vaccine.

In general, evidence about associations between naturopathy and pediatric vaccination is sparse, but "published reports suggest that only a minority of naturopathic physicians actively support full vaccination". In Washington state from 2000 to 2003, children were significantly less likely to receive immunizations if they had seen a naturopath. A survey of naturopathic students published in 2004 found that students at the Canadian College of Naturopathic Medicine became less likely to recommend vaccinations to their patients and became more distrustful of public health and conventional medicine as they advanced in the program.

The British Columbia Naturopathic Association lists several major concerns regarding the pediatric vaccine schedule and vaccines in general, and the group's policy is to not advocate for or against vaccines. The Oregon Association of Naturopathic Physicians reports that many naturopaths "customize" the pediatric vaccine schedule.

As of 2016, the American Association of Naturopathic Physicians, which is the largest professional organization for licensed naturopaths in the U.S., is "still discussing its stance on vaccinations."

Practitioners

Naturopaths represent a diverse group of practitioners. In general, they can be categorized into three groups: 1) those with a government issued license; 2) those who practice outside of an official status ("traditional naturopaths"); 3) those who are primarily another kind of health professional who also practices naturopathy.

In Switzerland, these divisions fall between those with a federal diploma, those recognized by health insurances, and those with neither federal diploma nor recognition by health insurances. Naturopaths with federal diploma can be divided into four categories: European traditional medicine, Chinese traditional medicine, ayurvedic medicine and homeopathy. The number of listed naturopaths (including traditional healers) in Switzerland rose from 223 in 1970 to 1835 in 2000.

Licensed Naturopaths

Licensed naturopaths may be referred to as "naturopathic doctors" or "naturopathic physicians" in 17 US states and 5 Canadian provinces. Licensed naturopaths present themselves as primary care providers. Licensed naturopaths do not receive comparable training to medical doctors in terms of the quality of education or quantity of hours. In British Columbia, licensed naturopaths are permitted to refer to themselves as simply "doctor" or "physician".

Education

Licensed naturopaths must pass the Naturopathic Physicians Licensing Examinations (NPLEX) administered by the North American Board of Naturopathic Examiners (NABNE) after graduating from a program accredited by the Council on Naturopathic Medical Education (CNME). Training in CNME-accredited programs includes basic medical diagnostics and procedures such as rudimentary physical exams and common blood tests, in addition to pseudoscientific modalities, such as homeopathy, acupuncture, and energy modalities. These accredited programs have been criticized for misrepresenting their medical rigor and teaching subjects that are antithetical to the best understandings of science and medicine. The CNME as an accrediting authority has been characterized as unreliable and suffering from conflicts of interest. The naturopathic licensing exam has been called a mystery by those outside the naturopathic profession and criticized for testing on homeopathic remedies, including for the use to treat pediatric emergencies.

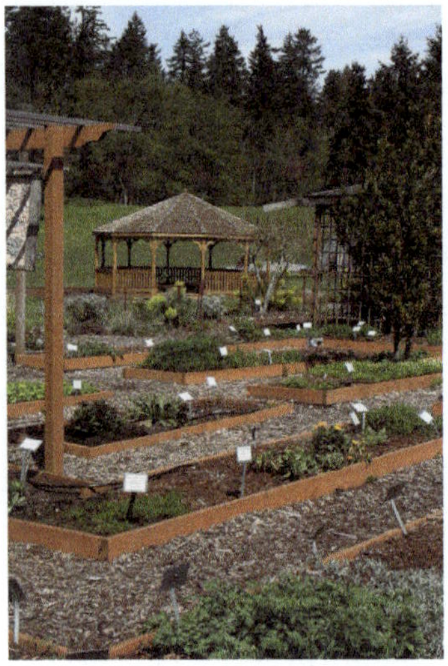

The herb garden at Bastyr University, another naturopathic program whose graduates can become licensed naturopaths in some North American jurisdictions.

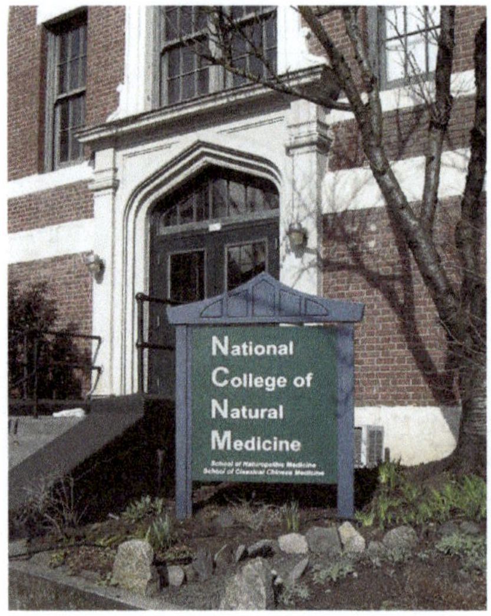

National University of Natural Medicine trains students in naturopathic medicine who are eligible to become licensed in some jurisdictions in North America.

Naturopathic doctors are not eligible for medical residencies, which are available exclusively for medical doctors and doctors of osteopathic medicine. There are limited post-graduate "residency" positions available to naturopathic doctors offered through naturopathic schools and naturopathic clinics approved by the CNME. Most naturopathic doctors do not complete such a residency, and naturopathic doctors are not mandated to complete one for licensure, except in the state of Utah. Continuing education in naturopathic modalities for health care professionals varies greatly.

Political Activity

Naturopaths affiliated with the CNME-accredited schools lobby state, provincial, and federal governments for medical licensure and participation in social health programs. The American Association of Naturopathic Physicians represents licensed naturopaths in the United States; the Canadian Association of Naturopathic Doctors represents licensed naturopaths in Canada. Naturopathic lobbying efforts are funded by vitamin and supplement makers and focus on portraying naturopathic education as comparable to medical education received by physicians and on having high professional standards. Medical societies and advocacy groups dispute these claims by citing evidence of licensed naturopaths using pseudoscientific methods without a sound evidence basis and lacking adequate clinical training to diagnose and treat disease competently according to the standard of care. Jann Bellamy has characterized the process by which naturopaths and other practitioners of pseudoscience convince lawmakers to provide them with medical licenses as "legislative alchemy."

Since 2005, the Massachusetts Medical Society has opposed licensure based on concerns that NDs are not required to participate in residency and concerns that the "practices" of naturopaths included many "erroneous and potentially dangerous claims." The Massachusetts Special Commission on Complementary and Alternative Medical Practitioners rejected their concerns and recommended licensure. The Massachusetts Medical Society states:

Naturopathic medical school is not a medical school in anything but the appropriation of the word medical. Naturopathy is not a branch of medicine. It is a hodge podge of nutritional advice, home remedies and discredited treatments...Naturopathic colleges claim accreditation but follow a true "alternative" accreditation method that is virtually meaningless. They are not accredited by the same bodies that accredit real medical schools and while some courses have similar titles to the curricula of legitimate medical schools the content is completely different.

In 2015, a former naturopathic doctor, Britt Marie Hermes, who graduated from Bastyr University and practiced as a licensed ND in Washington and Arizona, began advocating against naturopathic medicine. In addition to opposing further licensure, she believes that NDs should not be allowed to use the titles "doctor" or "physician," and be barred from treating children. She states:

Naturopaths aggressively lobby for laws to issue them medical licenses. I would characterize this political effort as a perverted redefinition of the words "physician," "doctor," "medical school," and "residency" in order to mask the inadequacy of the training provided in naturopathic programs. ND students do not realize that they are taking educational shortcuts and therefore do not possess any demonstrable competencies found in modern medicine.

Traditional Naturopaths

Traditional naturopaths are represented in the United States by the American Naturopathic Association (ANA), representing about 1,800 practitioners and the American Naturopathic Medical Association (ANMA).

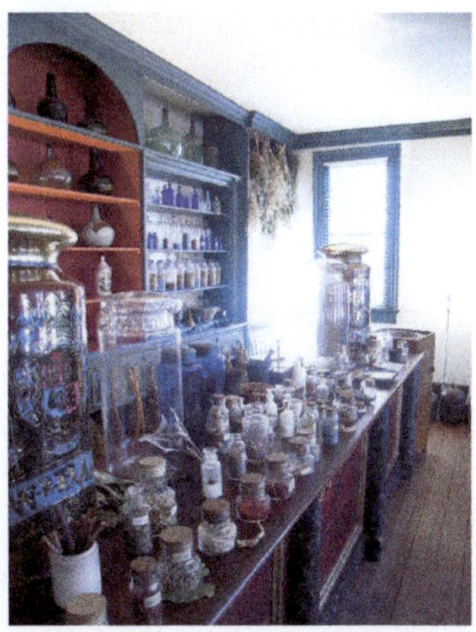

Hugh Mercer Apothecary in Fredericksburg, Virginia. Like all naturopaths, traditional naturopaths have a strong adversion to modern medicine and rely heavily on practices using herbs to treat diseases.

The level of naturopathic training varies among traditional naturopaths in the United States. Traditional naturopaths may complete non-degree certificate programs or undergraduate degree programs and generally refer to themselves as Naturopathic Consultants. These programs often offer online unaccredited degrees, but do not offer comprehensive biomedical education or clinical training.

Traditional naturopathic practitioners surveyed in Australia perceive evidence-based medicine to be an ideological assault on their beliefs in vitalistic and holistic principles. They advocate the integrity of natural medicine practice.

Naturopaths graduating from accredited programs argued in 2002 that their training used evidence-based scientific principles unlike traditional naturopathic programs, but this claim remains inaccurate.

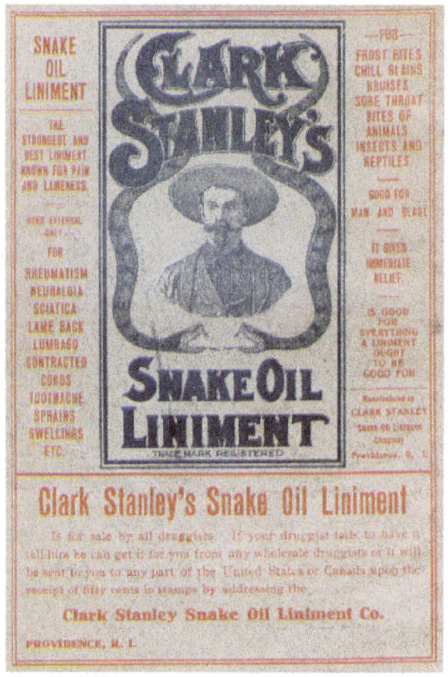

Clark Stanley's Snake Oil Liniment

Regulation

Naturopathy is practiced in many countries and is subject to different standards of regulation and levels of acceptance. The scope of practice varies widely between jurisdictions. The practice of naturopathy is illegal in two USA states.

Australia

In 1977, a committee reviewed all colleges of naturopathy in Australia and found that, although the syllabuses of many colleges were reasonable in their coverage of basic biomedical sciences on paper, the actual instruction bore little relationship to the documented course. In no case was any practical work of consequence available. The lectures which were attended by the committee varied from the dictation of textbook material to a slow, but reasonably methodical, exposition of the terminology of medical sciences, at a level of dictionary definitions, without the benefit of depth or the understanding of mechanisms or the broader significance of the concepts. The committee did not see any significant teaching of the various therapeutic approaches favoured by naturopaths. People reported to be particularly interested in homoeopathy, Bach's floral remedies or mineral salts were interviewed, but no systematic courses in the choice and use of these therapies were seen in the various colleges. The committee were left with the impression that the choice of therapeutic regime was based on the general whim of the naturopath and, since the suggested applications in the various textbooks and dispensations overlapped to an enormous extent, no specific indications were or could be taught.

The position of the Australian Medical Association is that "evidence-based aspects of complementary medicine can be part of patient care by a medical practitioner", but it has concerns that there is "limited efficacy evidence regarding most complementary medicine. Unproven complementary medicines and therapies can pose a risk to patient health either directly through misuse or indirectly if a patient defers seeking medical advice." The AMA's position on regulation is that "there should be appropriate regulation of complementary medicine practitioners and their activities."

In 2015, the Australian government found no clear evidence of effectiveness for naturopathy.

India

In India, naturopathy is overseen by the Department of Ayurveda, Yoga and Naturopathy, Unani, Siddha and Homoeopathy (AYUSH); there is a 5½-year degree in "Bachelor of Naturopathy and Yogic Sciences" (BNYS) degree that was offered by twelve colleges in India as of August 2010. The National Institute of Naturopathy in Pune that operates under AYUSH, which was established on December 22, 1986 and encourages facilities for standardization and propagation of the existing knowledge and its application through research in naturopathy throughout India.

North America

In five Canadian provinces, seventeen U.S. states, and the District of Columbia, naturopathic doctors who are trained at an accredited school of naturopathic medicine in North America, are entitled to use the designation ND or NMD. Elsewhere, the designations "naturopath", "naturopathic doctor", and "doctor of natural medicine" are generally unprotected or prohibited.

In North America, each jurisdiction that regulates naturopathy defines a local scope of practice for naturopathic doctors that can vary considerably. Some regions permit minor surgery, access to prescription drugs, spinal manipulations, midwifery (natural childbirth), and gynecology; other regions exclude these from the naturopathic scope of practice or prohibit the practice of naturopathy entirely.

Canada

Five Canadian provinces license naturopathic doctors: Ontario, British Columbia, Manitoba, Saskatchewan, and Alberta. British Columbia has the largest scope of practice in Canada allowing certified NDs to prescribe pharmaceuticals and perform minor surgeries.

United States

- U.S. jurisdictions that currently regulate or license naturopathy include Alaska, Arizona, California, Connecticut, Colorado, District of Columbia, Hawaii, Kansas, Maine, Maryland, Minnesota, Montana, New Hampshire, North Dakota, Oregon, Puerto Rico, US Virgin Islands, Utah, Vermont, and Washington. Additionally, Florida and Virginia license the practice of naturopathy under a grandfather clause.
    - U.S. jurisdictions that permit access to prescription drugs: Arizona, California, District of Columbia, Hawaii, Kansas, Maine, Montana, New Hampshire, Oregon, Utah, Vermont, and Washington.

  - U.S. jurisdictions that permit minor surgery: Arizona, District of Columbia, Kansas, Maine, Montana, Oregon, Utah, Vermont, and Washington.
- U.S. states which specifically prohibit the practice of naturopathy: South Carolina, and Tennessee.

United Kingdom

Naturopathy is not regulated in the United Kingdom. In 2012, publicly funded universities in the United Kingdom dropped their alternative medicine programs, including naturopathy.

Switzerland

The Swiss Federal Constitution defines the Swiss Confederation and the Cantons of Switzerland within the scope of their powers to oversee complementary medicine. In particular, the Federal authorities must set up diplomas for the practice of non-scientific medicine. The first of such diplomas has been validated in April 2015 for the practice of naturopathy. There is a long tradition for naturopathy and traditional medicine in Switzerland. The Cantons of Switzerland make their own public health regulations. Although the law in certain cantons is typically monopolistic, the authorities are relatively tolerant with regard to alternative practitioners.

Acupuncture

Acupuncture is a form of pseudoscience and alternative medicine involving thin needles being inserted into the body. It is a key component of traditional Chinese medicine (TCM). TCM theory and practice are not based upon scientific knowledge, and acupuncture is commonly described as without scientific basis. There is a diverse range of acupuncture theories, involving different philosophies. Techniques vary depending on the country. The method used in TCM is likely the most widespread in the US. It is most often used for pain relief, though it is also used for a wide range of other conditions. It is generally only used in combination with other forms of treatment.

The conclusions of many trials and numerous systematic reviews of acupuncture are largely inconsistent. An overview of Cochrane reviews found that acupuncture is not effective for a wide range of conditions, and they suggest it may be effective for only chemotherapy-induced nausea/vomiting, postoperative nausea/vomiting, and idiopathic headache. An overview of high-quality Cochrane reviews suggests that acupuncture may alleviate certain kinds of pain. A systematic review of systematic reviews found little evidence of acupuncture's effectiveness in treating pain. The evidence suggests that short-term treatment with acupuncture does not produce long-term benefits. Some research results suggest acupuncture can alleviate pain, though the majority of research suggests that acupuncture's effects are mainly due to placebo. A systematic review concluded that the analgesic effect of acupuncture seemed to lack clinical relevance and could not be clearly distinguished from bias.

Acupuncture is generally safe when done by an appropriately trained practitioner using clean needle technique and single-use needles. When properly delivered, it has a low rate of mostly minor adverse effects. Accidents and infections are associated with infractions of sterile technique or neglect of the practitioner. A review stated that the reports of infection transmission increased significantly in the prior decade. The most frequently reported adverse events were pneumothorax and infections. Since serious adverse events continue to be reported, it is recommended that acupuncturists be trained sufficiently to reduce the risk. A meta-analysis found that acupuncture for chronic low back pain was cost-effective as an adjunct to standard care, while a systematic review found insufficient evidence for the cost-effectiveness of acupuncture in the treatment of chronic low back pain.

Scientific investigation has not found any histological or physiological evidence for traditional Chinese concepts such as *qi*, meridians, and acupuncture points, and many modern practitioners no longer support the existence of life force energy (*qi*) flowing through meridians, which was a major part of early belief systems. Acupuncture is believed to have originated around 100 BC in China, around the time *The Yellow Emperor's Classic of Internal Medicine* (Huangdi Neijing) was published, though some experts suggest it could have been practiced earlier. Over time, conflicting claims and belief systems emerged about the effect of lunar, celestial and earthly cycles, yin and yang energies, and a body's "rhythm" on the effectiveness of treatment. Acupuncture grew and diminished in popularity in China repeatedly, depending on the country's political leadership and the favor of rationalism or Western medicine. Acupuncture spread first to Korea in the 6th century AD, then to Japan through medical missionaries, and then to Europe, starting with France. In the 20th century, as it spread to the United States and Western countries, the spiritual elements of acupuncture that conflict with Western beliefs were abandoned in favor of tapping needles into nerves.

Clinical Practice

Acupuncture is a form of alternative medicine. It is commonly used for pain relief, though it is also used to treat a wide range of conditions. The majority of people who seek out acupuncture do so for musculoskeletal problems, including low back pain, shoulder stiffness, and knee pain. Acupuncture is generally only used in combination with other forms of treatment. For example, American Society of Anesthesiologists states it may be considered in the treatment for nonspecific, noninflammatory low back pain only in conjunction with conventional therapy.

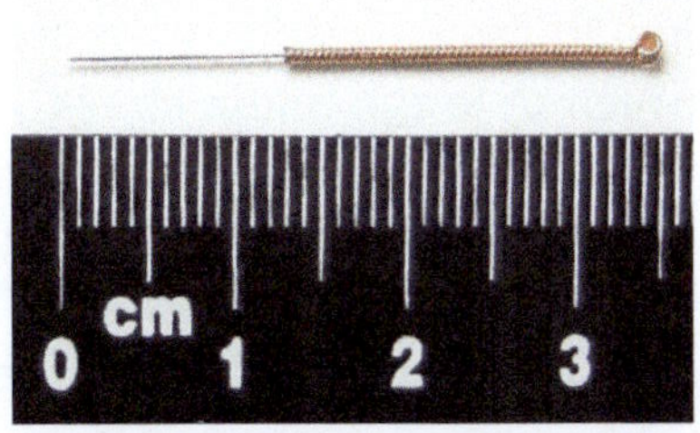

One type of acupuncture needle

Acupuncture is the insertion in the skin of thin needles. According to the Mayo Foundation for Medical Education and Research (Mayo Clinic), a typical session entails lying still while approximately five to twenty needles are inserted; for the majority of cases, the needles will be left in place for ten to twenty minutes. It can be associated with the application of heat, pressure, or laser light. Classically, acupuncture is individualized and based on philosophy and intuition, and not on scientific research. There is also a non-invasive therapy developed in early 20th century Japan using an elaborate set of "needles" for the treatment of children (*shōnishin* or *shōnihari*).

Clinical practice varies depending on the country. A comparison of the average number of patients treated per hour found significant differences between China (10) and the United States (1.2). Chinese herbs are often used. There is a diverse range of acupuncture approaches, involving different philosophies. Although various different techniques of acupuncture practice have emerged, the method used in traditional Chinese medicine (TCM) seems to be the most widely adopted in the US. Traditional acupuncture involves needle insertion, moxibustion, and cupping therapy, and may be accompanied by other procedures such as feeling the pulse and other parts of the body and examining the tongue. Traditional acupuncture involves the belief that a "life force" (*qi*) circulates within the body in lines called meridians. The main methods practiced in the UK are TCM and Western medical acupuncture. The term Western medical acupuncture is used to indicate an adaptation of TCM-based acupuncture which focuses less on TCM. The Western medical acupuncture approach involves using acupuncture after a medical diagnosis. Limited research has compared the contrasting acupuncture systems used in various countries for determining different acupuncture points and thus there is no defined standard for acupuncture points.

In traditional acupuncture, the acupuncturist decides which points to treat by observing and questioning the patient to make a diagnosis according to the tradition used. In TCM, the four diagnostic methods are: inspection, auscultation and olfaction, inquiring, and palpation. Inspection focuses on the face and particularly on the tongue, including analysis of the tongue size, shape, tension, color and coating, and the absence or presence of teeth marks around the edge. Auscultation and olfaction involves listening for particular sounds such as wheezing, and observing body odor. Inquiring involves focusing on the "seven inquiries": chills and fever; perspiration; appetite, thirst and taste; defecation and urination; pain; sleep; and menses and leukorrhea. Palpation is focusing on feeling the body for tender *"A-shi"* points and feeling the pulse.

Needles

The most common mechanism of stimulation of acupuncture points employs penetration of the skin by thin metal needles, which are manipulated manually or the needle may be further stimulated by electrical stimulation (electroacupuncture). Acupuncture needles are typically made of stainless steel, making them flexible and preventing them from rusting or breaking. Needles are usually disposed of after each use to prevent contamination. Reusable needles when used should be sterilized between applications. Needles vary in length between 13 to 130 millimetres (0.51 to 5.12 in), with shorter needles used near the face and eyes, and longer needles in areas with thicker tissues; needle diameters vary from 0.16 mm (0.006 in) to 0.46 mm (0.018 in), with thicker needles used on more robust patients. Thinner needles may be flexible and require tubes for insertion. The tip of the needle should not be made too sharp to prevent breakage, although blunt needles cause more pain.

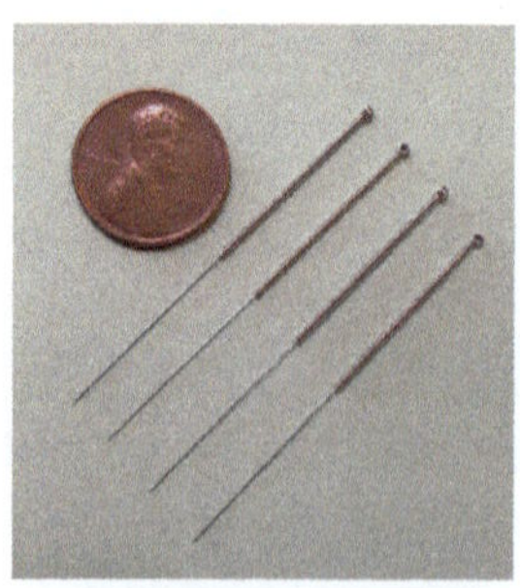

Acupuncture needles

Apart from the usual filiform needle, other needle types include three-edged needles and the Nine Ancient Needles. Japanese acupuncturists use extremely thin needles that are used superficially, sometimes without penetrating the skin, and surrounded by a guide tube (a 17th-century invention adopted in China and the West). Korean acupuncture uses copper needles and has a greater focus on the hand.

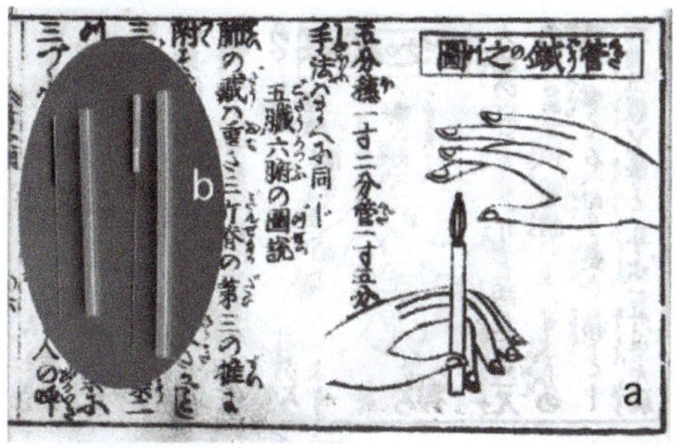

Traditional and modern Japanese guiding tube needles

Needling Technique

Insertion

The skin is sterilized and needles are inserted, frequently with a plastic guide tube. Needles may be manipulated in various ways, including spinning, flicking, or moving up and down relative to the skin. Since most pain is felt in the superficial layers of the skin, a quick insertion of the needle is recommended. Often the needles are stimulated by hand in order to cause a dull, localized, aching sensation that is called *de qi*, as well as "needle grasp," a tugging feeling felt by the acupuncturist and generated by a mechanical interaction between the needle and skin. Acupuncture can be painful. The skill level of the acupuncturist may influence how painful the needle insertion is, and a sufficiently skilled practitioner may be able to insert the needles without causing any pain.

De-qi Sensation

De-qi (Chinese: □□; pinyin: *dé qì*; "arrival of qi") refers to a sensation of numbness, distension, or electrical tingling at the needling site which might radiate along the corresponding meridian. If *de-qi* can not be generated, then inaccurate location of the acupoint, improper depth of needle insertion, inadequate manual manipulation, or a very weak constitution of the patient can be considered, all of which are thought to decrease the likelihood of successful treatment. If the *de-qi* sensation does not immediately occur upon needle insertion, various manual manipulation techniques can be applied to promote it (such as "plucking", "shaking" or "trembling").

Once *de-qi* is achieved, further techniques might be utilized which aim to "influence" the *de-qi*; for example, by certain manipulation the *de-qi* sensation allegedly can be conducted from the needling site towards more distant sites of the body. Other techniques aim at "tonifying" (Chinese: □; pinyin: *b□*) or "sedating" (Chinese: □; pinyin: *xiè*) *qi*. The former techniques are used in deficiency patterns, the latter in excess patterns. *De qi* is more important in Chinese acupuncture, while Western and Japanese patients may not consider it a necessary part of the treatment.

Related Practices

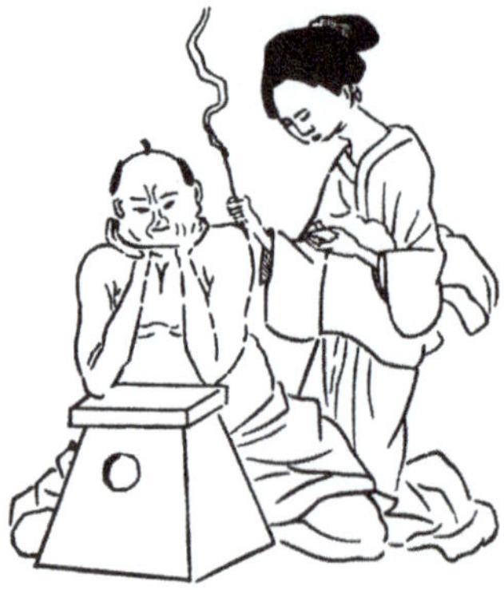

Japanese moxibustion

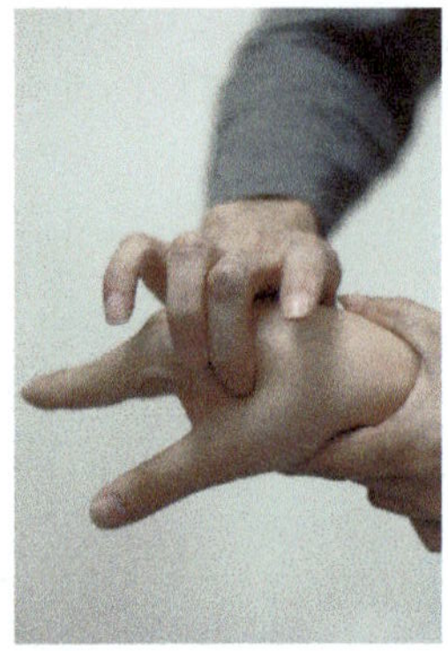

Acupressure being applied to a hand.

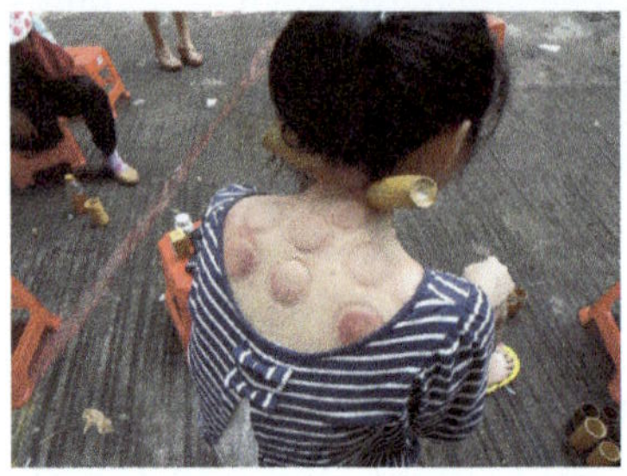

A woman receiving fire cupping in China.

- Acupressure, a non-invasive form of bodywork, uses physical pressure applied to acupressure points by the hand or elbow, or with various devices.
- Acupuncture is often accompanied by moxibustion, the burning of cone-shaped preparations of moxa (made from dried mugwort) on or near the skin, often but not always near or on an acupuncture point. Traditionally, acupuncture was used to treat acute conditions while moxibustion was used for chronic diseases. Moxibustion could be direct (the cone was placed directly on the skin and allowed to burn the skin, producing a blister and eventually a scar), or indirect (either a cone of moxa was placed on a slice of garlic, ginger or other vegetable, or a cylinder of moxa was held above the skin, close enough to either warm or burn it).
- Cupping therapy is an ancient Chinese form of alternative medicine in which a local suction is created on the skin; practitioners believe this mobilizes blood flow in order to promote healing.
- Tui na is a TCM method of attempting to stimulate the flow of *qi* by various bare-handed techniques that do not involve needles.
- Electroacupuncture is a form of acupuncture in which acupuncture needles are attached to a device that generates continuous electric pulses (this has been described as "essentially transdermal electrical nerve stimulation [TENS] masquerading as acupuncture").
- Fire needle acupuncture also known as fire needling is a technique which involves quickly inserting a flame-heated needle into areas on the body.

- Sonopuncture is a stimulation of the body similar to acupuncture using sound instead of needles. This may be done using purpose-built transducers to direct a narrow ultrasound beam to a depth of 6–8 centimetres at acupuncture meridian points on the body. Alternatively, tuning forks or other sound emitting devices are used.
- Acupuncture point injection is the injection of various substances (such as drugs, vitamins or herbal extracts) into acupoints.
- Auriculotherapy, commonly known as ear acupuncture, auricular acupuncture, or auriculoacupuncture, is considered to date back to ancient China. It involves inserting needles to stimulate points on the outer ear. The modern approach was developed in France during the early 1950s. There is no scientific evidence that it can cure disease; the evidence of effectiveness is negligible.
- Scalp acupuncture, developed in Japan, is based on reflexological considerations regarding the scalp. Hand acupuncture, developed in Korea, centers around assumed reflex zones of the hand. Medical acupuncture attempts to integrate reflexological concepts, the trigger point model, and anatomical insights (such as dermatome distribution) into acupuncture practice, and emphasizes a more formulaic approach to acupuncture point location.
- Cosmetic acupuncture is the use of acupuncture in an attempt to reduce wrinkles on the face.
- Bee venom acupuncture is a treatment approach of injecting purified, diluted bee venom into acupoints.
- A 2006 review of veterinary acupuncture found that there is insufficient evidence to "recommend or reject acupuncture for any condition in domestic animals". Rigorous evidence for complementary and alternative techniques is lacking in veterinary medicine but evidence has been growing.

Effectiveness

Sham Acupuncture and Research

It is difficult but not impossible to design rigorous research trials for acupuncture. Due to acupuncture's invasive nature, one of the major challenges in efficacy research is in the design of an appropriate placebo control group. For efficacy studies to determine whether acupuncture has specific effects, "sham" forms of acupuncture where the patient, practitioner, and analyst are blinded seem the most acceptable approach. Sham acupuncture uses non-penetrating needles or needling at non-acupuncture points, e.g. inserting needles on meridians not related to the specific condition being studied, or in places not associated with meridians. The under-performance of acupuncture in such trials may indicate that therapeutic effects are due entirely to non-specific effects, or that the sham treatments are not inert, or that systematic protocols yield less than optimal treatment.

A 2014 *Nature Reviews Cancer* review article found that "contrary to the claimed mechanism of redirecting the flow of *qi* through meridians, researchers usually find that it generally does not matter where the needles are inserted, how often (that is, no dose-response effect is observed), or even if needles are actually inserted. In other words, 'sham' or 'placebo' acupuncture generally produces the same effects as 'real' acupuncture and, in some cases, does better." A 2013 meta-analysis found little evidence that the effectiveness of acupuncture on pain (compared to sham) was modified by the location of the needles, the number of needles used, the experience or technique of the practitioner, or by the circumstances of the sessions. The same analysis also suggested that the number of needles and sessions is important, as greater numbers improved the outcomes of acupuncture compared to non-acupuncture controls. There has been little systematic investigation of which components of an acupuncture session may be important for any therapeutic effect, including needle placement and depth, type and intensity of stimulation, and number of needles used. The research seems to suggest that needles do not need to stimulate the traditionally specified acupuncture points or penetrate the skin to attain an anticipated effect (e.g. psychosocial factors).

A response to "sham" acupuncture in osteoarthritis may be used in the elderly, but placebos have usually been regarded as deception and thus unethical. However, some physicians and ethicists have suggested circumstances for applicable uses for placebos such as it might present a theoretical advantage of an inexpensive treatment without adverse reactions or interactions with drugs or other medications. As the evidence for most types of alternative medicine such as acupuncture is far from strong, the use of alternative medicine in regular healthcare can present an ethical question.

Using the principles of evidence-based medicine to research acupuncture is controversial, and has produced different results. Some research suggests acupuncture can alleviate pain but the majority of research suggests that acupuncture's effects are mainly due to placebo. Evidence suggests that any benefits of acupuncture are short-lasting. There is insufficient evidence to support use of acupuncture compared to mainstream medical treatments. Acupuncture is not better than mainstream treatment in the long term.

Publication Bias

Publication bias is cited as a concern in the reviews of randomized controlled trials (RCTs) of acupuncture. A 1998 review of studies on acupuncture found that trials originating in China, Japan, Hong Kong, and Taiwan were uniformly favourable to acupuncture, as were ten out of eleven studies conducted in Russia. A 2011 assessment of the quality of RCTs on TCM, including acupuncture, concluded that the methodological quality of most such trials (including randomization, experimental control, and blinding) was generally poor, particularly for trials published in Chinese journals (though the quality of acupuncture trials was better than the trials testing TCM remedies). The study also found that trials published in non-Chinese journals tended to be of higher quality. Chinese authors use more Chinese studies, which have been demonstrated to be uniformly positive. A 2012 review of 88 systematic reviews of acupuncture published in Chinese journals found that less than half of these reviews reported testing for publication bias, and that the majority of these reviews were published in journals with impact factors of zero.

Specific Conditions

Pain

The conclusions of many trials and numerous systematic reviews of acupuncture are largely inconsistent with each other. A 2011 overview of high-quality Cochrane reviews suggests that acupuncture is effective for certain types of pain. A 2011 systematic review of systematic reviews found that for reducing pain, real acupuncture was no better than sham acupuncture, and concluded that numerous reviews have shown little convincing evidence that acupuncture is an effective treatment for reducing pain. The same review found that neck pain was one of only four types of pain for which a positive effect was suggested, but cautioned that the primary studies used carried a considerable risk of bias. A 2009 overview of Cochrane reviews found acupuncture is not effective for a wide range of conditions, and suggested that it may be effective for only chemotherapy-induced nausea/vomiting, postoperative nausea/vomiting, and idiopathic headache.

A 2014 systematic review suggests that the nocebo effect of acupuncture is clinically relevant and that the rate of adverse events may be a gauge of the nocebo effect. According to the 2014 *Miller's Anesthesia* book, "when compared with placebo, acupuncture treatment has proven efficacy for relieving pain". A 2012 meta-analysis conducted by the Acupuncture Trialists' Collaboration found "relatively modest" efficiency of acupuncture (in comparison to sham) for the treatment of four different types of chronic pain (back and neck pain, knee osteoarthritis, chronic headache, and shoulder pain) and on that basis concluded that it "is more than a placebo" and a reasonable referral option. Commenting on this meta-analysis, both Edzard Ernst and David Colquhoun said the results were of negligible clinical significance. Edzard Ernst later stated that "I fear that, once we manage to eliminate this bias [that operators are not blind] ... we might find that the effects of acupuncture exclusively are a placebo response." Andrew Vickers, lead author of the original 2012 paper and chair of the *Acupuncture Trialists' Collaboration*, rejects that analysis, stating that the differences between acupuncture and sham acupuncture are statistically significant.

A 2010 systematic review suggested that acupuncture is more than a placebo for commonly occurring chronic pain conditions, but the authors acknowledged that it is still unknown if the overall benefit is clinically meaningful or cost-effective. A 2010 review found real acupuncture and sham acupuncture produce similar improvements, which can only be accepted as evidence against the efficacy of acupuncture. The same review found limited evidence that real acupuncture and sham acupuncture appear to produce biological differences despite similar effects. A 2009 systematic review and meta-analysis found that acupuncture had a small analgesic effect, which appeared to lack any clinical importance and could not be discerned from bias. The same review found that it remains unclear whether acupuncture reduces pain independent of a psychological impact of the needling ritual. A 2016 Cochrane review found moderate quality evidence that real acupuncture was more effective than sham acupuncture or inactive for short-term relief of neck pain measured either upon completion of treatment or at short-term follow-up.

Low Back

A 2013 meta-analysis found that acupuncture was better than no treatment for reducing lower back pain, but not better than sham acupuncture, and concluded that the effect of acupuncture "is likely to be produced by the nonspecific effects of manipulation". A 2013 systematic review found supportive evidence that real acupuncture may be more effective than sham acupuncture with respect to relieving lower back pain, but there were methodological limitations with the studies. A 2013 systematic review found that acupuncture may be effective for nonspecific lower back pain, but the authors noted there were limitations in the studies examined, such as heterogeneity in study characteristics and low methodological quality in many studies. A 2012 systematic review found some supporting evidence that acupuncture was more effective than no treatment for chronic non-specific low back pain; the evidence was conflicting comparing the effectiveness over other treatment approaches. A 2011 overview of Cochrane reviews found inconclusive evidence regarding acupuncture efficacy in treating low back pain. A 2011 systematic review of systematic reviews found that "for chronic low back pain, individualized acupuncture is not better in reducing symptoms than formula acupuncture or sham acupuncture with a toothpick that does not penetrate the skin." A 2010 review found that sham acupuncture was as effective as real acupuncture for chronic low back pain. The specific therapeutic effects of acupuncture were small, whereas its clinically relevant benefits were mostly due to contextual and psychosocial circumstances. Brain imaging studies have shown that traditional acupuncture and sham acupuncture differ in their effect on limbic structures, while at the same time showed equivalent analgesic effects. A 2005 Cochrane review found insufficient evidence to recommend for or against either acupuncture or dry needling for acute low back pain. The same review found low quality evidence for pain relief and improvement compared to no treatment or sham therapy for chronic low back pain only in the short term immediately after treatment. The same review also found that acupuncture is not more effective than conventional therapy and other alternative medicine treatments.

Headaches and Migraines

Two separate 2016 Cochrane reviews found that acupuncture could be useful in the prophylaxis of tension-type headaches and episodic migraines. The 2016 Cochrane review evaluating acupuncture for episodic migraine prevention concluded that true acupuncture had a small effect beyond sham acupuncture and found moderate-quality evidence to suggest that acupuncture is at least similarly effective to prophylactic medications for this purpose. A 2012 review found that acupuncture has demonstrated benefit for the treatment of headaches, but that safety needed to be more fully documented in order to make any strong recommendations in support of its use. A 2009 Cochrane review of the use of acupuncture for migraine prophylaxis treatment concluded that "true" acupuncture was no more efficient than sham acupuncture, but "true" acupuncture appeared to be as effective as, or possibly more effective than routine care in the treatment of migraines, with fewer adverse effects than prophylactic drug treatment. The same review stated that the specific points chosen to needle may be of limited importance. A 2009 Cochrane review found insufficient evidence to support acupuncture for tension-type headaches. The same review found evidence that suggested that acupuncture might be considered a helpful non-pharmacological approach for frequent episodic or chronic tension-type headache.

Osteoarthritis

A 2014 review concluded that "current evidence supports the use of acupuncture as an alternative to traditional analgesics in osteoarthritis patients." As of 2014, a meta-analysis showed that acupuncture may help osteoarthritis pain but it was noted that the effects were insignificant in comparison to sham needles. A 2013 systematic review and network meta-analysis found that the evidence suggests that acupuncture may be considered one of the more effective physical treatments for alleviating pain due to knee osteoarthritis in the short-term compared to other relevant physical treatments, though much of the evidence in the topic is of poor quality and there is uncertainty about the efficacy of many of the treatments. A 2012 review found "the potential beneficial action of acupuncture on osteoarthritis pain does not appear to be clinically relevant." A 2010 Cochrane review found that acupuncture shows statistically significant benefit over sham acupuncture in the treatment of peripheral joint osteoarthritis; however, these benefits were found to be so small that their clinical significance was doubtful, and "probably due at least partially to placebo effects from incomplete blinding".

Extremity Conditions

A 2014 systematic review found moderate quality evidence that acupuncture was more effective than sham acupuncture in the treatment of lateral elbow pain. A 2014 systematic review found that although manual acupuncture was effective at relieving short-term pain when used to treat tennis elbow, its long-term effect in relieving pain was "unremarkable". A 2007 review found that acupuncture was significantly better than sham acupuncture at treating chronic knee pain; the evidence was not conclusive due to the lack of large, high-quality trials.

A 2011 overview of Cochrane reviews found inconclusive evidence regarding acupuncture efficacy in treating shoulder pain and lateral elbow pain.

Nausea and Vomiting and Post-operative Pain

A 2014 overview of systematic reviews found insufficient evidence to suggest that acupuncture is an effective treatment for postoperative nausea and vomiting (PONV) in a clinical setting. A 2013 systematic review concluded that acupuncture might be beneficial in prevention and treatment of PONV. A 2009 Cochrane review found that stimulation of the P6 acupoint on the wrist was as effective (or ineffective) as antiemetic drugs and was associated with minimal side effects. The same review found "no reliable evidence for differences in risks of postoperative nausea or vomiting after P6 acupoint stimulation compared to antiemetic drugs."

A 2014 overview of systematic reviews found insufficient evidence to suggest that acupuncture is effective for surgical or post-operative pain. For the use of acupuncture for post-operative pain, there was contradictory evidence. A 2014 systematic review found supportive but limited evidence for use of acupuncture for acute post-operative pain after back surgery. A 2014 systematic review found that while the evidence suggested acupuncture could be an effective treatment for postoperative gastroparesis, a firm conclusion could not be reached because the trials examined were of low quality.

Allergies

Acupuncture is an unproven treatment for allergic-immunologic conditions. A 2015 meta-analysis suggests that acupuncture might be a good option for people with allergic rhinitis (AR), and a number of randomized clinical trials (RCTs) support the use of acupuncture for AR and itch. There is some evidence that acupuncture might have specific effects on perennial allergic rhinitis (PAR), though all of the efficacy studies were small and conclusions should be made with caution. There is mixed evidence for the symptomatic treatment or prevention of AR. For seasonal allergic rhinitis (SAR), the evidence failed to demonstrate specific effects for acupuncture. Using acupuncture to treat other allergic conditions such as contact eczema, drug rashes, or anaphylaxis is not recommended.

Cancer-related Conditions

A 2015 Cochrane review found that there is insufficient evidence to determine whether acupuncture is an effective treatment for cancer pain in adults. A 2014 systematic review found that acupuncture may be effective as an adjunctive treatment to palliative care for cancer patients. A 2013 overview of reviews found evidence that acupuncture could be beneficial for people with cancer-related symptoms, but also identified few rigorous trials and high heterogeneity between trials. A 2012 systematic review of randomised clinical trials (RCTs) using acupuncture in the treatment of cancer pain found that the number and quality of RCTs was too low to draw definite conclusions.

A 2014 systematic review reached inconclusive results with regard to the effectiveness of acupuncture for treating cancer-related fatigue. A 2013 systematic review found that acupuncture is an acceptable adjunctive treatment for chemotherapy-induced nausea and vomiting, but that further research with a low risk of bias is needed. A 2013 systematic review found that the quantity and quality of available RCTs for analysis were too low to draw valid conclusions for the effectiveness of acupuncture for cancer-related fatigue. A 2012 systematic review and meta-analysis found very limited evidence regarding acupuncture compared with conventional intramuscular injections for the treatment of hiccups in cancer patients. The methodological quality and amount of RCTs in the review was low.

Dyspepsia

A 2015 systematic review and meta-analysis found some evidence that acupuncture was effective for FD, but also called for further well-designed, long-term studies to be conducted to evaluate its efficacy for this condition. A 2014 Cochrane review found that "it remains unknown whether manual acupuncture or electroacupuncture is more effective or safer than other treatments" for functional dyspepsia (FD).

Fertility and Childbirth

A 2014 systematic review and meta-analysis found poor quality evidence for use of acupuncture in infertile men to improve sperm motility, sperm concentration, and the pregnancy rate; the evidence was rated as insufficient to draw any conclusion regarding efficacy. A 2013 Cochrane review found no evidence of acupuncture for improving the success of *in vitro* fertilization (IVF). A 2013 systematic review found no benefit of adjuvant acupuncture for IVF on pregnancy success rates. A 2012 systematic review found that acupuncture may be a useful adjunct to IVF, but its conclusions were rebutted after reevaluation using more rigorous, high quality meta-analysis standards. A 2012 systematic review and meta-analysis found that acupuncture did not significantly improve the outcomes of in vitro fertilization. A 2011 overview of systematic reviews found that the evidence that acupuncture was effective was not compelling for most gynecologic conditions. The exceptions to this conclusion included the use of acupuncture during embryo transfer as an adjunct to in vitro fertilization.

Rheumatological Conditions

A 2013 Cochrane review found low to moderate evidence that acupuncture improves pain and stiffness in treating people with fibromyalgia compared with no treatment and standard care. A

2012 review found "there is insufficient evidence to recommend acupuncture for the treatment of fibromyalgia." A 2010 systematic review found a small pain relief effect that was not apparently discernible from bias; acupuncture is not a recommendable treatment for the management of fibromyalgia on the basis of this review.

A 2012 review found that the effectiveness of acupuncture to treat rheumatoid arthritis is "sparse and inconclusive." A 2005 Cochrane review concluded that acupuncture use to treat rheumatoid arthritis "has no effect on ESR, CRP, pain, patient's global assessment, number of swollen joints, number of tender joints, general health, disease activity and reduction of analgesics." A 2010 overview of systematic reviews found insufficient evidence to recommend acupuncture in the treatment of most rheumatic conditions, with the exceptions of osteoarthritis, low back pain, and lateral elbow pain.

Stroke

A 2014 overview of systematic reviews and meta-analyses found that the evidence does not demonstrate acupuncture helps reduce the rates of death or disability after a stroke or improve other aspects of stroke recovery, such as poststroke motor dysfunction, but the evidence suggests it may help with poststroke neurological impairment and dysfunction such as dysphagia, which would need to be confirmed with future rigorous studies. A 2012 review found evidence of benefit for acupuncture combined with exercise in treating shoulder pain after stroke. A 2010 systematic review found that acupuncture was not effective as a treatment for functional recovery after a stroke. A 2012 overview of systematic reviews found inconclusive evidence supporting the effectiveness of acupuncture for stroke.

A 2015 systematic review found limited evidence that the method of *Xingnao Kaiqiao* needling had a better effect than *Xingnao Kaiqiao* alone or combined with other treatments in reducing disability rate for ischemic stroke, and that the long-term effect was better than traditional acupuncture or combination treatment. A 2014 meta-analysis found tentative evidence for acupuncture in cerebral infarction, a type of ischemic stroke, but the authors noted the trials reviewed were often of poor quality. A 2008 Cochrane review found that evidence was insufficient to draw any conclusion about the effect of acupuncture on dysphagia after acute stroke. A 2006 Cochrane review found no clear evidence for acupuncture on subacute or chronic stroke. A 2005 Cochrane review found no clear evidence of benefit for acupuncture on acute stroke.

Sleep

A 2016 systematic review and meta-analysis found that acupuncture was "associated with a significant reduction in sleep disturbances in women experiencing menopause-related sleep disturbances."

Other Conditions

For the following conditions, the Cochrane Collaboration or other reviews have concluded there is no strong evidence of benefit: alcohol dependence, angina pectoris, ankle sprain, Alzheimer's disease, attention deficit hyperactivity disorder, autism, asthma, bell's palsy, traumatic brain injury, carpal tunnel syndrome, chronic obstructive pulmonary disease, cardiac arrhythmias, cerebral hemorrhage, cocaine dependence, constipation, depression, diabetic peripheral neuropathy, drug detoxification, dry eye, primary dysmenorrhoea, enuresis, endometriosis, epilepsy, erectile dysfunction, essential hypertension, glaucoma, gynaecological conditions (except possibly fertility and nausea/vomiting), hot flashes, hypoxic ischemic encephalopathy in neonates, insomnia, induction of childbirth, irritable bowel syndrome, labor pain, lumbar spinal stenosis, major depressive disorders in pregnant women, musculoskeletal disorders of the extremities, myopia, obesity, obstetrical conditions, Parkinson's disease, polycystic ovary syndrome, premenstrual syndrome, preoperative anxiety, psychological symptoms associated with opioid addiction, restless legs syndrome, schizophrenia, sensorineural hearing loss, smoking cessation, stress urinary incontinence, acute stroke, stroke rehabilitation, temporomandibular joint dysfunction, tennis elbow, labor induction, tinnitus, uremic itching, uterine fibroids, vascular dementia, and whiplash.

Moxibustion and Cupping

A 2010 overview of systematic reviews found that moxibustion was effective for several conditions but the primary studies were of poor quality, so there persists ample uncertainty, which limits the conclusiveness of their findings. A 2012 systematic review suggested that cupping therapy seems to be effective for herpes zoster and various other conditions but due to the high risk of publication bias, larger studies are needed to draw definitive conclusions.

Safety

Adverse Events

Acupuncture is generally safe when administered by an experienced, appropriately trained practitioner using clean-needle technique and sterile single-use needles. When improperly delivered it can cause adverse effects. Accidents and infections are associated with infractions of sterile technique or neglect on the part of the practitioner. To reduce the risk of serious adverse events after acupuncture, acupuncturists should be trained sufficiently. People with serious spinal disease, such as cancer or infection, are not good candidates for acupuncture. Contraindications to acupuncture (conditions that should not be treated with acupuncture) include coagulopathy disorders (e.g. hemophilia and advanced liver disease), warfarin use, severe psychiatric disorders (e.g. psychosis), and skin infections or skin trauma (e.g. burns). Further, electroacupuncture should be avoided at the spot of implanted electrical devices (such as pacemakers).

A 2011 systematic review of systematic reviews (internationally and without language restrictions) found that serious complications following acupuncture continue to be reported. Between 2000 and 2009, ninety-five cases of serious adverse events, including five deaths, were reported. Many such events are not inherent to acupuncture but are due to malpractice of acupuncturists. This might be why such complications have not been reported in surveys of adequately-trained acupuncturists. Most such reports originate from Asia, which may reflect the large number of treatments performed there or a relatively higher number of poorly trained Asian acupuncturists. Many serious adverse events were reported from developed countries. These included Australia, Austria, Canada, Croatia, France, Germany, Ireland, the Netherlands, New Zealand, Spain, Sweden, Switzerland, the UK, and the US. The number of adverse effects reported from the UK appears particularly unusual, which may indicate less under-reporting in the UK than other countries. Reports included 38 cases of infections and 42 cases of organ trauma. The most frequent adverse events included pneumothorax, and bacterial and viral infections.

A 2013 review found (without restrictions regarding publication date, study type or language) 295 cases of infections; mycobacterium was the pathogen in at least 96%. Likely sources of infection include towels, hot packs or boiling tank water, and reusing reprocessed needles. Possible sources of infection include contaminated needles, reusing personal needles, a person's skin containing mycobacterium, and reusing needles at various sites in the same person. Although acupuncture is generally considered a safe procedure, a 2013 review stated that the reports of infection transmission increased significantly in the prior decade, including those of mycobacterium. Although it is recommended that practitioners of acupuncture use disposable needles, the reuse of sterilized needles is still permitted. It is also recommended that thorough control practices for preventing infection be implemented and adapted.

The *Xingnao Kaiqiao* approach appears to be a safe form of treatment. Fainting was the most frequent adverse event. Fainting while being treated, hematoma, and pain while being treated are associated with individual physical differences and with needle manipulation.

English-language

A 2013 systematic review of the English-language case reports found that serious adverse events associated with acupuncture are rare, but that acupuncture is not without risk. Between 2000 and 2011 the English-language literature from 25 countries and regions reported 294 adverse events. The majority of the reported adverse events were relatively minor, and the incidences were low. For example, a prospective survey of 34,000 acupuncture treatments found no serious adverse events and 43 minor ones, a rate of 1.3 per 1000 interventions. Another survey found there were 7.1% minor adverse events, of which 5 were serious, amid 97,733 acupuncture patients. The most common adverse effect observed was infection (e.g. mycobacterium), and the majority of infections were bacterial in nature, caused by skin contact at the needling site. Infection has also resulted from skin contact with unsterilized equipment or with dirty towels in an unhygienic clinical setting. Other adverse complications included five reported cases of spinal-cord injuries (e.g. migrating broken needles or needling too deeply), four brain injuries, four peripheral nerve injuries, five heart injuries, seven other organ and tissue injuries, bilateral hand edema, epithelioid granuloma, pseudolymphoma, argyria, pustules, pancytopenia, and scarring due to hot-needle technique. Adverse reactions from acupuncture, which are unusual and uncommon in typical acupuncture practice, included syncope, galactorrhoea, bilateral nystagmus, pyoderma gangrenosum, hepatotoxicity, eruptive lichen planus, and spontaneous needle migration.

A 2013 systematic review found 31 cases of vascular injuries caused by acupuncture, three resulting in death. Two died from pericardial tamponade and one was from an aortoduodenal fistula. The same review found vascular injuries were rare, bleeding and pseudoaneurysm were most prevalent. A 2011 systematic review (without restriction in time or language), aiming to summarize all reported case of cardiac tamponade after acupuncture, found 26 cases resulting in 14 deaths, with little doubt about causality in most fatal instances. The same review concluded cardiac tamponade was a serious, usually fatal, though theoretically avoidable complication following acupuncture, and urged training to minimize risk.

A 2012 review found a number of adverse events were reported after acupuncture in the UK's National Health Service (NHS) but most (95%) were not severe, though miscategorization and under-reporting may alter the total figures. From January 2009 to December 2011, 468 safety incidents were recognized within the NHS organizations. The adverse events recorded included retained needles (31%), dizziness (30%), loss of consciousness/unresponsive (19%), falls (4%), bruising or soreness at needle site (2%), pneumothorax (1%) and other adverse side effects (12%). Acupuncture practitioners should know, and be prepared to be responsible for, any substantial harm from treatments. Some acupuncture proponents argue that the long history of acupuncture suggests it is safe. However, there is an increasing literature on adverse events (e.g. spinal-cord injury).

Acupuncture seems to be safe in people getting anticoagulants, assuming needles are used at the correct location and depth. Studies are required to verify these findings. The evidence suggests that acupuncture might be a safe option for people with allergic rhinitis.

Chinese, South Korean, and Japanese-language

A 2010 systematic review of the Chinese-language literature found numerous acupuncture-related adverse events, including pneumothorax, fainting, subarachnoid hemorrhage, and infection as the most frequent, and cardiovascular injuries, subarachnoid hemorrhage, pneumothorax, and recurrent cerebral hemorrhage as the most serious, most of which were due to improper technique. Between 1980 and 2009, the Chinese-language literature reported 479 adverse events. Prospective surveys show that mild, transient acupuncture-associated adverse events ranged from 6.71% to 15%. In a study with 190,924 patients, the prevalence of serious adverse events was roughly 0.024%. Another study showed a rate of adverse events requiring specific treatment of 2.2%, 4,963 incidences among 229,230 patients. Infections, mainly hepatitis, after acupuncture are reported often in English-language research, though are rarely reported in Chinese-language research, making it plausible that acupuncture-associated infections have been underreported in China. Infections were mostly caused by poor sterilization of acupuncture needles. Other adverse events included spinal epidural hematoma (in the cervical, thoracic and lumbar spine), chylothorax, injuries of abdominal organs and tissues, injuries in the neck region, injuries to the eyes, including orbital hemorrhage, traumatic cataract, injury of the oculomotor nerve and retinal puncture, hemorrhage to the cheeks and the hypoglottis, peripheral motor-nerve injuries and subsequent motor dysfunction, local allergic reactions to metal needles, stroke, and cerebral hemorrhage after acupuncture.

A causal link between acupuncture and the adverse events cardiac arrest, pyknolepsy, shock, fever, cough, thirst, aphonia, leg numbness, and sexual dysfunction remains uncertain. The same review concluded that acupuncture can be considered inherently safe when practiced by properly trained practitioners, but the review also stated there is a need to find effective strategies to minimize the health risks. Between 1999 and 2010, the Republic of Korean-literature contained reports of 1104 adverse events. Between the 1980s and 2002, the Japanese-language literature contained reports of 150 adverse events.

Children and Pregnancy

Although acupuncture has been practiced for thousands of years in China, its use in pediatrics in the United States did not become common until the early 2000s. In 2007, the National Health Interview Survey (NHIS) conducted by the National Center For Health Statistics (NCHS) estimated that approximately 150,000 children had received acupuncture treatment for a variety of conditions.

Acupuncture can potentially improve a number of common pediatric issues, including gastrointestinal issues, reflux, colic, asthma, allergies, ADHD, and headaches, however, its safety has been debated. In 2008 a study determined that the use of acupuncture-needle treatment on children was "questionable" due to the possibility of adverse side-effects and the pain manifestation differences in children versus adults. The study also includes warnings against practicing acupuncture on infants, as well as on children who are over-fatigued, very weak, or have over-eaten.

When used on children, acupuncture is considered safe when administered by well-trained, licensed practitioners using sterile needles; however, a 2011 review found there was limited research to draw definite conclusions about the overall safety of pediatric acupuncture. The same review found 279 adverse events, 25 of them serious. The adverse events were mostly mild in nature (e.g. bruising or bleeding). The prevalence of mild adverse events ranged from 10.1% to 13.5%, an estimated 168 incidences among 1,422 patients. On rare occasions adverse events were serious (e.g. cardiac rupture or hemoptysis); many might have been a result of substandard practice. The incidence of serious adverse events was 5 per one million, which included children and adults.

When used during pregnancy, the majority of adverse events caused by acupuncture were mild and transient, with few serious adverse events. The most frequent mild adverse event was needling or unspecified pain, followed by bleeding. Although two deaths (one stillbirth and one neonatal death) were reported, there was a lack of acupuncture-associated maternal mortality. Limiting the evidence as certain, probable or possible in the causality evaluation, the estimated incidence of adverse events following acupuncture in pregnant women was 131 per 10,000. Although acupuncture is not contraindicated in pregnant women, some specific acupuncture points are particularly sensitive to needle insertion; these spots, as well as the abdominal region, should be avoided during pregnancy.

Moxibustion and Cupping

Four adverse events associated with moxibustion were bruising, burns and cellulitis, spinal epidural abscess, and large superficial basal cell carcinoma. Ten adverse events were associated with cupping. The minor ones were keloid scarring, burns, and bullae; the serious ones were acquired hemophilia A, stroke following cupping on the back and neck, factitious panniculitis, reversible cardiac hypertrophy, and iron deficiency anemia.

Cost-effectiveness

A 2013 meta-analysis found that acupuncture for chronic low back pain was cost-effective as a complement to standard care, but not as a substitute for standard care except in cases where comorbid depression presented. The same meta-analysis found there was no difference between sham and non-sham acupuncture. A 2011 systematic review found insufficient evidence for the cost-effectiveness of acupuncture in the treatment of chronic low back pain. A 2010 systematic review found that the cost-effectiveness of acupuncture could not be concluded. A 2012 review found that acupuncture seems to be cost-effective for some pain conditions.

Risk of Forgoing Conventional Medical Care

As with other alternative medicines, unethical or naïve practitioners may induce patients to exhaust financial resources by pursuing ineffective treatment. Profession ethical codes set by accrediting organizations such as the National Certification Commission for Acupuncture and Oriental Medicine require practitioners to make "timely referrals to other health care professionals as may be appropriate." Stephen Barrett states that there is a "risk that an acupuncturist whose approach to diagnosis is not based on scientific concepts will fail to diagnose a dangerous condition".

Conceptual Basis

Traditional

Acupuncture is a substantial part of traditional Chinese medicine (TCM). Early acupuncture beliefs relied on concepts that are common in TCM, such as a life force energy called *qi*. *Qi* was believed to flow from the body's primary organs (zang-fu organs) to the "superficial" body tissues of the skin, muscles, tendons, bones, and joints, through channels called meridians. Acupuncture points where needles are inserted are mainly (but not always) found at locations along the meridians. Acupuncture points not found along a meridian are called extraordinary points and those with no designated site are called "A-shi" points.

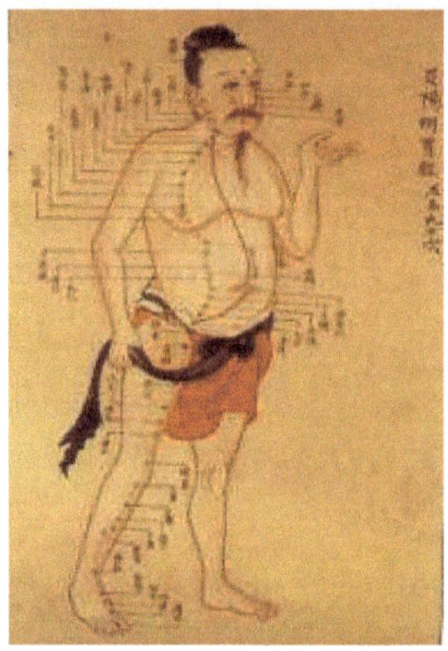

Old Chinese medical chart of acupuncture meridians

In TCM, disease is generally perceived as a disharmony or imbalance in energies such as yin, yang, *qi*, xuě, zàng-f?, meridians, and of the interaction between the body and the environment. Therapy is based on which "pattern of disharmony" can be identified. For example, some diseases are believed to be caused by meridians being invaded with an excess of wind, cold, and damp. In order to determine which pattern is at hand, practitioners examine things like the color and shape of the tongue, the relative strength of pulse-points, the smell of the breath, the quality of breathing, or the sound of the voice. TCM and its concept of disease does not strongly differentiate between the cause and effect of symptoms.

Purported Scientific Basis

Scientific research has not supported the existence of *qi*, meridians, or yin and yang. A *Nature* editorial described TCM as "fraught with pseudoscience", with the majority of its treatments having no logical mechanism of action. Quackwatch states that "TCM theory and practice are not based upon the body of knowledge related to health, disease, and health care that has been widely accepted by the scientific community. TCM practitioners disagree among themselves about how to diagnose patients and which treatments should go with which diagnoses. Even if they could agree, the TCM theories are so nebulous that no amount of scientific study will enable TCM to offer rational care."

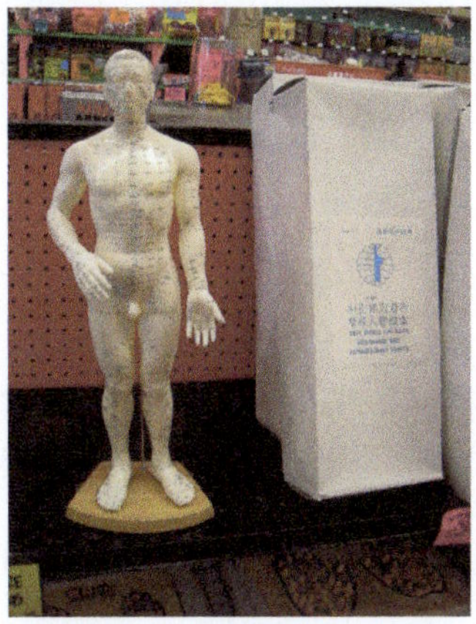

Modern acupuncture model

Some modern practitioners support the use of acupuncture to treat pain, but have abandoned the use of *qi*, meridians, *yin*, *yang* and other energies based in mysticism, as explanatory frameworks. The use of *qi* as an explanatory framework has been decreasing in China, even as it becomes more prominent during discussions of acupuncture in the US. Academic discussions of acupuncture still make reference to pseudoscientific concepts such as *qi* and meridians despite the lack of scientific evidence. Many within the scientific community consider attempts to rationalize acupuncture in science to be quackery, pseudoscience and "theatrical placebo". Academics Massimo Pigliucci and Maarten Boudry describe it as a "borderlands science" lying between science and pseudoscience.

Many acupuncturists attribute pain relief to the release of endorphins when needles penetrate, but no longer support the idea that acupuncture can affect a disease. It is a generally held belief within the acupuncture community that acupuncture points and meridians structures are special conduits for electrical signals but no research has established any consistent anatomical structure or function for either acupuncture points or meridians. Human tests to determine whether electrical continuity was significantly different near meridians than other places in the body have been inconclusive.

Some studies suggest acupuncture causes a series of events within the central nervous system, and that it is possible to inhibit acupuncture's analgesic effects with the opioid antagonist naloxone. Mechanical deformation of the skin by acupuncture needles appears to result in the release of adenosine. The anti-nociceptive effect of acupuncture may be mediated by the adenosine A1 receptor. A 2014 *Nature Reviews Cancer* review article found that since the key mouse studies that suggested acupuncture relieves pain via the local release of adenosine, which then triggered close-by A1 receptors "caused more tissue damage and inflammation relative to the size of the animal in mice than in humans, such studies unnecessarily muddled a finding that local inflammation can result in the local release of adenosine with analgesic effect."

It has been proposed that acupuncture's effects in gastrointestinal disorders may relate to its effects on the parasympathetic and sympathetic nervous system, which have been said to be the "Western medicine" equivalent of "yin and yang". Another mechanism whereby acupuncture may be effective for gastrointestinal dysfunction involves the promotion of gastric peristalsis in subjects with low initial gastric motility, and suppressing peristalsis in subjects with active initial motility. Acupuncture has also been found to exert anti-inflammatory effects, which may be mediated by the activation of the vagus nerve and deactivation of inflammatory macrophages. Neuroimaging studies suggest that acupuncture stimulation results in deactivation of the limbic brain areas and the default mode network.

History

Origins

Acupuncture, along with moxibustion, is one of the oldest practices of Traditional Chinese Medicine. Most historians believe the practice began in China, though there are some conflicting narratives on when it originated. Academics David Ramey and Paul Buell said the exact date acupuncture was founded depends on the extent dating of ancient texts can be trusted and the interpretation of what constitutes acupuncture.

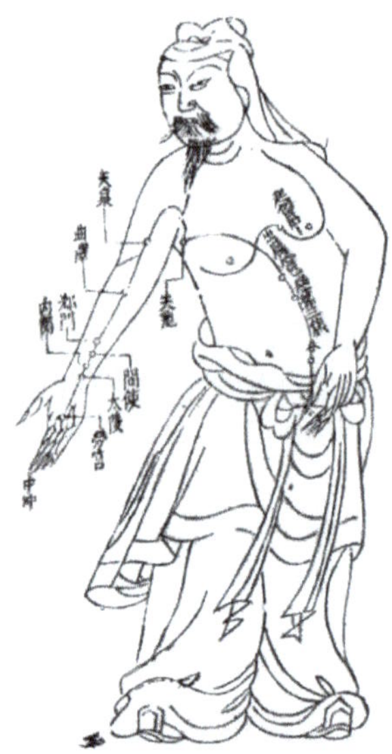

Acupuncture chart from the Ming dynasty (c. 1368–1644)

According to an article in *Rheumatology*, the first documentation of an “organized system of diagnosis and treatment” for acupuncture was in *The Yellow Emperor’s Classic of Internal Medicine* (Huangdi Neijing) from about 100 BC. Gold and silver needles found in the tomb of Liu Sheng from around 100 BC are believed to be the earliest archeological evidence of acupuncture, though it is unclear if that was their purpose. According to Dr. Plinio Prioreschi, the earliest known historical record of acupuncture is the Shih-Chi (“Record of History”), written by a historian around 100 BC. It is believed that this text was documenting what was established practice at that time.

Alternate Theories

The 5,000-year-old mummified body of Ötzi the Iceman was found with 15 groups of tattoos, many of which were located at points on the body where acupuncture needles are used for abdominal or lower back problems. Evidence from the body suggests Otzi suffered from these conditions. This has been cited as evidence that practices similar to acupuncture may have been practiced elsewhere in Eurasia during the early Bronze Age; however, *The Oxford Handbook of the History of Medicine* calls this theory "speculative". It is considered unlikely that acupuncture was practiced before 2000 BC. The Ötzi the Iceman's tattoo marks suggest to some experts that an acupuncture-like treatment was previously used in Europe 5 millennia ago.

Acupuncture may have been practiced during the Neolithic era, near the end of the stone age, using sharpened stones called Bian shi. Many Chinese texts from later eras refer to sharp stones called "plen", which means "stone probe", that may have been used for acupuncture purposes. The ancient Chinese medical text, Huangdi Neijing, indicates that sharp stones were believed at-the-time to cure illnesses at or near the body's surface, perhaps because of the short depth a stone could penetrate. However, it is more likely that stones were used for other medical purposes, such as puncturing a growth to drain its pus. The *Mawangdui* texts, which are believed to be from the 2nd century BC, mention the use of pointed stones to open abscesses, and moxibustion, but not for acupuncture. It is also speculated that these stones may have been used for bloodletting, due to the ancient Chinese belief that illnesses were caused by demons within the body that could be killed or released. It is likely bloodletting was an antecedent to acupuncture.

According to historians Lu Gwei-djen and Joseph Needham, there is substantial evidence that acupuncture may have begun around 600 BC. Some hieroglyphs and pictographs from that era suggests acupuncture and moxibustion were practiced. However, historians Gwei-djen and Needham said it was unlikely a needle could be made out of the materials available in China during this time period. It is possible Bronze was used for early acupuncture needles. Tin, copper, gold and silver are also possibilities, though they are considered less likely, or to have been used in fewer cases. If acupuncture was practiced during the Shang dynasty (1766 to 1122 BC), organic materials like thorns, sharpened bones, or bamboo may have been used. Once methods for producing steel were discovered, it would replace all other materials, since it could be used to create a very fine, but sturdy needles. Gwei-djen and Needham noted that all the ancient materials that could have been used for acupuncture and which often produce archeological evidence, such as sharpened bones, bamboo or stones, were also used for other purposes. An article in *Rheumatology* said that the absence of any mention of acupuncture in documents found in the tomb of Ma-Wang-Dui from 198 BC suggest that acupuncture was not practiced by that time.

Belief Systems

Several different and sometimes conflicting belief systems emerged regarding acupuncture. This may have been the result of competing schools of thought. Some ancient texts referred to using acupuncture to cause bleeding, while others mixed the ideas of blood-letting and spiritual ch'i energy. Over time, the focus shifted from blood to the concept of puncturing specific points on the body, and eventually to balancing Yin and Yang energies as well. According to Dr. David Ramey, no single "method or theory" was ever predominantly adopted as the standard. At the time, scientific knowledge of medicine was not yet developed, especially because in China dissection of the deceased was forbidden, preventing the development of basic anatomical knowledge.

It is not certain when specific acupuncture points were introduced, but the autobiography of Pien Chhio from around 400–500 BC references inserting needles at designated areas. Bian Que believed there was a single acupuncture point at the top of one's skull that he called the point "of the hundred meetings." Texts dated to be from 156–186 BC document early beliefs in channels of life force energy called meridians that would later be an element in early acupuncture beliefs.

Ramey and Buell said the "practice and theoretical underpinnings" of modern acupuncture were introduced in the *The Yellow Emperor's Classic* (Huangdi Neijing) around 100 BC. It introduced the concept of using acupuncture to manipulate the flow of life energy (*qi*) in a network of meridian (channels) in the body. The network concept was made up of acu-tracts, such as a line down the arms, where it said acupoints were located. Some of the sites acupuncturists use needles at today still have the same names as those given to them by the *Yellow Emporer's Classic*. Numerous additional documents were published over the centuries introducing new acupoints. By the 4th century AD, most of the acupuncture sites in use today had been named and identified.

Early Development in China

Establishment and Growth

In the first half of the 1st century AD, acupuncturists began promoting the belief that acupuncture's effectiveness was influenced by the time of day or night, the lunar cycle, and the season. The Science of the Yin-Yang Cycles (*Yün Chhi Hsüeh*) was a set of beliefs that curing diseases relied on the alignment of both heavenly (thien) and earthly (ti) forces that were attuned to cycles like that of the sun and moon. There were several different belief systems that relied on a number of celestial and earthly bodies or elements that rotated and only became aligned at certain times. According to Needham and Gwei-djen, these "arbitrary predictions" were depicted by acupuncturists in complex charts and through a set of special terminology.

Acupuncture needles during this period were much thicker than most modern ones and often resulted in infection. Infection is caused by a lack of sterilization, but at that time it was believed to be caused by use of the wrong needle, or needling in the wrong place, or at the wrong time. Later, many needles were heated in boiling water, or in a flame. Sometimes needles were used while they were still hot, creating a cauterizing effect at the injection site. Nine needles were recommended in the *Chen Chiu Ta Chheng* from 1601, which may have been because of an ancient Chinese belief that nine was a magic number.

Other belief systems were based on the idea that the human body operated on a rhythm and acupuncture had to be applied at the right point in the rhythm to be effective. In some cases a lack of balance between Yin and Yang were believed to be the cause of disease.

In the 1st century AD, many of the first books about acupuncture were published and recognized acupuncturist experts began to emerge. The *Zhen Jiu Jia Yi Jing*, which was published in the mid-3rd century, became the oldest acupuncture book that is still in existence in the modern era. Other books like the *Yu Kuei Chen Ching*, written by the Director of Medical Services for China, were also influential during this period, but were not preserved. In the mid 7th century, Sun Simiao published acupuncture-related diagrams and charts that established standardized methods for finding acupuncture sites on people of different sizes and categorized acupuncture sites in a set of modules.

Acupuncture became more established in China as improvements in paper led to the publication of more acupuncture books. The Imperial Medical Service and the Imperial Medical College, which both supported acupuncture, became more established and created medical colleges in every province. The public was also exposed to stories about royal figures being cured of their diseases by prominent acupuncturists. By time *The Great Compendium of Acupuncture and Moxibustion* was published during the Ming dynasty (1368–1644 AD), most of the acupuncture practices used in the modern era had been established.

Decline

By the end of the Song dynasty (1279 AD), acupuncture had lost much of its status in China. It became rarer in the following centuries, and was associated with less prestigious professions like alchemy, shamanism, midwifery and moxibustion. Additionally, by the 18th century, scientific rationality was becoming more popular than traditional superstitious beliefs. By 1757 a book documenting the history of Chinese medicine called acupuncture a "lost art". Its decline was attributed in part to the popularity of prescriptions and medications, as well as its association with the lower classes.

In 1822, the Chinese Emperor signed a decree excluding the practice of acupuncture from the Imperial Medical Institute. He said it was unfit for practice by gentlemen-scholars. In China acupuncture was increasingly associated with lower-class, illiterate practitioners. It was restored for a time, but banned again in 1929 in favor of science-based Western medicine. Although acupuncture declined in China during this time period, it was also growing in popularity in other countries.

International Expansion

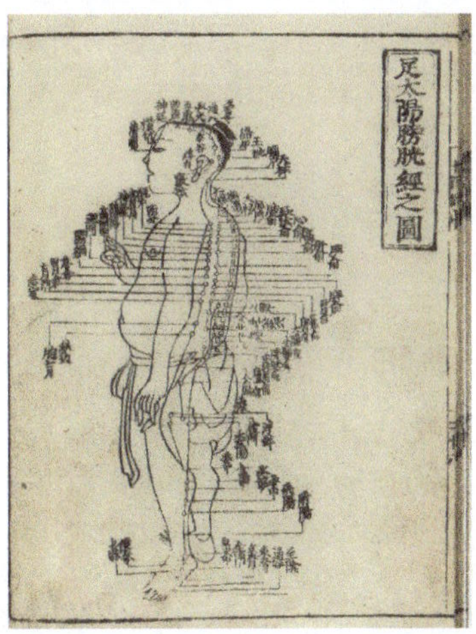

Acupuncture chart from *Shisi jing fahui* (Expression of the Fourteen Meridians) written by Hua Shou (fl. 1340s, Ming dynasty). Japanese reprint by Suharaya Heisuke (Edo, 1. year Kyōhō = 1716).

Korea is believed to be the first country in Asia that acupuncture spread to outside of China. Within Korea there is a legend that acupuncture was developed by emperor Dangun, though it is more likely to have been brought into Korea from a Chinese colonial prefecture in 514 AD. Acupuncture use was commonplace in Korea by the 6th century. It spread to Vietnam in the 8th and 9th centuries. As Vietnam began trading with Japan and China around the 9th century, it was influenced by their acupuncture practices as well. China and Korea sent "medical missionaries" that spread traditional Chinese medicine to Japan, starting around 219 AD. In

553, several Korean and Chinese citizens were appointed to re-organize medical education in Japan and they incorporated acupuncture as part of that system. Japan later sent students back to China and established acupuncture as one of five divisions of the Chinese State Medical Administration System.

Acupuncture began to spread to Europe in the second half of the 17th century. Around this time the surgeon-general of the Dutch East India Company met Japanese and Chinese acupuncture practitioners and later encouraged Europeans to further investigate it. He published the first in-depth description of acupuncture for the European audience and created the term "acupuncture" in his 1683 work *De Acupunctura*. France was an early adopter among the West due to the influence of Jesuit missionaries, who brought the practice to French clinics in the 16th century. The French doctor Louis Berlioz (the father of the composer Hector Berlioz) is usually credited with being the first to experiment with the procedure in Europe in 1810, before publishing his findings in 1816.

By the 19th century, acupuncture had become commonplace in many areas of the world. Americans and Britains began showing interest in acupuncture in the early 20th century. Western practitioners abandoned acupuncture's traditional beliefs in spiritual energy, pulse diagnosis, and the cycles of the moon, sun or the body's rhythm. Diagrams of the flow of spiritual energy, for example, conflicted with the West's own anatomical diagrams. It adopted a new set of ideas for acupuncture based on tapping needles into nerves. In Europe it was speculated that acupuncture may allow or prevent the flow of electricity in the body, as electrical pulses were found to make a frog's leg twitch after death.

The West eventually created a belief system based on Travell trigger points that were believed to inhibit pain. They were in the same locations as China's spiritually identified acupuncture points, but under a different nomenclature. The first elaborate Western treatise on acupuncture was published in 1683 by Willem ten Rhijne.

Modern Era

In China, the popularity of acupuncture rebounded in 1949 when Mao Zedong took power and sought to unite China behind traditional cultural values. It was also during this time that many Eastern medical practices were consolidated under the name Traditional Chinese Medicine (TCM).

New practices were adopted in the 20th century, such as using a cluster of needles, electrified needles, or leaving needles inserted for up to a week. A lot of emphasis developed on using acupuncture on the ear. Acupuncture research organizations were founded in the 1950s and acupuncture services became available in modern hospitals. China, where acupuncture was believed to have originated, was increasingly influenced by Western medicine. Meanwhile, acupuncture grew in popularity in the US. The US Congress created the Office of Alternative Medicine in 1992 and the National Institutes of Health (NIH) declared support for acupuncture for some conditions in November 1997. In 1999, the National Center for Complementary and Alternative Medicine was created within the NIH. Acupuncture became the most popular alternative medicine in the US.

Politicians from the Chinese Communist Party said acupuncture was superstitious and conflicted with the party's commitment to science. Communist Party Chairman Mao Zedong later reversed this position, arguing that the practice was based on scientific principles.

In 1971, a *New York Times* reporter published an article on his acupuncture experiences in China, which led to more investigation of and support for acupuncture. The US President Richard Nixon visited China in 1972. During one part of the visit, the delegation was shown a patient undergoing major surgery while fully awake, ostensibly receiving acupuncture rather than anesthesia. Later it was found that the patients selected for the surgery had both a high pain tolerance and received heavy indoctrination before the operation; these demonstration cases were also frequently receiving morphine surreptitiously through an intravenous drip that observers were told contained only fluids and nutrients. One patient receiving open heart surgery while awake was ultimately found to have received a combination of three powerful sedatives as well as large injections of a local anesthetic into the wound. After the National Institute of Health expressed support for acupuncture for a limited number of conditions, adoption in the US grew further. In 1972 the first legal acupuncture center in the US was established in Washington DC and in 1973 the American Internal Revenue Service allowed acupuncture to be deducted as a medical expense.

In 2006, a BBC documentary *Alternative Medicine* filmed a patient undergoing open heart surgery allegedly under acupuncture-induced anesthesia. It was later revealed that the patient had been given a cocktail of anesthetics.

Adoption

Acupuncture is popular in China, the US, Australia, and Europe including all five Nordic countries, though less so in Finland. It is most heavily practiced in China and is one of the most common alternative medicine practices in Europe. In Switzerland, acupuncture has become the most frequently used alternative medicine since 2004. In the United Kingdom, a total of 4 million acupuncture treatments were administered in 2009. Acupuncture is used in most pain clinics and hospices in the UK. An estimated 1 in 10 adults in Australia used acupuncture in 2004. In Japan, it is estimated that 25 percent of the population will try acupuncture at some point, though in most cases it is not covered by public health insurance. Users of acupuncture in Japan are more likely to be elderly and to have a limited education. Approximately half of users surveyed indicated a likelihood to seek such remedies in the future, while 37% did not. Less than one percent of the US population reported having used acupuncture in the early 1990s. By the early 2010s, more than 14 million Americans reported having used acupuncture as part of their health care.

In the US, acupuncture is increasingly (as of 2014) used at academic medical centers, and is usually offered through CAM centers or anesthesia and pain management services. Examples include those at Harvard University, Stanford University, Johns Hopkins University, and UCLA. This usage has been criticized owing to there being little scientific evidence for explicit effects, or the mechanisms for its supposed effectiveness, for any condition that is discernible from placebo. Acupuncture has been called 'theatrical placebo', and David Gorski argues that when acupuncture proponents advocate 'harnessing of placebo effects' or work on developing 'meaningful placebos', they essentially concede it is little more than that.

The use of acupuncture in Germany increased by 20% in 2007, after the German acupuncture trials supported its efficacy for certain uses. In 2011, there were more than one million users, and insurance companies have estimated that two-thirds of German users are women. As a result of the trials, German public health insurers began to cover acupuncture for chronic low back pain and osteoarthritis of the knee, but not tension headache or migraine. This decision was based in part on socio-political reasons. Some insurers in Germany chose to stop reimbursement of acupuncture because of the trials. For other conditions, insurers in Germany were not convinced that acupuncture had adequate benefits over usual care or sham treatments. Highlighting the results of the placebo group, researchers refused to accept a placebo therapy as efficient.

Regulation

There are various government and trade association regulatory bodies for acupuncture in the United Kingdom, the United States, Saudi Arabia, Australia, Japan, Canada, and in European countries and elsewhere. The World Health Organization recommends that before being licensed or certified, an acupuncturist receive 200 hours of specialized training if they are a physician and 2,500 hours for non-physicians; many governments have adopted similar standards.

In China, the practice of acupuncture is regulated by the Chinese Medicine Council that was formed in 1999 by the Legislative Council. It includes a licensing exam and registration, as well as degree courses approved by the board. Canada has acupuncture licensing programs in the provinces of British Columbia, Ontario, Alberta and Quebec; standards set by the Chinese Medicine and Acupuncture Association of Canada are used in provinces without government regulation. Regulation in the US began in the 1970s in California, which was eventually followed by every state but Wyoming and Idaho. Licensing requirements vary greatly from state to state. The needles used in acupuncture are regulated in the US by the Food and Drug Administration. In some states acupuncture is regulated by a board of medical examiners, while in others by the board of licensing, health or education.

In Japan, acupuncturists are licensed by the Minister of Health, Labour and Welfare after passing an examination and graduating from a technical school or university. Australia regulates Chinese medical traditions through the Chinese Medicine Board of Australia and the Public Health (Skin Penetration) Regulation of 2000. It restricts the use of words like "Acupuncture" and "Registered Acupuncturist". At least 28 countries in Europe have professional associations for acupuncturists. In France, the Académie Nationale de Médecine (National Academy of Medicine) has regulated acupuncture since 1955.

Ozone Therapy

Ozone therapy is a form of alternative medicine treatment that purports to increase the amount of oxygen in the body through the introduction of ozone. Various techniques have been suggested, with purported benefits including the treatment of cancer, AIDS, and multiple sclerosis, among others. There is no credible, peer reviewed evidence to support the use of ozone as a type of medical therapy.

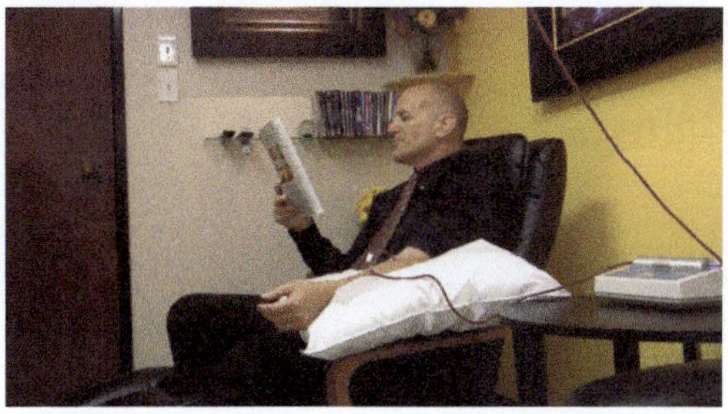

Person undergoing ozone IV therapy

Proposed Uses

Ozone therapy consists of the introduction of ozone into the body via various methods, usually involving its mixture with various gases and liquids before injection, with potential routes including the vagina, rectum, intramuscular (in a muscle), subcutaneously (under the skin), or intravenously (directly into veins). Ozone can also be introduced via autohemotherapy, in which blood is drawn from the patient, exposed to ozone and re-injected into the patient.

This therapy has been proposed for use in various diseases, including cancer, AIDS, multiple sclerosis, arthritis, heart disease, Alzheimer's dementia, Lyme disease, though supportive evidence for these applications is limited. Theories about the ability of ozone to kill tumor cells with oxygen have no credible scientific basis. For treatment of HIV/AIDS, although ozone deactivates the viral particles outside the body, there is no evidence of benefit for living patients.

The United States Food and Drug Administration initially stated in 1976, and reiterated its position in 2006, that when inhaled, ozone is a toxic gas which has no demonstrated safe medical application, though their position statements primarily deal with its potential for causing inflammation and pulmonary edema in the lungs. Their second major contention is that in order for ozone to be effective as a germicide, it must be present in a concentration far greater than can be safely tolerated by humans or other animals.

Ozone has been suggested for use in dentistry, but existing evidence does not support its use.

One review found tentative evidence that ozone injection is an effective treatment for herniated discs.

There is some controversy about its use by athletes in an attempt to increase performance; although its use is not disallowed in and of itself, it can be mixed with other banned substances for administration prior to injection.

Safety

Much of the concern related to ozone therapy revolves around the safety of blood ozonation. It is well established that when inhaled by mammals, ozone reacts with compounds in tissues lining the lungs and triggers a cascade of pathological effects including pulmonary edema. Saul Green has argued that since ozone has the capacity to oxidize organic compounds in an atmospheric environment, it should also logically oxidize blood components and endogenous human tissues. High levels of inhaled ozone are known to be toxic, though single-dose inhalation of lower levels is not. Proponents suggest that its effects are tissue dependent, though the subject is still debated.

Serious complications reported from the use of this therapy include the development of hepatitis and also include five reported fatalities. There is some concern about an association with heart attacks after autohemotherapy, though this association has been contested as well.

History

In 1856, just 16 years after its discovery, ozone was first used in a health care setting to disinfect operating rooms and sterilize surgical instruments. By the end of the 19th century the use of ozone to disinfect drinking water of bacteria and viruses was well established in mainland Europe. In 1892 *The Lancet* published an article describing the administration of ozone for treatment of tuberculosis. Ozone was used during the First World War to for disinfection of wounds.

Grape Therapy

Grape therapy, also known as ampelotherapy is a form of naturopathic alternative medicine that involves heavy consumption of grapes, including seeds, and parts of the vine, including leaves. Although there is some limited evidence of positive benefits from the use of grape therapy for health purposes, extreme claims, such as its ability to cure cancer, have been widely derided as "quackery".

Background

Grapes have been associated with health for many centuries. They contain organic acids (tartaric, malic, citric, tannic), B group vitamins, vitamins P, PP, and C, calcium, carotene, magnesium salts, phosphorus and potassium, as well as trace elements such as copper, iron, manganese, sulphur and zinc. Proanthocyanidins, first extracted from grape seeds in 1970, and resveratrol, found in grape skins, are currently being studied for possible uses in the prevention and treatment of cancer and other illnesses, and for anti-ageing. Proanthocyanidins are powerful antioxidants that can block the action of free radicals. Advocates of grape therapy argue that these antioxidants inhibit the development of cancer, and can be used in treating a variety of other medical conditions such as arthritis and diabetes. Grapes are said to be beneficial for protecting against cardiovascular disease and, because of their potassium and glucose content, they are argued to be useful for treatment of heart disease by strengthening muscle tone, improving heart function and having a positive impact on convalescence. Alternative medicine practitioners have at times also recommended grapes and parts of the vine for high blood pressure, menopause, varicose veins, high cholesterol, skin rashes, and urination problems. The grape diet was promoted in the past as a treatment to flush toxins from the body. The grape cure is also prescribed for a decline in nutrition, especially with patients with early stage of tuberculosis, for diseases of the liver, kidneys and lungs and for gout and secondary anaemia and, in addition, for mental disease, nervous disorders, and sexual problems. Recent research by scientists at UCLA has found that combining resveratrol with benzoyl peroxide may improve that drug's ability to kill the bacteria associated with acne. The presence of resveratrol on the skin of red grapes has prompted some doctors to recommend that adults drink reasonable quantities of red wine to combat heart disease. Resveratrol in red wine is suggested as an explanation for the disputed "French paradox," i.e. the apparent low occurrence of heart disease among the French, even though they eat a high-fat diet.

History

The documentation of grape cures was first seen in a publication by V.N. Dmitriev called "Treatment With Grapes in Yalta on the Southern Crimean Shore" (1878). In the USSR, the principles of the grape cure were developed in the 1920s by a group of physicians of the Semashko Institute (Yalta), headed by A.V. D'iakov. Ampelotherapy continues to be offered in health clinics and spas, particularly in Europe, together with vinotherapy, a cosmetic treatment that involves rubbing grapes into the skin. Johanna Brandt, a South African doctor, popularized the grape diet as a treatment for cancer from 1925. She published about twenty pamphlets on the subject of natural remedies for health problems with her best-known publication being *The Grape Cure*, which is said to have been written after Brandt had cured herself of stomach cancer by following the diet. The book was republished in 1989 as *How to Conquer Cancer, Naturally*, including an endorsement of Brandt's work by Benedict Lust, who is commonly referred to as "the father of naturopathy". The book may have been inspired by Arnold Ehret, a contemporary, who taught a Grape Cure course.

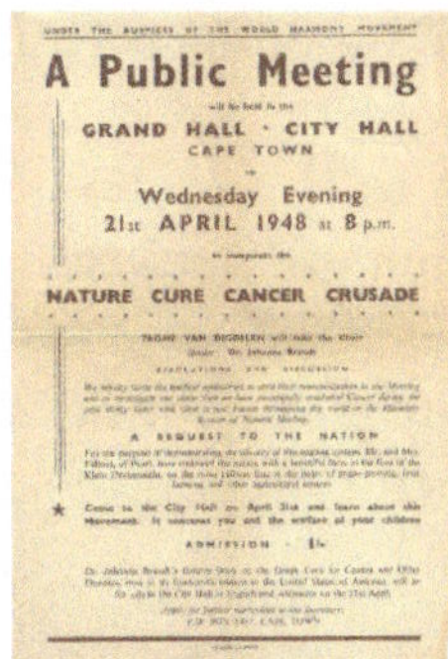
A Public Meeting
GRAND HALL · CITY HALL
CAPE TOWN
Wednesday Evening
21st APRIL 1948 at 8 p.m.
NATURE CURE CANCER CRUSADE
A REQUEST TO THE NATION
ADMISSION · 1/-

Johanna Brandt - Notice

Treatments

The leaves, stems, and grape itself, including seeds and skins, are used in herbal remedies. Most recommended diets involve large quantities of grapes, together with other foods. Treatments offered have varied from a diet that consists of eating large quantities of grapes together with other food to those that involve consuming nothing but grapes. One recommended course of ampelotherapy has to last 1-2 months. It is recommended to eat 2 kilos of grapes with their seed three times per week. This intake should be accompanied by a diet that limits the intake of smoked meat, milk and all dairy products and alcohol. The diet proposed by Johanna Brandt recommended fasting for two or three days, consuming only cold water, followed by a diet of only grapes and water for one to two weeks, with seven meals a day. Fresh fruits, tomatoes, and sour milk or cottage cheese are then introduced to the diet followed by raw vegetables.

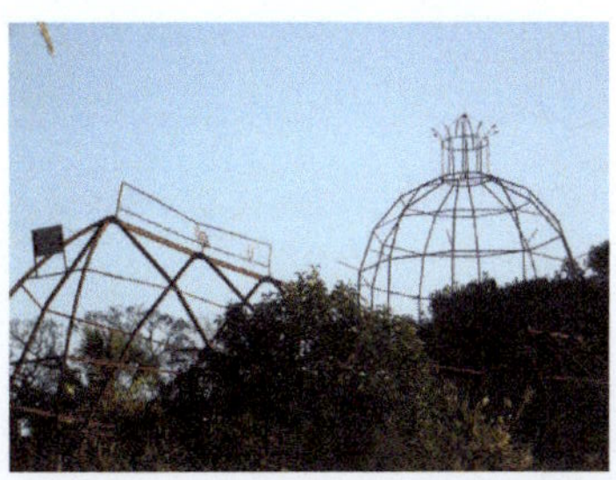

An abandoned Ampelotherapy clinic on the outskirts of Rome, Italy

Criticisms

Available scientific evidence does not support claims that a diet of grapes is alone effective for treating cancer or any other disease. Some laboratory evidence suggests that certain chemicals in grapes, their seeds and skins may help prevent heart disease and cancer, and are effective in treating diabetes but more research is needed on humans to understand the possible long-term benefits. The Brandt diet, in particular, has been described as "quackery" by Barrett who notes that the American Cancer Society reviewed the *The Grape Cure* in 1965, 1971, 1974, and 2000 and found no evidence of benefit against human cancer or any other disease.

Orthomolecular Medicine

Orthomolecular medicine, a form of alternative medicine, aims to maintain human health through nutritional supplementation. The concept builds on the idea of an optimum nutritional environment in the body and suggests that diseases reflect deficiencies in this environment. Treatment for disease, according to this view, involves attempts to correct "imbalances or deficiencies based on individual biochemistry" by use of supposedly "natural" substances such as vitamins, minerals, amino acids, trace elements and fatty acids. The notions behind orthomolecular medicine are not supported by sound medical evidence and the therapy is not effective; even the accuracy of calling the orthomolecular approach a form of medicine has been questioned since the 1970s.

The approach is sometimes referred to as megavitamin therapy because its practice evolved out of, and in some cases still uses, doses of vitamins and minerals many times higher than the recommended dietary intake. Orthomolecular practitioners may also incorporate a variety of other styles of treatment into their approaches, including dietary restriction, megadoses of non-vitamin nutrients and mainstream pharmaceutical drugs. Proponents argue that non-optimal levels of certain substances can cause health issues beyond simple vitamin deficiency and see balancing these substances as an integral part of health.

Linus Pauling coined the term "orthomolecular" in the 1960s to mean "the right molecules in the right amounts" (*ortho-* in Greek implies "correct"). Proponents of orthomolecular medicine hold that treatment must be based on each patient's individual biochemistry.

The scientific and medical consensus holds that the broad claims of efficacy advanced by advocates of orthomolecular medicine are not adequately tested as drug therapies. It has been described as a form of food faddism and as quackery. Proponents point to mainstream sources that have published research supporting the benefits of nutrient supplementation and to instances where conventional medicine uses vitamins as treatments for some diseases.

Some vitamins in large doses have been linked to increased risk of cardiovascular disease, of cancer and of death. The scientific consensus view is that for normal individuals, a balanced diet contains all necessary vitamins and minerals, and that routine supplementation is not necessary absent specific diagnosed deficiencies.

History and Development

In the early 20th century, some doctors hypothesised that vitamins could cure disease, and supplements were prescribed in megadoses by the 1930s. Their effects on health were disappointing, though, and in the 1950s and 1960s, nutrition was de-emphasised in standard medical curricula. Riordon's organization cite figures from this period as founders of their movement, although the word "orthomolecular" was coined by Linus Pauling only in 1967.

Amongst the individuals described posthumously as orthomolecularists are Max Gerson, who developed a diet that he claimed could treat diseases, which the American Medical Association's 1949 Council on Pharmacy and Chemistry found ineffective; and the Shute brothers, who attempted to treat heart disease with vitamin E. Several concepts now cited by orthomolecularists, including individual biochemical variation and inborn errors of metabolism, debuted in scientific papers early in the 20th century.

In 1948, William McCormick theorized that vitamin C deficiency played an important role in many diseases and began to use large doses in patients. In the 1950s, Fred R. Klenner also tried vitamin C megadosage as a therapy for a wide range of illnesses, including polio. Irwin Stone stated that organisms that do not synthesise their own vitamin C due to a loss-of-function mutation have a disease he called "hypoascorbemia". This term is not used by the medical community, and the idea of an organism-wide lack of a biosynthetic pathway as a disease was not endorsed by Stone's contemporaries.

In the 1950s, some individuals believed that vitamin deficiencies caused mental illness. Psychiatrists Humphry Osmond and Abram Hoffer gave people having acute schizophrenic episodes high doses of niacin, while William Kaufman used niacinamide. While niacin has no known efficacy in psychiatric disease, the use of niacin in combination with statins and other medical therapies has become one of several medical treatments for cardiovascular disease.

In the late 1960s, Linus Pauling introduced the expression "orthomolecular" to express the idea of *the right molecules in the right amounts*. Since the first claims of medical breakthroughs with vitamin C by Pauling and others, findings on the health effects of vitamin C have been controversial and contradictory. Pauling's claims have been criticised as overbroad.

Later research branched out into nutrients besides niacin and vitamin C, including essential fatty acids.

Scope

According to Abram Hoffer, orthomolecular medicine does not purport to treat all diseases, nor is it "a replacement for standard treatment. A proportion of patients will require orthodox treatment, a proportion will do much better on orthomolecular treatment, and the rest will need a skillful blend of both." Nevertheless, advocates have said that nutrients can prevent, treat, and sometimes cure a wide range of medical conditions, including: acne, alcoholism, allergies, arthritis, autism, bee stings, bipolar disorder, burns, cancer, the common cold, depression, drug addiction, drug overdose, epilepsy, heart diseases, heavy metal toxicity, acute hepatitis, herpes, hyperactivity, hypertension, hypoglycemia, influenza, learning disabilities, mental and metabolic disorders, migraine, mononucleosis, mushroom poisoning, neuropathy & polyneuritis (including multiple sclerosis), osteoporosis, polio, an hypothesised condition called "pyroluria", radiation sickness, Raynaud's disease, mental retardation, schizophrenia, shock, skin problems, snakebite, spider bite, tetanus toxin and viral pneumonia.

Orthomolecular Psychiatry

Hoffer believed that particular nutrients could cure mental illness. In the 1950s, he attempted to treat schizophrenia with niacin, although proponents of orthomolecular psychiatry say that the ideas behind their approach predate Hoffer. According to Hoffer and others who called themselves "orthomolecular psychiatrists", psychiatric syndromes result from biochemical deficiencies, allergies, toxicities or several hypothetical contributing conditions which they termed pyroluria, histadelia and histapenia. These purported causes were said to be found during an "individual biochemical workup" and treated with megavitamin therapy and dietary changes including fasting. These diagnoses and treatments are not accepted by evidence-based medicine.

Principles

According to Abram Hoffer, "primitive" peoples do not consume processed foods and do not have "degenerative" diseases. In contrast, typical "Western" diets are said to be insufficient for long-term health, necessitating the use of megadose supplements of vitamins, dietary minerals, proteins, antioxidants, amino acids, ω-3 fatty acids, ω-6 fatty acids, medium-chain triglycerides, dietary fiber, short and long chain fatty acids, lipotropes, systemic and digestive enzymes, other digestive factors, and prohormones to ward off hypothetical metabolism anomalies at an early stage, before they cause disease.

Orthomolecularists say that they provide prescriptions for optimal amounts of micronutrients after individual diagnoses based on blood tests and personal histories. Lifestyle and diet changes may also be recommended. The battery of tests ordered includes many that are not considered useful by medicine.

Prevalence

Orthomolecular medicine is practiced by few medical practitioners.

A survey released in May, 2004 by the National Center for Complementary and Alternative Medicine focused on who used alternative medicine, what was used, and why it was used in the United States by adults age 18 years and over during 2003. The survey reported uses in the previous twelve months that include orthomolecular related uses: Nonvitamin, nonmineral, natural products 18.9%, Diet-based therapies 3.5%, Megavitamin therapy 2.8%.

Another recent CAM survey reported that 12% of liver disease patients used the antioxidant silymarin, more than 6% used vitamins, and that "in all, 74% of patients reported using CAM in addition to the medications prescribed by their physician, but 26% did not inform their physician of their CAM use."

Even though the health benefits are not established, the use of high doses of vitamins is also common in people who have been diagnosed with cancer. According to Cancer Research UK, cancer patients should always seek professional advice before taking such supplements, and using them as a substitute for conventional treatment "could be harmful to [their] health and greatly reduce the chance of curing or controlling [their] cancer".

Medical and Scientific Reception

Methodology

Orthomolecular therapies have been criticized as lacking a sufficient evidence base for clinical use: their scientific foundations are too weak, the studies that have been performed are too few and too open to interpretation, and reported positive findings in observational studies are contradicted by the results of more rigorous clinical trials. Accordingly, "there is no evidence that orthomolecular medicine is effective". Proponents of orthomolecular medicine strongly dispute this statement by citing studies demonstrating the effectiveness of treatments involving vitamins, though this ignores the belief that a normal diet will provide adequate nutrients to avoid deficiencies, and that orthomolecular treatments are not actually related to vitamin deficiency. The lack of scientifically rigorous testing of orthomolecular medicine has led to its practices being classed with other forms of alternative medicine and regarded as unscientific. It has been described as food faddism and quackery, with critics arguing that it is based upon an "exaggerated belief in the effects of nutrition upon health and disease." Orthomolecular practitioners will often use dubious diagnostic methods to define what substances are "correct"; one example is hair analysis, which produces spurious results when used in this fashion.

Proponents of orthomolecular medicine contend that, unlike some other forms of alternative medicine such as homeopathy, their ideas are at least biologically based, do not involve magical thinking, and are capable of generating testable hypotheses. *Orthomolecular* is not a standard medical term, and clinical use of specific nutrients is considered a form of chemoprevention (to prevent or delay development of disease) or chemotherapy (to treat an existing condition).

Despite a lack of evidence for its efficacy, interest in intravenous high dose vitamin C therapy has not been permanently extinguished, and some research groups continue to investigate whether it has an effect as a possible cancer treatment.

Views on Safety and Efficacy

In general, the vitamin megadoses advocated by orthomolecular medicine are unsupported by scientific consensus. Some vitamins are toxic in high doses, including niacin (B_3), cholecalciferol (D) and tocopherol (E). The view of the medical community is that there is no evidence for the efficacy of Orthomolecular medicine as a treatment for cancer, and that high vitamin doses may – on the contrary – increase overall mortality. Nutritional treatments are not generally accepted as being helpful for psychological health. Its claims have been criticized by most medical organizations, including the American Cancer Society, the American Psychiatric Association, the National Institute of Mental Health, the American Academy of Pediatrics, CHAMPUS, and the Canadian Paediatric Society. The American Medical Association describes as "myths" the ideas that adequate nutrition is not readily achievable with normal food, all food grown with pesticide is poisonous, all food additives are poisonous, vitamin and mineral deficiencies are common, that the cause of most disease is poor diet, which can be prevented by nutritional supplements.

Similarly, the American Cancer Society comments that the current scientific evidence does not "support use of orthomolecular therapy for most of the conditions for which it is promoted." Some supplements have exhibited benefits for specific conditions, while a few have been confirmed to be harmful; the consumption of nutritious foods is the best recognized method to obtain vitamins, minerals, and nutrients crucial for good health. Barrie Cassileth, an adviser on alternative medicine to the National Institutes of Health, stated that "scientific research has found no benefit from orthomolecular therapy for any disease," and medical textbooks also report that there is "no evidence that megavitamin or orthomolecular therapy is effective in treating any disease."

A 1973 task force of the American Psychiatric Association unanimously concluded:

This review and critique has carefully examined the literature produced by megavitamin proponents and by those who have attempted to replicate their basic and clinical work. It concludes in this regard that the credibility of the megavitamin proponents is low. Their credibility is further diminished by a consistent refusal over the past decade to perform controlled experiments and to report their new results in a scientifically acceptable fashion. Under these circumstances this Task Force considers the massive publicity which they promulgate via radio, the lay press and popular books, using catch phrases which are really misnomers like "megavitamin therapy" and "orthomolecular treatment," to be deplorable.

In response to claims that orthomolecular medicine could cure childhood psychoses and learning disorders, the American Academy of Pediatrics labelled orthomolecular medicine a "cult" in 1976.

Proponents of orthomolecular medicine counter that some vitamins and nutrients are now used in medicine as treatments for specific diseases, such as megadose niacin and fish oil for dyslipidemias, and megavitamin therapies for a group of rare inborn errors of metabolism. A review in the *Annals of Internal Medicine* concluded that while some therapies might be beneficial, others might be harmful or interfere with effective medical therapy. A recent study of over 161,000 individuals provided, in the words of the authors, "convincing evidence that multivitamin use has little or no influence on the risk of common cancers, cardiovascular disease, or total mortality in postmenopausal women." A recent meta-analysis in *JAMA* suggested that supplementation with combinations of antioxidant vitamins (beta-carotene, vitamin A, and vitamin E) may increase mortality, although with respect to beta-carotene this conclusion may be due to the known harmful effect in smokers.

Safety

In the United States, pharmaceuticals must be proven safe and effective to the satisfaction of the FDA before they can be marketed, whereas dietary supplements must be proven *unsafe* before regulatory action can be taken. A number of orthomolecular supplements are available in the US in pharmaceutical versions that are sometimes quite similar in strength and general content, or in other countries are regulated as pharmaceuticals. The US regulations also have provisions to recognize a general level of safety for established nutrients that can forgo new drug safety tests. Proponents of orthomolecular medicine argue that supplements are less likely to cause dangerous side-effects or harm, since they are normally present in the body. Some vitamins are toxic in high doses and nearly all (with the possible exception of Vitamin C) will cause adverse effects given high levels of overdosing for prolonged periods as recommended by orthomolecular practitioners. Forgoing medical care in favor of orthomolecular treatments can lead to adverse health outcomes.

Health professionals see orthomolecular medicine as encouraging individuals to dose themselves with large amounts of vitamins and other nutrients without conventional supervision, which they worry might be damaging to health. Potential risks of inappropriate vitamin and supplement regimes include an increased risk of coronary heart disease, hypertension, thrombophlebitis, peripheral neuropathy, ataxia, neurological effects, liver toxicity, congenital abnormalities, spontaneous abortion, gouty arthritis, jaundice, kidney stones, and diarrhea. In their book *Trick or Treatment*, Edzard Ernst and Simon Singh conclude that "The concepts of orthomolecular medicine are not biologically plausible and not supported by the results of rigorous clinical trials. These problems are compounded by the fact that orthomolecular medicine can cause harm and is often very expensive."

Example: Vitamin E

Orthomolecular proponents claim that even large doses of vitamin E pose no risk to health and are useful for the treatment and prevention of a broad list of conditions, including heart and circulatory diseases, diabetes and nephritis. Initial hopes for the usefulness of vitamin E in orthomolecular medicine were based on epidemiological studies suggesting that people who consumed more vitamin E had lower risks of chronic disease, such as coronary heart disease. These observational studies could not distinguish between whether the higher levels of vitamin E improved health themselves, or whether confounding variables (such as other dietary factors or exercise) were responsible. To distinguish between these possibilities, a number of randomized controlled trials were performed and meta-analysis of these controlled clinical trials have not shown any clear benefit from any form of vitamin E supplementation for preventing chronic disease. Further clinical studies show no benefit of vitamin E supplements for cardiovascular disease. The current position of the American National Institutes of Health is that there is no convincing evidence that vitamin E supplements can prevent or treat any disease.

Beyond the lack of apparent benefit, a series of three meta-analyses reported that vitamin E supplementation is associated with an increased risk of death; one of the meta-analyses performed by the Cochrane Collaboration also found significantly increased mortality for the antioxidant vitamins A and beta-carotene. A subsequent meta-analysis found no mortality benefit from vitamin E, but also no increase in mortality either.

Use in AIDS

Several articles in the alternative-medicine literature have suggested that orthomolecular-related dietary supplementation might be helpful for patients with HIV/AIDS. A study using 250 mg and 1000 mg doses of vitamin C along with other antioxidants to treat people with AIDS did not find any benefit. However, these doses are far smaller than the ones used by orthomolecular physicians for treatment of AIDS.

A meta analysis in 2010 found that micronutrient supplementation decreased the risk of death and improved outcomes in pregnant women with HIV in Africa. Vitamin A in children with HIV may also be beneficial. Vitamin A deficiency is found in children with HIV infection who may or may not have symptoms of AIDS. Vitamin A supplementation reduces morbidity and mortality in AIDS symptomatic children, but has no effect on asymptomatic children. It does not prevent HIV infection, cannot treat the chronic HIV infection, and will not cure AIDS.

Deaths Resulting from Illegal Vitamin Trials in South Africa

Matthias Rath has been extensively criticized for presenting his vitamin supplements as a treatment for AIDS and for testing them in illegal trials in South Africa. A former associate of Linus Pauling, Rath has promoted vitamins as a treatment for HIV infection, describing treatment with effective antiretroviral drugs as toxic and part of a global conspiracy serving the financial interests of the pharmaceutical industry. In a lawsuit that found against Rath, the South African Medical Association blamed his vitamin products for several deaths. The World Health Organization and two health agencies of the United Nations also described Rath's advertisements as "wrong and misleading" and "an irresponsible attack on ARV (antiretroviral) therapy." The South African Centre for Social Science Research described the trials as "state sponsored pseudo-science". Rath's trials, conducted with the aid of AIDS denialist David Rasnick, were declared unlawful by the Cape High Court; Rath, Rasnick and their foundation were barred from conducting further unauthorised clinical trials and from advertising their products.

Alleged Institutional Bias

Advocates of orthomolecular medicine, including Pauling, Hoffer and Ewan Cameron have claimed that their findings are actively suppressed by the medical and pharmaceutical industry. Hoffer wrote "There is no conspiracy led and directed by a single person or by a single organization. There is no Mafia in psychiatry. However, there is a conspiracy led and directed by a large number of professionals and their associations who have a common aim to protect their hard-earned orthodoxy, no matter what the cost to their opponent colleagues or to their patients.".

The *Journal of Orthomolecular Medicine*, founded in 1967 as the *Journal of Schizophrenia*, is a major publication of orthomolecular medicine. As Abram Hoffer wrote:

> We had to create our own journals because it was impossible to obtain entry into the official journals of psychiatry and medicine. Before 1967 I had not found it difficult to publish reports in these journals, and by then I had about 150 articles and several books in the establishment press.

Other members of the medical community deny the existence of such an institutional prejudice. A review in the *Journal of Clinical Oncology* denied that physicians collude against unconventional treatments. Despite claims of conspiracy, the Linus Pauling Institute's funding comes primarily from the National Institutes of Health, and in 1995 some orthomolecular therapies were reported as being sanctioned in Japan.

References

- Williams, William (2002). Encyclopedia of Pseudoscience: From Alien Abductions to Zone Therapy. New York: Routledge. p. 229. ISBN 978-0816050802.
- Sarris, Jerome; Wardle, Jon (2010). Clinical Naturopathy: An evidence-based guide to practice. Sydney: Churchill Livingstone / Elsevier Health Sciences. pp. 32–36. ISBN 9780729579261. Retrieved 2013-09-01.

- Pizzorno, Joseph E. (1999). "Naturopathy: Practice Issues". In Clark, Carolyn C.; Gordon, Rena J. Encyclopedia of Complementary Health Practice. Springer Publishing. pp. 57–59. ISBN 9780826117229. Retrieved 2013-09-03.
- Young, Jacqueline (2007). "Chapters 8 & 13". Complementary Medicine for Dummies. Chichester, England: Wiley. ISBN 9780470026250. OCLC 174043853.
- Herbert, Victor; Barrett, Stephen (1994). The Vitamin Pushers: How the "Health Food" Industry is Selling America a Bill of Goods. Buffalo, NY: Prometheus Books. ISBN 9780879759094.
- Barrett, Stephen; Raso, Jack (1993). Mystical Diets: Paranormal, Spiritual, and Occult Nutrition Practices. Buffalo, New York: Prometheus Books. ISBN 0879757612.
- Swartout, Kristy A.; Thomson Gale (Firm), eds. (2006). Encyclopedia of Associations (44 ed.). Thomson Gale. pp. 1777–1778. ISBN 9780787682866. Retrieved 2013-09-04.
- de las Peñas, César Fernández; Arendt-Nielsen, Lars; Gerwin, Robert D (2010). Tension-type and cervicogenic headache: pathophysiology, diagnosis, and management. Jones & Bartlett Learning. pp. 251–254. ISBN 9780763752835.
- Williams, WF (2013). Encyclopedia of Pseudoscience: From Alien Abductions to Zone Therapy. Encyclopedia of Pseudoscience. Routledge. pp. 3–4. ISBN 1135955220.
- Gwei-Djen Lu; Joseph Needham (October 25, 2002). Celestial Lancets: A History and Rationale of Acupuncture and Moxa. ISBN 0700714588.
- Porter, S.B. (2013). Tidy's Physiotherapy15: Tidy's Physiotherapy. Churchill Livingstone. Elsevier. p. 403. ISBN 978-0-7020-4344-4. Retrieved July 14, 2015.
- Jackson, M. (2011). The Oxford Handbook of the History of Medicine. Oxford Handbooks in History. OUP Oxford. p. 610. ISBN 978-0-19-954649-7. Retrieved July 14, 2015.
- Thomas Wernicke (2014). The Art of Non-Invasive Paediatric Acupuncture. Jessica Kingsley Publishers. ISBN 978-1848191600.
- Adrian White; Mike Cummings; Jacqueline Filshie (2008). "2". An Introduction to Western Medical Acupuncture. Churchill Livingstone. p. 7. ISBN 978-0-443-07177-5.
- Angela Hicks (2005). The Acupuncture Handbook: How Acupuncture Works and How It Can Help You (1 ed.). Piatkus Books. p. 41. ISBN 978-0749924720.
- Collinge, William J. (1996). The American Holistic Health Association Complete guide to alternative medicine. New York: Warner Books. ISBN 0-446-67258-0.
- Steven Aung; William Chen (10 January 2007). Clinical Introduction to Medical Acupuncture. Thieme. p. 116. ISBN 9781588902214. Retrieved 20 September 2012.
- Cui-lan Yan (January 1997). The Treatment of External Diseases with Acupuncture and Moxibustion. Blue Poppy Enterprises, Inc. pp. 112–. ISBN 978-0-936185-80-4.
- "Sonopuncture". American Cancer Society's Guide to complementary and alternative cancer methods. American Cancer Society. 2000. p. 158. ISBN 9780944235249.
- Alvarez, L. (2015). "Chapter 18: Acupuncture". In James S. Gaynor & William W. Muir III. Handbook of Veterinary Pain Management (3rd edition). Elsevier. ISBN 978-0323089357.
- Lee Goldman; Andrew I. Schafer (21 April 2015). Goldman-Cecil Medicine: Expert Consult - Online. Elsevier Health Sciences. pp. 98–. ISBN 978-0-323-32285-0.
- Barrett, Stephen (2013). "'Alternative' Medicine: More Hype Than Hope". In Humber, James M.; Almeder, Robert F. Alternative Medicine and Ethics. Springer Science & Business Media. p. 10. ISBN 978-1-4757-2774-6.

3

Anthroposophic Medicine: An Integrated Study

Anthroposophic medicine includes treatment techniques such as massages, exercises and counseling. It tends to explain health and natural medicine in terms of spirituality and science both. The philosophy behind anthroposophic medicine is known as anthroposophy. This text will provide an integrated understanding of anthroposophic medicine.

Anthroposophic Medicine

Anthroposophic medicine (or anthroposophical medicine) is a form of pseudoscience and alternative medicine. Devised in the 1920s by Rudolf Steiner (1861–1925) in conjunction with Ita Wegman (1876–1943), anthroposophical medicine is based on occult notions and draws on Steiner's spiritual philosophy, which he called anthroposophy. Practitioners employ a variety of treatment techniques based upon anthroposophic precepts, including massage, exercise, counselling, and substances.

Many drug preparations used in anthroposophic medicine are ultra-diluted substances, similar to those used in homeopathy. Homeopathic remedies are not medically effective and are generally considered harmless, except when used as a substitute for a scientifically proven and effective cure. In certain European countries, people with cancer are sometimes prescribed remedies made from specially harvested mistletoe, but research has found no convincing evidence of clinical benefit. Some anthroposophic doctors oppose childhood vaccination, and this has led to preventable outbreaks of disease. Professor of complementary medicine Edzard Ernst and other critics have characterized anthroposophic medicine as having no basis in science, pseudoscientific, and quackery.

Anthroposophic medicine departs from fundamental biological principles in several respects. For example, it claims that the heart does not pump blood but that blood propels itself along. Anthroposophic medicine also proposes that a patient's past lives may influence their illness and that the course of an illness is subject to karmic destiny.

History

The first steps towards an anthroposophic approach to medicine were made before 1920, when homeopathic physicians and pharmacists began working with Rudolf Steiner, who recommended new medicinal substances as well as specific methods for preparation along with an anthroposophic concept of man. In 1921, Ita Wegman opened the first anthroposophic medical clinic, now known as the Klinik Arlesheim, in Arlesheim, Switzerland. Wegman was soon joined by a number of other doctors. They then began to train the first anthroposophic nurses for the clinic.

At Wegman's request, Steiner regularly visited the clinic and suggested treatment regimes for particular patients. Between 1920 and 1925, he also gave several series of lectures on medicine. In 1925, Wegman and Steiner wrote the first book on the anthroposophic approach to medicine, *Fundamentals of Therapy*.

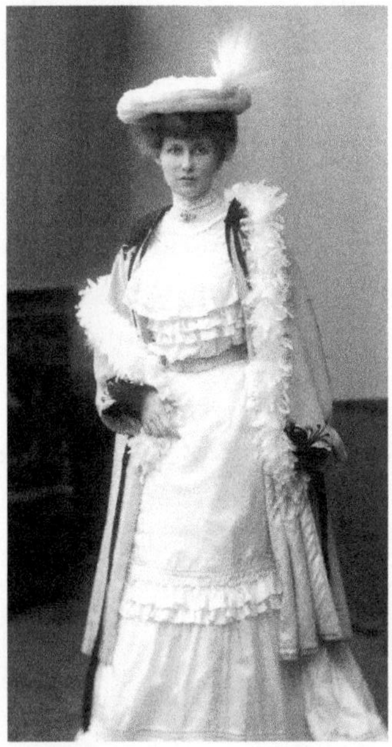

Ita Wegman, co-founder of the medical approach, before 1900 in Berlin.

The clinic expanded and soon opened a branch in Ascona. Wegman lectured widely, visiting the Netherlands and England particularly frequently, and an increasing number of doctors began to include the anthroposophic approach in their practices. A cancer clinic, the Lukas Clinic, opened in Arlesheim in 1963.

In 1976 anthroposophic medicine in Germany got regulated by law as a specific therapeutic system ("Besondere Therapierichtung") by the Medicines Act-Arzneimittelgesetz (AMG) and by the Code of Social Law (Sozialgesetzbuch V)

In the 1990s the Witten/Herdecke University in Germany established a chair in anthroposophical medicine. The press described the appointment as a "death sentence" and the perception that pseudoscience was being taught damaged the university's reputation, bringing it close to financial collapse. It was ultimately saved by a cash injection from Software AG, a technology corporation with a history of funding anthroposophic projects.

In 2006, anthroposophical medicine was practised in 80 countries.

In 2012 the University of Aberdeen considered establishing a chair in holistic health jointly funded by Software AG, and by the Anthroposophic Health, Education, and Social Care Movement, each of which would provide £1.5 million of endowment. Edzard Ernst commented "that any decent university should even consider an anthroposophical medicine unit seems incomprehensible. The fact that it would be backed by people who have a financial interest in this bogus approach makes it even worse." The University's governance and nominations committee eventually decided not to proceed with the appointment.

Categorization and Conceptual Basis

The categorization of anthroposophical medicine is complex since in part it complements conventional medicine, and in part it substitutes for it. In 2008, Ernst wrote that it was being promoted as an "extension to conventional medicine".

Ernst writes that Steiner used imagination and insight as a basis for his ideas, drawing mystical knowledge from the occult Akashic Records, a work which is supposedly situated on the astral plane, and which Steiner said was accessible to him via his intuitive powers. On this basis, Steiner proposed "associations between four postulated dimensions of the human body (physical body, etheric body, astral body, and ego), plants, minerals, and the cosmos". Steiner also proposed a connection betweens planets, metals and organs so that, for example, the planet Mercury, the element mercury and the lung were all somehow associated. These propositions form the basis of anthroposophical medicine.

Ernst has said that anthroposophical medicine "includes some of the least plausible theories one could possibly imagine", categorized it as "pure quackery", and said that it "has no basis in science". According to Quackwatch, anthroposophical medicine practitioners regard illness as a "rite of passage" necessary to purge spiritual impurities carried over from past lives, according to the precepts of "karmic destiny".

Methods

In anthroposophic pharmacy drugs are prepared according to ancient notions of alchemy and homeopathy which are not related to the science underlying modern pharmacology. During the preparation process, patterns formed by crystallization are interpreted to see which "etheric force" they most closely resemble. Most anthroposophic preparations are highly diluted, like homeopathic remedies. This means that, while they are completely harmless in themselves, using them in place of conventional medicine to treat serious illness carries a risk of severe adverse consequences.

As well as drug remedies, anthroposophical medicine also includes:

- Anthroposophic nursing
- Counselling
- Eurythmy – claimed to have an effect on «inner life functions» leading to a «re-integration of body, soul, and spirit».
- External applications
- Rhythmic massages

Plant-derived Treatments

To select an anthroposophic substance for a particular illness, practitioners consider the source of the substances used. The character of a mineral, plant or animal is hypothesised to have been formed by the substances that are most active within it, in the belief that this character may also influence what the substance will accomplish when given to treat another organism. This is related to Samuel Hahnemann's Doctrine of signatures. Willow, for example, is considered to have an unusual character:

... plants that grow near water are usually heavy, with big, dark green leaves that wilt and break easily. An exception is ... the white willow, a tree that always grows near water and loves light. However, unlike other "watery" plants, the willow has fine, almost dry leaves and looks very light ... Its branches are unbelievably tough. They are elastic and cannot be broken. They bend easily and form "joints" rather than break. These few signatures can give us the clue to what salix can be used for therapeutically: arthritis, deformation of joints, swollen joints ...

There is no scientific evidence that the shape of plants has ever caused a new medical property to be discovered.

Heart

Steiner described the heart not as a pump, but as a regulator of flow, such that the heartbeat itself can be distinguished from the circulation of blood. Anthroposophic medicine claims the flow in the blood of the circulatory system is, as Marinelli put it, *"propelled with its own biological momentum, as can be seen in the embryo, and boosts itself with* induced *momenta from the heart"*.

This view of the heart is not based on any scientific theory and has been characterized as "crank science".

Mistletoe Treatment for Cancer

Rudolf Steiner hypothesised that mistletoe could cure cancer, on the basis of the observation that the plant was a parasite which eventually killed its host, a process which he claimed paralleled the progression of cancer. Steiner believed the plant's medical potential was influenced by the position of the sun, moon and planets and that it therefore was important to harvest the plant at the right time. Some mistletoe preparations are ultra-diluted; others are made from fermented mistletoe. The most commonly used trade names for mistletoe drugs are Iscador and Helixor.

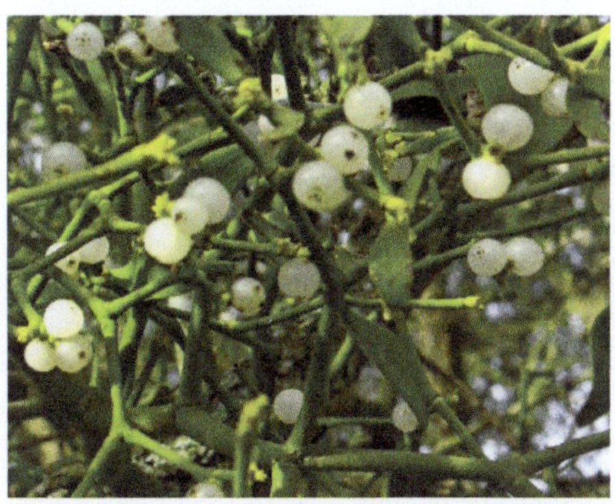

Mistletoe – Steiner said that harvesting it when the planets were aligned would yield a cancer treatment

Although laboratory experiments have suggested that mistletoe extract may affect the immune system and be able to kill some kinds of cancer cells, there is little evidence of its benefit to people with cancer. Most of the clinical research claiming that mistletoe therapy is effective is published in Germany, and it is generally considered unreliable because of major lapses in quality. Edzard Ernst wrote that research by anthroposophic doctors often reached positive conclusions on mistletoe therapy because it drew on unreliable material; independent researchers tended instead to find no evidence of benefit. The American Cancer Society says that "available evidence from well-designed clinical trials does not support claims that mistletoe can improve length or quality of life".

Mistletoe-based cancer drugs are widely used in Europe, especially in German-speaking countries. In 2002 nearly half a million prescriptions were paid for by German health insurance and in 2006 there were reportedly around 30 types of mistletoe extract on the market. Mistletoe extracts have been used as an unconventional treatment for cancer patients in the Netherlands, and in Germany the treatment has been approved as palliative therapy to treat the symptoms of patients with malignant tumors. In Sweden, controversially, mistletoe therapy has been approved for use in the treatment of cancer symptoms.

In other countries mistletoe therapy is virtually unknown. The United States Food and Drug Administration has not approved mistletoe-based drugs for any purpose; mistletoe extracts may not be distributed in or imported into the US except for research purposes. As of 2015 no mistletoe-based drugs are licensed for use in the United Kingdom.

A 2013 article on mistletoe in *Lancet Oncology* invoked Ben Goldacre's observation that a geographical preference for certain therapies was a hallmark of quackery, and proposed that the continuing use of this "apparently ineffectual therapy" in a small cluster of countries was based on sociological rather than medical reasons, indicating a need for a more informed consent from patients.

Regulation

In 2008 anthroposophic medicines which are not homeopathic have been required in the Netherlands to get marketing certification as any other ordinary medicines. This means that these will be unavailable until such certification is obtained.

Immunization

The risks arising from using anthroposophical medicine as a substitute for evidence-based medicine are exemplified by several cases of low vaccination levels in anthroposophic schools, since some anthroposophical doctors oppose immunization. A 1999 study of children in Sweden showed that in anthroposophical schools, only 18% had received MMR vaccination, compared to a level of 93% in other schools nationally.

A 2003 report of a widespread measles outbreak around Coburg, Germany, identified an anthroposophical school as the origin. At the time the town's mayor had condemned homeopathic doctors who had discouraged vaccination, saying "Their stronghold is the Waldorf School, which actively encourages people not to have their children vaccinated. Now we have an epidemic."

Paul Offit writes that Steiner believed vaccination "interferes with karmic development and the cycles of reincarnation", and that adherence to this belief led to a 2008 pertussis outbreak in a Californian Waldorf school, causing its temporary closure.

Anthroposophy

Anthroposophy is a philosophy founded by Rudolf Steiner that postulates the existence of an objective, intellectually comprehensible spiritual world that is accessible by direct experience through inner development. More specifically, it aims to develop faculties of perceptive imagination, inspiration and intuition through the cultivation of a form of thinking independent of sensory experience, and to present the results thus derived in a manner subject to rational verification. Anthroposophy aims to attain in its study of spiritual experience the precision and clarity attained by the natural sciences in their investigations of the physical world. The philosophy has double roots in German idealism and German mysticism and was initially expressed in language drawn from Theosophy.

Anthroposophical ideas have been applied practically in many areas including Steiner/Waldorf education, special education (most prominently through the Camphill Movement), biodynamic agriculture, medicine, ethical banking, organizational development, and the arts. The Anthroposophical Society has its international center at the Goetheanum in Dornach, Switzerland.

Modern critics, particularly Michael Shermer, have termed anthroposophy's application in areas such as medicine, biology, and biodynamic agriculture to be pseudoscience. Anthroposophy has also been termed "the most important esoteric society in European history."

History

The early work of the founder of anthroposophy, Rudolf Steiner, culminated in his *Philosophy of Freedom* (also translated as *The Philosophy of Spiritual Activity* and *Intuitive Thinking as a Spiritual Path*). Here, Steiner developed a concept of free will based on inner experiences, especially those that occur in the creative activity of independent thought.

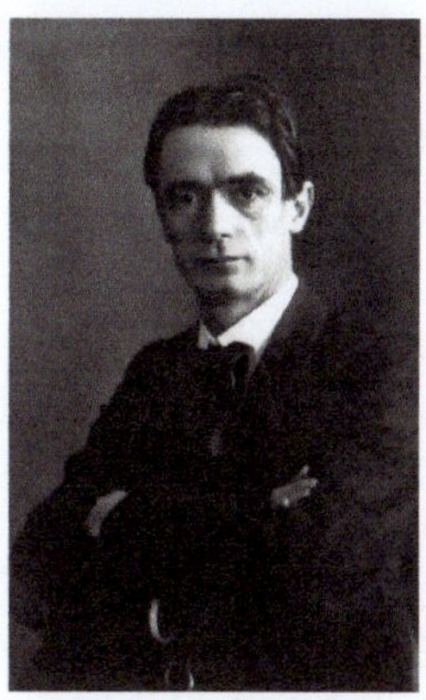

Rudolf Steiner

By the beginning of the twentieth century, Steiner's interests turned to explicitly spiritual areas of research. His work began to interest others interested in spiritual ideas; among these was the Theosophical Society. From 1900 on, thanks to the positive reception given to his ideas, Steiner focused increasingly on his work with the Theosophical Society becoming the secretary of its section in Germany in 1902. During the years of his leadership, membership increased dramatically, from a few individuals to sixty-nine Lodges.

By 1907, a split between Steiner and the mainstream Theosophical Society had begun to become apparent. While the Society was oriented toward an Eastern and especially Indian approach, Steiner was trying to develop a path that embraced Christianity and natural science. The split became irrevocable when Annie Besant, then president of the Theosophical Society, began to present the child Jiddu Krishnamurti as the reincarnated Christ. Steiner strongly objected and considered any comparison between Krishnamurti and Christ to be nonsense; many years later, Krishnamurti also repudiated the assertion. Steiner's continuing differences with Besant led him to separate from the Theosophical Society Adyar; he was followed by the great majority of the membership of the Theosophical Society's German Section, as well as members of other national sections.

By this time, Steiner had reached considerable stature as a spiritual teacher. He spoke about what he considered to be his direct experience of the Akashic Records (sometimes called the "Akasha Chronicle"), thought to be a spiritual chronicle of the history, pre-history, and future of the world and mankind. In a number of works, Steiner described a path of inner development he felt would let anyone attain comparable spiritual experiences. Sound vision could be developed, in part, by practicing rigorous forms of ethical and cognitive self-discipline, concentration, and meditation; in particular, a person's moral development must precede the development of spiritual faculties.

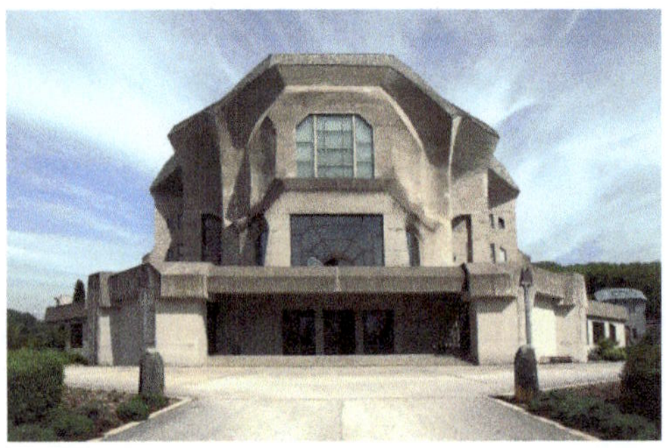

Second Goetheanum, seat of the Anthroposophical Society

In 1912, the Anthroposophical Society was founded. After World War I, the Anthroposophical movement took on new directions. Projects such as schools, centers for those with special needs, organic farms and medical clinics were established, all inspired by anthroposophy.

In 1923, faced with differences between older members focusing on inner development and younger members eager to become active in the social transformations of the time, Steiner refounded the Society in an inclusive manner and established a School for Spiritual Science. As a spiritual basis for the refounded movement, Steiner wrote a "Foundation Stone Meditation" which remains a central meditative expression of anthroposophical ideas.

Steiner died just over a year later, in 1925. The Second World War temporarily hindered the anthroposophical movement in most of Continental Europe, as the Anthroposophical Society and most of its daughter movements (e.g. Steiner/Waldorf education) were banned by the National Socialists (Nazis); virtually no anthroposophists ever joined the National Socialist Party.

By 2007, national branches of the Anthroposophical Society had been established in fifty countries, and about 10,000 institutions around the world were working on the basis of anthroposophy. In the same year, the Anthroposophical Society was called the "most important esoteric society in European history."

Etymology

Steiner began using the term in the early 1900s as an alternative to the term *theosophy* (divine wisdom), a term central to the Theosophical Society, with which Steiner was associated at the time, and to a long tradition of European esotericists. Steiner probably first encountered the word "anthroposophy" in the work of Zimmermann, some of whose lectures in the University of Vienna he had attended while a student.

Central Ideas

Spiritual Knowledge and Freedom

Anthroposophical proponents aim to extend the clarity of the scientific method to phenomena of human soul-life and to spiritual experiences. This requires developing new faculties of objective spiritual perception, which Steiner maintained was possible for humanity today. The steps of this process of inner development he identified as consciously achieved *imagination*, *inspiration* and *intuition*. Steiner believed results of this form of spiritual research should be expressed in a way that can be understood and evaluated on the same basis as the results of natural science: "The anthroposophical schooling of thinking leads to the development of a non-sensory, or so-called supersensory consciousness, whereby the spiritual researcher brings the experiences of this realm into ideas, concepts, and expressive language in a form which people can understand who do not yet have the capacity to achieve the supersensory experiences necessary for individual research."

Steiner hoped to form a spiritual movement that would free the individual from any external authority: "The most important problem of all human thinking is this: to comprehend the human being as a personality grounded in him or herself." For Steiner, the human capacity for rational thought would allow individuals to comprehend spiritual research on their own and bypass the danger of dependency on an authority.

Steiner contrasted the anthroposophical approach with both conventional mysticism, which he considered lacking the clarity necessary for exact knowledge, and natural science, which he considered arbitrarily limited to investigating the outer world.

Nature of The Human Being

In *Theosophy*, Steiner suggested that human beings unite a physical body of substances gathered from (and that ultimately return to) the inorganic world; a life body (also called the etheric body), in common with all living creatures (including plants); a bearer of sentience or consciousness (also called the astral body), in common with all animals; and the ego, which anchors the faculty of self-awareness unique to human beings.

Anthroposophy describes a broad evolution of human consciousness. Early stages of human evolution possess an intuitive perception of reality, including a clairvoyant perception of spiritual realities. Humanity has progressively evolved an increasing reliance on intellectual faculties and a corresponding loss of intuitive or clairvoyant experiences, which have become atavistic. The increasing intellectualization of consciousness, initially a progressive direction of evolution, has led to an excessive reliance on abstraction and a loss of contact with both natural and spiritual realities. However, to go further requires new capacities that combine the clarity of intellectual thought with the imagination, and beyond this with consciously achieved inspiration and intuitive insights.

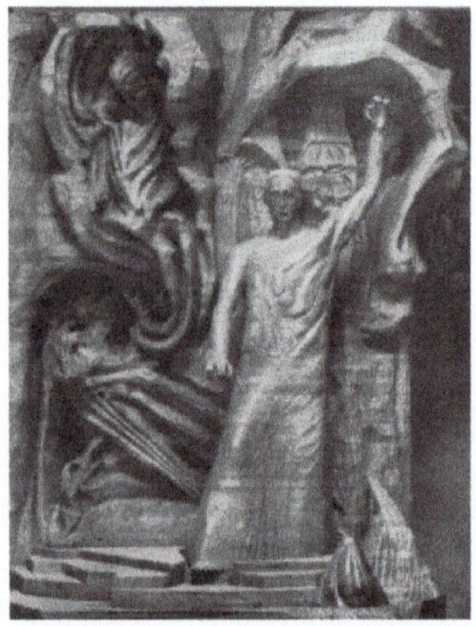

The Representative of Humanity, detail of a sculpture in wood by Rudolf Steiner and Edith Maryon.

Anthroposophy speaks of the reincarnation of the human spirit: that the human being passes between stages of existence, incarnating into an earthly body, living on earth, leaving the body behind and entering into the spiritual worlds before returning to be born again into a new life on earth. After the death of the physical body, the human spirit recapitulates the past life, perceiving its events as they were experienced by the objects of its actions. A complex transformation takes place between the review of the past life and the preparation for the next life. The individual's karmic condition eventually leads to a choice of parents, physical body, disposition, and capacities that provide the challenges and opportunities that further development requires, which includes karmically chosen tasks for the future life.

Steiner described some conditions that determine the interdependence of a person's lives, or karma.

Evolution

The anthroposophical view of evolution considers all animals to have evolved from an early, unspecialized form. As the least specialized animal, human beings have maintained the closest connection to the archetypal form; contrary to the Darwinian conception of human evolution, all other animals *devolve* from this archetype. The spiritual archetype originally created by spiritual beings was devoid of physical substance; only later did this descend into material existence on Earth. In this view, human evolution has accompanied the Earth's evolution throughout the existence of the Earth.

The evolution of man, Steiner said, has consisted in the gradual incarnation of a spiritual being into a material body. It has been a true "descent" of man from a spiritual world into a world of matter. The evolution of the animal kingdom did not precede, but rather *accompanied* the process of human incarnation. Man is thus not the end result of the evolution of the animals, but is rather in a certain sense their *cause*. In the succession of types which appears in the fossil record-the fishes, reptiles, mammals, and finally fossil remains of man himself — the stages of this process of incarnation are reflected.

Anthroposophy took over from Theosophy a complex system of cycles of world development and human evolution. The evolution of the world is said to have occurred in cycles. The first phase of the world consisted only of heat. In the second phase, a more active condition, light, and a more condensed, gaseous state separate out from the heat. In the third phase, a fluid state arose, as well as a sounding, forming energy. In the fourth (current) phase, solid physical matter first exists. This process is said to have been accompanied by an evolution of consciousness which led up to present human culture.

Ethics

The anthroposophical view is that good is found in the balance between two polar influences on world and human evolution. These are often described through their mythological embodiments as spiritual adversaries which endeavour to tempt and corrupt humanity, Lucifer and his counterpart Ahriman. These have both positive and negative aspects. Lucifer is the light spirit, which "plays on human pride and offers the delusion of divinity", but also motivates creativity and spirituality; Ahriman is the dark spirit that tempts human beings to "...deny [their] link with divinity and to live entirely on the material plane", but that also stimulates intellectuality and technology. Both figures exert a negative effect on humanity when their influence becomes misplaced or one-sided, yet their influences are necessary for human freedom to unfold.

Each human being has the task to find a balance between these opposing influences, and each is helped in this task by the mediation of the *Representative of Humanity*, also known as the Christ being, a spiritual entity who stands between and harmonizes the two extremes.

Applications

The applications of anthroposophy to practical fields include:

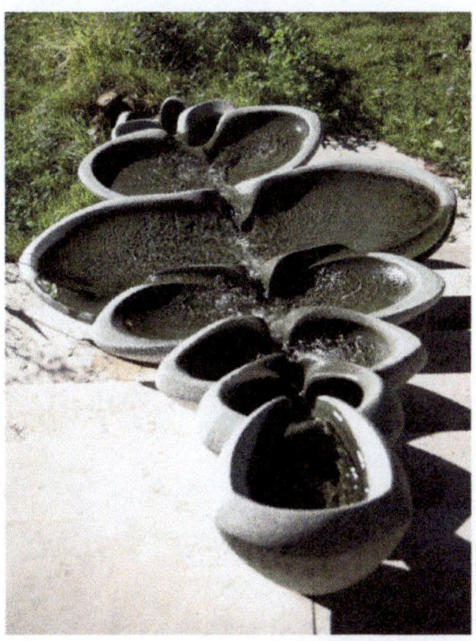

Flowforms in Darmstadt, Germany

Steiner/Waldorf Education

This is a pedagogical movement with over 1000 Steiner or Waldorf schools (the latter name stems from the first such school, founded in Stuttgart in 1919) located in some 60 countries; the great majority of these are independent (private) schools. Sixteen of the schools have been affiliated with the United Nations' UNESCO Associated Schools Project Network, which sponsors education projects that foster improved quality of education throughout the world. Waldorf schools receive full or partial governmental funding in some European nations, Australia and in parts of the United States (as Waldorf method public or charter schools).

The schools have been founded in a variety of communities: for example in the *favelas* of São Paulo to wealthy suburbs of major cities; in India, Egypt, Australia, the Netherlands, Mexico and South Africa. Though most of the early Waldorf schools were teacher-founded, the schools today are usually initiated and later supported by a parent community. Waldorf schools are among the most visible anthroposophical institutions.

Biodynamic Agriculture

Biodynamic agriculture, the first intentional form of organic farming, began in 1924, when Rudolf Steiner gave a series of lectures published in English as *The Agriculture Course*. Steiner is considered one of the founders of the modern organic farming movement.

Anthroposophical Medicine

Steiner gave several series of lectures to physicians and medical students. Out of those grew a complementary medical movement intending to "extend the knowledge gained through the methods of the natural sciences of the present age with insights from spiritual science." This movement now includes hundreds of M.D.s, chiefly in Europe and North America, and has its own clinics, hospitals, and medical schools.

One of the most studied applications has been the use of mistletoe extracts in cancer therapy. The extracts are generally no longer used to reduce or inhibit tumor growth, for which verifiable results have been found in vitro and in animal studies but not in humans, but instead to improve the patients' quality of life and to reduce tumor-induced symptoms and the side-effects of chemotherapy and radiotherapy. According to the National Cancer Institute, "Mistletoe extract has been shown to kill cancer cells in the laboratory and to affect the immune system. However, there is limited evidence that mistletoe's effects on the immune system help the body fight cancer.... At present, the use of mistletoe cannot be recommended outside the context of well-designed clinical trials."

Several pharmaceutical companies have grown out of anthroposophical medicine, including Weleda, Wala, and Dr. Hauschka.

Special Needs Education and Services

In 1922, Ita Wegman founded an anthroposophical center for special needs education, the Sonnenhof, in Switzerland. In 1940, Karl König founded the Camphill Movement in Scotland. The latter in particular has spread widely, and there are now over a hundred Camphill communities and other anthroposophical homes for children and adults in need of special care in about 22 countries around the world. Both Karl König, Thomas Weihs and others have written extensively on these ideas underlying Special education.

Architecture

Steiner designed around thirteen buildings in an organic—expressionist architectural style. Foremost among these are his designs for the two Goetheanum buildings in Dornach, Switzerland. Thousands of further buildings have been built by later generations of anthroposophic architects.

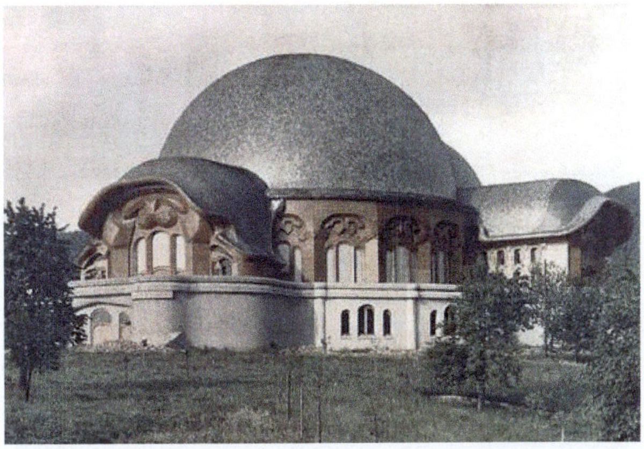

The First Goetheanum, designed by Steiner in 1920, Dornach, Switzerland.

Architects who have been strongly influenced by the anthroposophic style include Imre Makovecz in Hungary, Hans Scharoun and Joachim Eble in Germany, Erik Asmussen in Sweden, Kenji Imai in Japan, Thomas Rau, Anton Alberts and Max van Huut in the Netherlands, Christopher Day and Camphill Architects in the UK, Thompson and Rose in America, Denis Bowman in Canada, and Walter Burley Griffin and Gregory Burgess in Australia.

ING House in Amsterdam is a contemporary building by an anthroposophical architect which has received awards for its ecological design and approach to a self-sustaining ecology as an autonomous building and example of sustainable architecture.

Eurythmy

Together with Marie von Sivers, Steiner developed eurythmy, a performance art combining dance, speech, and music.

Social Finance

Around the world today are a number of banks, companies, charities, and schools for developing co-operative forms of business using Steiner's ideas about economic associations, aiming at harmonious and socially responsible roles in the world economy. The first anthroposophic bank was the *Gemeinschaftsbank für Leihen und Schenken* in Bochum, Germany, founded in 1974. Socially responsible banks founded out of anthroposophy in the English-speaking world include Triodos Bank, founded in 1980 and active in the UK, Netherlands, Germany, Belgium, and Spain. Cultura Sparebank dates from 1982 when a group of Norwegian anthroposophists start to grow the idea of having ethical banking but only in the late 90s the bank starts to operate as a savings bank in Norway. La Nef in France and RSF Social Finance in San Francisco are other examples.

Organizational Development, Counselling and Biography Work

Bernard Lievegoed, a psychiatrist, founded a new method of individual and institutional development oriented towards humanizing organizations and linked with Steiner's ideas of the threefold social order. This work is represented by the NPI Institute for Organizational Development in the Netherlands and sister organizations in many other countries. Various forms of biographic and counselling work have been developed on the basis of anthroposophy.

Speech and Drama

There are also anthroposophical movements to renew speech and drama, the most important of which are based in the work of Marie Steiner-von Sivers (*speech formation*, also known as *Creative Speech*) and the *Chekhov Method* originated by Michael Chekhov (nephew of Anton Chekhov).

Art

Anthroposophic painting, a style inspired by Rudolf Steiner, featured prominently in the first Goetheanum's cupola. The technique frequently begins by filling the surface to be painted with color, out of which forms are gradually developed, often images with symbolic-spiritual significance. Paints that allow for many transparent layers are preferred, and often these are derived from plant materials.

Other

Other applications include:

- Phenomenological approaches to science,
- New approaches to painting and sculpture.
- John Wilkes' fountain-like flowforms, sculptural forms that guide water into rhythmic movement and are used both in water-purification projects and decoratively.

Social Goals

For a period after World War I, Steiner was extremely active and well known in Germany, in part because he lectured widely proposing social reforms. Steiner was a sharp critic of nationalism, which he saw as outdated, and a proponent of achieving social solidarity through individual freedom. A petition proposing a radical change in the German constitution and expressing his basic social ideas (signed by Herman Hesse, among others) was widely circulated. His main book on social reform is *Toward Social Renewal*.

Anthroposophy continues to aim at reforming society through maintaining and strengthening the independence of the spheres of cultural life, human rights and the economy. It emphasizes a particular ideal in each of these three realms of society:

1. Freedom in cultural life
2. Equality of rights, the sphere of legislation
3. Fraternity in the economic sphere

Esoteric Path

Paths of Spiritual Development

According to Steiner, a real spiritual world exists,evolving along with the material one. Steiner held that the spiritual world can be researched in the right circumstances through direct experience, by persons practicing rigorous forms of ethical and cognitive self-discipline. Steiner described many exercises he said were suited to strengthening such self-discipline; the most complete exposition of these is found in his book *How To Know Higher Worlds*. The aim of these exercises is to develop higher levels of consciousness through meditation and observation. Details about the spiritual world, Steiner suggested, could on such a basis be discovered and reported, though no more infallibly than the results of natural science.

Anthroposophy is a path of knowledge, to guide the spiritual in the human being to the spiritual in the universe.... Anthroposophists are those who experience, as an essential need of life, certain questions on the nature of the human being and the universe, just as one experiences hunger and thirst.

Steiner regarded his research reports as being important aids to others seeking to enter into spiritual experience. He suggested that a combination of spiritual exercises (for example, concentrating on an object such as a seed), moral development (control of thought, feelings and will combined with openness, tolerance and flexibility) and familiarity with other spiritual researchers' results would best further an individual's spiritual development. He consistently emphasised that any inner, spiritual practice should be undertaken in such a way as not to interfere with one's responsibilities in outer life. Steiner distinguished between what he considered were true and false paths of spiritual investigation.

In anthroposophy, artistic expression is also treated as a potentially valuable bridge between spiritual and material reality.

Prerequisites to and Stages of Inner Development

A person seeking inner development must first of all make the attempt to give up certain formerly held inclinations. Then, new inclinations must be acquired by constantly holding the thought of such inclinations, virtues or characteristics in one's mind. They must be so incorporated into one's being that a person becomes enabled to alter his soul by his own will-power. This must be tried as objectively as a chemical might be tested in an experiment. A person who has never endeavored to change his soul, who has never made the initial decision to develop the qualities of endurance, steadfastness and calm logical thinking, or a person who has such decisions but has given up because he did not succeed in a week, a month, a year or a decade, will never conclude anything inwardly about these truths.

—*Rudolf Steiner, "On the Inner Life",*

Steiner's stated prerequisites to beginning on a spiritual path include a willingness to take up serious cognitive studies, a respect for factual evidence, and a responsible attitude. Central to progress on the path itself is a harmonious cultivation of the following qualities:

- Control over one's own thinking
- Control over one's will
- Composure
- Positivity
- Impartiality

Steiner sees meditation as a concentration and enhancement of the power of thought. By focusing consciously on an idea, feeling or intention the meditant seeks to arrive at pure thinking, a state exemplified by but not confined to pure mathematics. In Steiner's view, conventional sensory-material knowledge is achieved through relating perception and concepts. The anthroposophic path of esoteric training articulates three further stages of supersensory knowledge, which do not necessarily follow strictly sequentially in any single individual's spiritual progress.

- By focusing on symbolic patterns, images, and poetic mantras, the meditant can achieve consciously directed Imaginations that allow sensory phenomena to appear as the expression of underlying beings of a soul-spiritual nature.
- By transcending such imaginative pictures, the meditant can become conscious of the meditative activity itself, which leads to experiences of expressions of soul-spiritual beings unmediated by sensory phenomena or qualities. Steiner calls this stage Inspiration.
- By intensifying the will-forces through exercises such as a chronologically reversed review of the day's events, the meditant can achieve a further stage of inner independence from sensory experience, leading to direct contact, and even union, with spiritual beings ("Intuition") without loss of individual awareness.

Spiritual Exercises

Steiner described numerous exercises he believed would bring spiritual development; other anthroposophists have added many others. A central principle is that "for every step in spiritual perception, three steps are to be taken in moral development." According to Steiner, moral development reveals the extent to which one has achieved control over one's inner life and can exercise it in harmony with the spiritual life of other people; it shows the real progress in spiritual development, the fruits of which are given in spiritual perception. It also guarantees the capacity to distinguish between false perceptions or illusions (which are possible in perceptions of both the outer world and the inner world) and true perceptions: i.e., the capacity to distinguish in any perception between the influence of subjective elements (i.e., viewpoint) and objective reality.

Place in Western Philosophy

Steiner built upon Goethe's conception of an imaginative power capable of synthesizing the sense-perceptible form of a thing (an image of its outer appearance) and the concept we have of that thing (an image of its inner structure or nature). Steiner added to this the conception that a further step in the development of thinking is possible when the thinker observes his or her own thought processes. "The organ of observation and the observed thought process are then identical, so that the condition thus arrived at is simultaneously one of perception through thinking and one of thought through perception."

Thus, in Steiner's view, we can overcome the subject-object divide through inner activity, even though all human experience begins by being conditioned by it. In this connection, Steiner examines the step from thinking determined by outer impressions to what he calls sense-free thinking. He characterizes thoughts he considers without sensory content, such as mathematical or logical thoughts, as free deeds. Steiner believed he had thus located the origin of free will in our thinking, and in particular in sense-free thinking.

Some of the epistemic basis for Steiner's later anthroposophical work is contained in the seminal work, Philosophy of Freedom. In his early works, Steiner sought to overcome what he perceived as the dualism of Cartesian idealism and Kantian subjectivism by developing Goethe's conception of the human being as a natural-supernatural entity, that is: natural in that humanity is a product of nature, supernatural in that through our conceptual powers we extend nature's realm, allowing it to achieve a reflective capacity in us as philosophy, art and science. Steiner was one of the first European philosophers to overcome the subject-object split in Western thought. Though not well known among philosophers, his philosophical work was taken up by Owen Barfield (and through him influenced the Inklings, an Oxford group of Christian writers that included J. R. R. Tolkien and C. S. Lewis).

Christian and Jewish mystical thought have also influenced the development of anthroposophy.

Union of Science and Spirit

Steiner believed in the possibility of applying the clarity of scientific thinking to spiritual experience, which he saw as deriving from an objectively existing spiritual world. Steiner identified mathematics, which attains certainty through thinking itself, thus through inner experience rather than empirical observation, as the basis of his epistemology of spiritual experience.

Relationship to Religion

Christ as The Center of Earthly Evolution

Steiner's writing, though appreciative of all religions and cultural developments, emphasizes Western tradition as having evolved to meet contemporary needs. He describes Christ and his mission on earth of bringing individuated consciousness as having a particularly important place in human evolution, whereby:

- Christianity has evolved out of previous religions;
- The being which manifests in Christianity also manifests in all faiths and religions, and each religion is valid and true for the time and cultural context in which it was born;
- All historical forms of Christianity need to be transformed considerably to meet the continuing evolution of humanity.

Spiritual science does not want to usurp the place of Christianity; on the contrary it would like to be instrumental in making Christianity understood. Thus it becomes clear to us through spiritual science that the being whom we call Christ is to be recognized as the center of life on earth, that the Christian religion is the ultimate religion for the earth's whole future. Spiritual science shows us particularly that the pre-Christian religions outgrow their one-sidedness and come together in the Christian faith. It is not the desire of spiritual science to set something else in the place of Christianity; rather it wants to contribute to a deeper, more heartfelt understanding of Christianity.

Thus, anthroposophy considers there to be a being who unifies all religions, and who is not represented by any particular religious faith. This being is, according to Steiner, not only the Redeemer of the Fall from Paradise, but also the unique pivot and meaning of earth's evolutionary processes and of human history. To describe this being, Steiner periodically used terms such as the "Representative of Humanity" or the "good spirit" rather than any denominational term.

Divergence from Conventional Christian Thought

Steiner's views of Christianity diverge from conventional Christian thought in key places, and include gnostic elements:

- One central point of divergence is Steiner's views on reincarnation and karma.
- Steiner differentiated three contemporary paths by which he believed it possible to arrive at Christ:
    - Through heart-filled experiences of the Gospels; Steiner described this as the historically dominant path, but becoming less important in the future.
    - Through inner experiences of a spiritual reality; this Steiner regarded as increasingly the path of spiritual or religious seekers today.
    - Through initiatory experiences whereby the reality of Christ's death and resurrection are experienced; Steiner believed this is the path people will increasingly take.
- Steiner also believed that there were two different Jesus children involved in the Incarnation of the Christ: one child descended from Solomon, as described in the Gospel of Matthew, the other child from Nathan, as described in the Gospel of Luke. (The genealogies given in the two gospels diverge some thirty generations before Jesus' birth, and 'Jesus' was a common name in biblical times.)
- His view of the second coming of Christ is also unusual; he suggested that this would not be a physical reappearance, but that the Christ being would become manifest in non-physical form, visible to spiritual vision and apparent in community life for increasing numbers of people beginning around the year 1933.
- He emphasized his belief that in the future humanity would need to be able to recognize the *Spirit of Love* in all its genuine forms, regardless of what name would be used to describe this being. He also warned that the traditional name of the *Christ* might be misused, and the true essence of this being of love ignored.

Judaism

Rudolf Steiner wrote and lectured on Judaism and Jewish issues for much of his life. In the 1880s and 1890s, he took part in debates on anti-semitism and on assimilation. He was a fierce opponent of anti-semitism and supported the unconditional acceptance and integration of the Jews in Europe. He also supported Émile Zola's position in the Dreyfus affair. In his later life, Steiner was accused by the Nazis of being a Jew, and Adolf Hitler called anthroposophy "Jewish methods". The anthroposophical institutions in Germany were banned during Nazi rule and several anthroposophists sent to concentration camps.

Steiner emphasized Judaism's central importance to the constitution of the modern era in the West but suggested that to appreciate the spirituality of the future it would need to overcome its tendency toward abstraction. Important early anthroposophists who were Jewish included two central members on the executive boards of the precursors to the modern Anthroposophical Society, and Karl König, the founder of the Camphill movement. Martin Buber and Hugo Bergmann, who viewed Steiner's social ideas as a solution to the Arab–Jewish conflict, were also influenced by anthroposophy.

There are several anthroposophical organisations in Israel, including the anthroposophical kibbutz Harduf, founded by Jesaiah Ben-Aharon. A number of these organizations are striving to foster positive relationships between the Arab and Jewish populations: The Harduf Waldorf school includes both Jewish and Arab faculty and students, and has extensive contact with the surrounding Arab communities. In Hilf near Haifa, there is a joint Arab-Jewish Waldorf kindergarten, the first joint Arab-Jewish kindergarten in Israel.

Christian Community

Towards the end of Steiner's life, a group of theology students (primarily Lutheran, with some Roman Catholic members) approached Steiner for help in reviving Christianity, in particular "to bridge the widening gulf between modern science and the world of spirit." They approached a notable Lutheran pastor, Friedrich Rittelmeyer, who was already working with Steiner's ideas, to join their efforts. Out of their co-operative endeavor, the *Movement for Religious Renewal*, now generally known as The Christian Community, was born. Steiner emphasized that he considered this movement, and his role in creating it, to be independent of his anthroposophical work, as he wished anthroposophy to be independent of any particular religion or religious denomination.

Reception

Supporters

Anthroposophy's supporters include Pulitzer Prize-winning and Nobel Laureate Saul Bellow, Nobel prize winner Selma Lagerlöf, Andrei Bely, Joseph Beuys, Owen Barfield, architect Walter Burley Griffin, Wassily Kandinsky, Andrei Tarkovsky, Bruno Walter, and Right Livelihood Award winners Sir George Trevelyan and Ibrahim Abouleish. Albert Schweitzer was a friend of Steiner's and was supportive of his ideals for cultural renewal.

Scientific Basis

Though Rudolf Steiner studied natural science at the Vienna Technical University at the undergraduate level, his doctorate was in epistemology and very little of his work is directly concerned with the empirical sciences. In his mature work, when he did refer to science it was often to present phenomenological or Goethean science as an alternative to what he considered the materialistic science of his contemporaries.

His primary interest was in applying the methodology of science to realms of inner experience and the spiritual worlds (Steiner's appreciation that the essence of science is its method of inquiry is unusual among esotericists), and Steiner called anthroposophy *Geisteswissenschaft* (lit.: Science of the mind, or cultural or spiritual science), a term generally used in German to refer to the humanities and social sciences; in fact, the term "science" is used more broadly in Europe as a general term that refers to any exact knowledge.

[Anthroposophy's] methodology is to employ a scientific way of thinking, but to apply this methodology, which normally excludes our inner experience from consideration, instead to the human being proper.

Whether this is a sufficient basis for anthroposophy to be considered a spiritual science has been a matter of controversy. As Freda Easton explained in her study of Waldorf schools, "Whether one accepts anthroposophy as a science depends upon whether one accepts Steiner's interpretation of a science that extends the consciousness and capacity of human beings to experience their inner spiritual world." Sven Ove Hansson has disputed anthroposophy's claim to a scientific basis, stating that its ideas are not empirically derived and neither reproducible nor testable.

Carlo Willmann points out that as, on its own terms, anthroposophical methodology offers no possibility of being falsified except through its own procedures of spiritual investigation, no intersubjective validation is possible by conventional scientific methods; it thus cannot stand up to positivistic science's criticism. Peter Schneider calls such objections untenable on the grounds that if a non-sensory, non-physical realm exists, then according to Steiner the experiences of pure thinking possible within the normal realm of consciousness would already be experiences of that, and it would be impossible to exclude the possibility of empirically grounded experiences of other supersensory content.

Olav Hammer suggests that anthroposophy carries scientism "to lengths unparalleled in any other Esoteric position" due to its dependence upon claims of clairvoyant experience, its subsuming natural science under "spiritual science", and its development of what Hammer calls "fringe" sciences such as anthroposophical medicine and biodynamic agriculture justified partly on the basis of the ethical and ecological values they promote, rather than purely on a scientific basis.

Though Steiner saw that spiritual vision itself is difficult for others to achieve, he recommended open-mindedly exploring and rationally testing the results of such research; he also urged others to follow a spiritual training that would allow them directly to apply the methods he used eventually to achieve comparable results. Some results of Steiner's research have been investigated and supported by scientists working to further and extend scientific observation in directions suggested by an anthroposophical approach.

Anthony Storr stated about Rudolf Steiner's Anthroposophy: "His belief system is so eccentric, so unsupported by evidence, so manifestly bizarre, that rational skeptics are bound to consider it delusional.... But, whereas Einstein's way of perceiving the world by thought became confirmed by experiment and mathematical proof, Steiner's remained intensely subjective and insusceptible of objective confirmation."

Religious Nature

As an explicitly spiritual movement, anthroposophy has sometimes been called a religious philosophy. In 2005, a California federal court ruled that a group alleging that anthroposophy is a religion for Establishment Clause purposes did not provide any legally admissible evidence in support of this view; the case is under appeal. In 2000, a French court ruled that a government minister's description of anthroposophy as a cult was defamatory.

Statements on Race

Anthroposophical ideas have been criticized from both sides in the race debate:

- From the mid-1930s on, National Socialist ideologues attacked the anthroposophical world-view as being opposed to Nazi racist and nationalistic principles; anthroposophy considered "Blood, Race and Folk" as primitive instincts that must be overcome.
- "A naive version of the evolution of consciousness, a theory foundational to both Steiner's anthroposophy and Waldorf education, sometimes places one race below another in one or another dimension of development".

The Anthroposophical Society in America has stated:

We explicitly reject any racial theory that may be construed to be part of Rudolf Steiner's writings. The Anthroposophical Society in America is an open, public society and it rejects any purported spiritual or scientific theory on the basis of which the alleged superiority of one race is justified at the expense of another race.

Eurythmy

Eurythmy is an expressive movement art originated by Rudolf Steiner in conjunction with Marie von Sivers in the early 20th century. Primarily a performance art, it is also used in education, especially in Waldorf schools, and – as part of anthroposophic medicine – for claimed therapeutic purposes.

Movement Repertoire

The gestures in the eurythmist's movement repertoire relate to the sounds and rhythms of speech, to the tones and rhythms of music and to soul experiences, such as joy and sorrow. Once these fundamental repertoire elements are learned, they can be composed into free artistic expressions. The eurythmist also cultivates a feeling for the qualities of straight lines and curves, the directions of movement in space (forward, backward, up, down, left, right), contraction and expansion, and color. The element of color is also emphasized both through the costuming, usually given characteristic colors for a piece or part and formed of long, loose fabrics that accentuate the movements rather than the bodily form, and through the lighting, which saturates the space and changes with the moods of the piece.

Eurythmy's aim is to bring the artists' expressive movement and both the performers' and audience's feeling experience into harmony with a piece's content; eurythmy is thus sometimes called "visible music" or "visible speech", expressions that originate with its founder, Rudolf Steiner, who described eurythmy as an "art of the soul".

Most eurythmy today is performed to classical (concert) music or texts such as poetry or stories. Silent pieces are also sometimes performed.

Eurythmy with Music

When performing eurythmy with music (also called *tone eurythmy*), the three major elements of music, melody, harmony and rhythm, are all expressed. The melody is primarily conveyed through expressing its rise and fall; the specific pitches; and the intervallic qualities present. Harmony is expressed through movement between tension and release, as expressions of dissonance and consonance, and between the more inwardly directed minor mood and the outwardly directed major mood. Rhythm is chiefly conveyed through livelier and more contoured movements for quick notes, slower, dreamier movements for longer notes; in addition, longer tones move into the more passive (listening) back space, quicker tones into the more active front space.

Breaths or pauses are expressed through a larger or smaller movement in space, giving new impulse to what follows. Beat is conveyed through greater emphasis of downbeats, or those beats upon which stress is normally placed. Beat is generally treated as a subsidiary element. Eurythmy has only occasionally been done to popular music, in which beat plays a large role.

The timbre of individual instruments is brought into the quality both of the tonal gestures and of the whole movement of the eurythmist. Usually there will be a different eurythmist or group of eurythmists expressing each instrument, for example in chamber or symphonic music.

A piece's choreography usually expresses elements such as the major or minor key, the shape of the melody line, the interplay between voices or instruments and the relative dominance of one or another voice or instrument. Thus, musicians can often follow even the finest details of their part in the movements of the eurythmists on stage. Particular musical forms (e.g. the sonata) can have special characteristic choreographic expressions.

Eurythmy with Spoken Texts

Eurythmy is often performed with spoken texts such as poetry, stories or plays. *Speech eurythmy* includes such elements as the sounds of speech, rhythms, poetic meters, grammar and mood. In speech eurythmy, all the sounds of language have characteristic gestural qualities: the sound of an 'A' is open due to the position of the articulators during the vowel. A 'k' sounds sharper due to the manner of articulation of the consonant, that it is a plosive. Note that it is the audible sounds themselves, not the letters of the written language, that are expressed.

History

Eurythmy was conceived in 1911 when a widow brought her young daughter, Lory Smits, who was interested in movement and dance, to the Austrian philosopher Rudolf Steiner. Due to the recent loss of her father, it was necessary for the girl to find a career. Steiner's advice was sought; he suggested that the girl begin working on a new art of movement. As preparation for this, she began to study human anatomy, to explore the human step, to contemplate the movement implicit in Greek sculpture and dance, and to find movements that would express spoken sentences using the sounds of speech. Soon a number of other young people became interested in this form of expressive movement.

During these years, Steiner was writing a new drama each year for performance at the Anthroposophical Society's summer gatherings; beginning in 1912, he began to incorporate the new art of movement into these dramas. When the Society decided to build an artistic center in Dornach, Switzerland (this later became known as the Goetheanum) a small stage group began work and offered weekly performances of the developing art. Marie Steiner-von Sivers, Steiner's wife, who was a trained actress and speech artist, was given responsibility for training and directing this ensemble. This first eurythmy ensemble went on tour in 1919, performing across Switzerland, the Netherlands and Germany.

Steiner saw eurythmy as a unique expression of the anthroposophical impulse:

It is the task of Anthroposophy to bring a greater depth, a wider vision and a more living spirit into the other forms of art. But the art of Eurythmy could only grow up out of the soul of Anthroposophy; could only receive its inspiration through a purely Anthroposophical conception.

—*Rudolf Steiner*

According to Steiner: *In eurythmy we present in the form and movement of the human organism a direct external proof of a man's share in the life of the supersensible world. When people do eurythmy they are linked directly with the supersensible world. Whenever art is formed from a truly artistic conviction it bears witness to the connection of the human being with the supersensible world.* (Dornach, 12 September 1920)

In 1924, Steiner gave two intensive workshops on different aspects of eurythmy; transcripts of his talks during these workshops are published as *Eurythmy as Visible Speech* and *Eurythmy as Visible Singing*.

Eurythmy ensembles in Stuttgart, Germany and at the Goetheanum soon became established parts of the cultural life of Europe. The Goetheanum ensemble was recognized with a gold medal at the Paris Expo of 1937/8. The Stuttgart training and ensemble, led by Else Klink, had to close in the Nazi period but reopened shortly after the close of World War II. There are now training centers and artistic ensembles in many countries.

Etymology

The word *eurythmy* stems from Greek roots meaning *beautiful* or *harmonious rhythm*. The term was used by Ancient Greek and Roman architects to refer to the harmonious proportions of a design or building; The English word *eurythmy* was used from the 17th to 19th century to refer not only to harmonious architectural proportions, but also to "rhythmical order or movement" and "a graceful proportion and carriage of the body".

Eurythmy as A Performing Art

There are notable eurythmy ensembles in Dornach, Switzerland; Stuttgart, Germany; The Hague, Netherlands; London, England; Järna, Sweden, and Chestnut Ridge, New York (near New York City). All of these groups both perform locally and tour internationally. Many smaller performing groups also exist. High schools that have their own performing ensembles include the San Francisco Waldorf High School ensemble.

Pedagogical Eurythmy

When the first Waldorf School was founded in 1919, Eurythmy was included in the curriculum. It was quickly recognized as a successful complement to gymnastics in the school's movement program and is now taught in most Waldorf schools, as well as in many non-Waldorf pre-school centers, kindergartens and schools. It is taught to all ages from pre-schools through high school and into college. Its purpose is to awaken and strengthen the expressive capacities of children through movement, stimulating the child to bring imagination, ideation and conceptualization to the point where they can manifest these as "vital, moving forms" in physical space. It is also thought to improve balance, coordination, concentration, rhythm, and form an awareness of patterns.

Eurythmy pedagogical exercises begin with the straight line and curve and proceed through successively more complicated geometric figures and choreographed forms, developing a child's coordination and concentration. An extensive set of special exercises has also been developed for pedagogical purposes. These include metamorphosing geometric patterns and dynamic movement sequences.

Rods or balls are sometimes used in exercises to develop precision in movement, to expand the experience of space, develop precise balance, and to objectify the movement experience. The rods are usually approximately the length of an arm; the balls are of a size to fit comfortably in one hand. Both are generally made of copper, a material receptive to warmth.

Though there are some independent post-graduate trainings for pedagogical eurythmy, this aspect is frequently included in courses focusing on artistic work.

Therapeutic Eurythmy

Eurythmy is a component of anthroposophic medicine, a system of alternative medicine which has been characterized by some critics as unscientific, pseudoscientific and as "pure quackery".

According to the precepts of anthroposophic medicine, a human has four aspects which need to be treated: spirit, soul, life and matter. Eurythmy is one of the practices said to act on the "life" aspect, and is claimed to effect an "improvement of health related life functions". A person receiving earthymy therapy moves under the guidance of a eurythmy therapist, who will have been trained two years beyond the four-year fundamental course in eurythmy. The movements may be adapted to the condition of the person being treated; for example, they may be done while either sitting or even lying down. Therapeutic eurythmy is claimed to bring about a "re-integration of body, soul, and spirit."

A 2008 review in *BMC Complementary and Alternative Medicine* said that eurythmy was a "potentially relevant add-on" to a therapeutic program, but though the studies reviewed reported improvement in symptoms, limitations in the underlying data and in the review methods means these conclusions "warrant cautious interpretation".

Anthroposophical View of the Human Being

The anthroposophical view of humans includes:

Threefold and Fourfold View

Rudolf Steiner often described humans as consisting of an eternal spirit, an evolving soul and a temporal body, giving a detailed analysis of each of these three realms.

Spirit: anthroposophical teachings describe the human spirit as eternal yet becoming progressively more individualized and consciously experienced. Steiner believed that humans pass between stages of existence, incarnating into an earthly body, living a life, leaving the body behind and entering into the spiritual worlds before returning to be born again into a new life on earth. In earthly life, the individuality or ego awakens to self-consciousness through its experience of its reflection in the deeds and suffering of a physical body.

Soul: We also have a framework of consciousness that includes our set feelings, concepts and intentions. As each human soul evolves through its experiences, the earth itself and civilization as a whole also evolve; thus, new types of experience are available at each successive incarnation.

Body: Steiner uses the term body to describe the aspects of human existence that endure for a single lifetime. The physical body is the most obvious of these. Permeating our physical existence are forces of life, growth and metamorphosis that maintain and develop the physical body; as it is an aspect of a lifetime that falls away after death, Steiner called this the life or etheric body. Steiner called that which receives sensory impressions the body of consciousness or sentient body.

A fourfold articulation of the human body often applied to contexts such as medicine and education includes:

- the physical body as physical-material structure, held in common with the mineral world;
- the life or etheric body, the source of life and growth, held in common with the plant world;
- the consciousness or astral body, held in common with the animal world;
- the ego or "I" of the human being, the faculty of self-awareness unique to humanity

Physical Body

In the physical body, Steiner differentiated three primary functional areas, each supporting a particular psychological activity:

- the nerve/sense system, primarily centered in the nervous system, supporting thinking and perception
- the rhythmic system, including the breathing and the circulatory system, supporting feeling
- the motor-metabolic system, including the organs below the diaphragm and the limbs, supporting willing

In his mature work, Steiner identified twelve senses: balance, or equilibrioception; movement, or proprioception; pain/well-being, or nociception, also called life sense; touch, or tactition; taste, or gustation; smell, or olfaction; warmth, or thermoception; sight, or vision; hearing, or audition; word / speech; thought / concept; ego / self.

Life or Etheric Body

All that lives has, in addition to a physical body, a permeating life organization. Steiner cites as proof of this the physical identity of a dead and living organism; what is lacking in the former is the element of life itself. Plant life is the embodiment of this.

Astral or Feeling Body

Animal life adds an element of sentience to the living world of plants. Steiner points to sleep life, when the physical body and life organization are identical with waking life, yet sentience is withdrawn, as proof that sentience is not purely a function of the physical and life bodies. Our instincts (and prejudices), emotions and will impulses reside here; these are relatively fixed, in contrast with our more fluid and active soul life.

Ego or "I"

Human existence includes an element distinct from animate life, the ego. This awakens to self-awareness through its experience of the physical body; Steiner points to the lack of a true biography, more particularly of autobiography in animal existence as an indication that the ego is particular to humans and each human has its own distinct 'concept'. The capacity for self-direction and full responsibility are connected to the ego, which anthroposophical researchers describe as only becoming independent around twenty-one years after conception.

Sevenfold View

In Steiner's sevenfold and ninefold descriptions, a human is composed of physical-body, life-body, astral-body, ego, spirit-self, life-spirit, and spirit-man.

- the physical body, *material structure*
- the life body, *life processes,*
- the astral body, *bearer of consciousness,*

- the ego, *self-awareness,*
- the spirit-self, *intuition and self,*
- the life-spirit, *enduring spirit-soul content,*
- the spirit-man, *the fully individuated spirit.*

The ego experiences itself through all three of the unconscious elements (consciousness, life and physicality) in specific ways: through the astral body, bearer of sentience, in the dreamier experience of the *sentient soul*; through the life body as rationality in the *intellectual soul*; through the physical body as fully conscious, autonomous egoity in the *consciousness soul*. Through differentiating ego consciousness into its experience as mediated through these unconscious organs, this gives a ninefold articulation of a human: physicality, life, consciousness; sentient, intellectual and consciousness soul; spirit self, life spirit, spirit man.

Anthroposophic Pharmacy

Anthroposophic pharmacy is the discipline related to conceiving, developing and producing medicinal products according to the anthroposophic understanding of man, nature, substance and pharmaceutical processing. One of the most characteristic features of anthroposophic medicine is the attempt to describe health and natural medicine in scientific as well as in spiritual terms. Anthroposophic pharmacy utilises vegetable, mineral and animal materials, manufactured according to particular principles and is sometimes potentised.

Anthroposophic medicines should be considered as complementary to conventional medicines and are often used in combination with them.

In 2005, a health technology assessment (HTA) produced the first systematic review of the efficacy, utility, costs and safety of anthroposophic medicine as part of the Swiss Government's evaluation of complementary medicine (PEK). The report concluded that there are many studies that show positive outcomes for anthroposophic medicine, although the methodological quality of the studies is very variable. In terms of safety almost all studies emphasise the good tolerability of anthroposophic medicinal therapies.

The conclusion of the PEK process was that there was insufficient evidence to support reimbursement of any of the five therapies investigated, including both anthroposophic medicine and homeopathy.

Origin and Development

The manufacture and use of anthroposophic medicines dates back to Rudolf Steiner (1861–1925), who together with Dr Ita Wegman (1876–1943) invented anthroposophic medicine at the beginning of the 20th century. Steiner and Wegman's ideas were extended by the chemist Dr Oskar Schmiedel (1887–1959), who manufactured anthroposophic medicines from 1920 onwards and introduced the newly conceived formulations and manufacturing processes into pharmaceutical practice. A second important pioneer of anthroposophic pharmacy was Dr Rudolf Hauschka (1891–1969).

Anthroposophic medicine is now practised in over 60 countries, and for example in Germany is recognised as a special therapy system in the Medicinal Product Act (Arzneimittelgesetz) and in the Code of Social Law (Sozialgesetzbuch) V (Paragraph 34, section 3). There are approximately 15,000 doctors in 22 European countries who prescribe anthroposophic medicinal products, e.g. in Austria, Denmark, France, Germany, Italy. It is estimated that in Germany some 6 million patients use anthroposophic medicine. According to the German Pharmaceutical Industry Association (BPI), for example, anthroposophicals reached a turnover in 2011 of 52.8 million Euro (Data March 2013).

There are about 1,700 different anthroposophic medicinal products on the market in the European Union. Within the EU there are differing rules as to whether or not an anthroposophic medicine must be prescribed by a doctor. In Germany, for example, most preparations are not prescription-only, and since 2004 must be paid for by the patient himself.

Theory and Background

Anthroposophic medicinal products rely on anthroposophical ideas of the relationship between man and nature: "The starting materials of these products come from minerals, plants and animal substances. They are developed and manufactured in accordance with the anthroposophic perception of human beings and nature".

The philosophy posits four levels of the human being and three systems by which they interact. The following table explains the correlation between the four different levels of the human being and the realms of nature as it is understood in anthroposophic pharmacy:

Human being	**Realm of Nature**
Physical constitution is related to ...	mineral world
Life or etheric body (maintenance of biological identity, regeneration and physiological functions) is related to ...	plant world
Psychological level or astral body (passion, feeling, movement) is related to ...	animal world
"Ego" as individual level and self-consciousness is unique to humanity	no correlations

Pharmaceutical Processing

Anthroposophic pharmaceutical processing involves specific anthroposophic and some typical homoeopathic pharmaceutical procedures. The ingredients of anthroposophic medicines are all of natural origin: used are mineral/metallic, vegetable or mineral raw materials e.g. quartz, sulphur, gold, copper, silver, arnica, chamomile or marigold. Animal testing is not used in the development of anthroposophic medicinal products.

Anthroposophic medicines are manufactured principally using rhythmical processes and/or heat. Examples of typical anthroposophic pharmaceutical processes using raw materials of botanical origin are:

Pharmaceutical process	Temperature	Raw material
Cold maceration	2-8 °C	fresh or dried plants, all parts
Maceration	ca. 15-20 °C	fresh plants, all parts
Rhythmic processing	4 / 37 °C	fresh plants, all parts
Digestion	37 °C	fresh plants, leaves, flowers
Infusion	60-90 °C	dried leaves, flowers
Decoction	ca 100 °C	dried roots, barks, seeds
Distillation	steam, ca 100 °C	fresh or dried plants, all parts

These pharmaceutical processes are specified in the European Pharmacopoeia, the Pharmacopoeia Helvetica (Ph.Helv.), the German Homoeopathic Pharmacopoeia (GHP/HAB), the Anthroposophic Pharmaceutical Codex (APC), and the British Homoeopathic Pharmacopoeia (B.Hom.P.).

Another pharmaceutical process often used in anthroposophic pharmacy is *potentisation*, which is also widely used in homoeopathy. Potentised preparations are gradually diluted substances, whereby at each diluting step a rhythmic shaking and striking against a resilient surface ("succussion") are involved. The principle of potentisation is not supported by any significant body of scientific evidence.

Production and Quality Control

"Anthroposophic medicinal products are produced in accordance with the modern standards of Good Manufacturing Practice GMP. Their quality is controlled by the criteria and parameters of official pharmacopoeia (e.g. European Pharmacopoeia (Ph.Eur.), German Homoeopathic Pharmacopoeia (GHP/HAB), French Pharmacopoeia (Ph.fr.), Pharmacopoeia Helvetica (Ph.Helv.), and the Anthroposophic Pharmaceutical Codex (APC)".

Detailed pharmaceutical information for quality control and regulatory needs is provided in the Anthroposophic Pharmaceutical Codex that is issued by the International Association of Anthroposophic Pharmacists (IAAP), the umbrella organisation for the national professional anthroposophic pharmacists' associations in Europe.

References

- DIANE Publishing Company (1 July 1995). Alternative Medicine: Expanding Medical Horizons. DIANE Publishing. p. 86. ISBN 978-0-7881-1820-3.
- Dugan, Dan (2002-01-01). Michael Shermer, ed. Anthroposophy and Anthroposophical Medicine. The Skeptic Encyclopedia of Pseudoscience. ABC-CLIO. pp. 31–32. ISBN 978-1-57607-653-8.
- Paul A. Offit (2011). Deadly Choices: How the Anti-Vaccine Movement Threatens Us All. Basic Books. p. 13. ISBN 978-0-465-02356-1.
- Gunver Sophia Kienle; Helmut Kiene; Hans Ulrich Albonico (2006). Anthroposophic Medicine: Effectiveness, Utility, Costs, Safety. Schattauer Verlag. ISBN 978-3-7945-2495-2.
- James S. Olson (5 January 2005). Bathsheba's Breast: Women, Cancer, and History. JHU Press. p. 452. ISBN 978-0-8018-8064-3. Retrieved 1 September 2013.
- Christian Clement (ed.), Rudolf Steiner: Schriften über Mystik, Mysterienwesen und Religionsgeschichte. Frommann-holzboog Verlag, Stuttgart-Bad Cannstatt, 2013. ISBN 978-3-7728-2635-1.

- Ruse, Michael (2013-09-25). The Gaia Hypothesis: Science on a Pagan Planet. University of Chicago Press. pp. 128–. ISBN 9780226060392. Retrieved 21 June 2015.
- Robert A. McDermott, "Rudolf Steiner and Anthroposophy", in Faivre and Needleman, Modern Esoteric Spirituality, ISBN 0-8245-1444-0.
- Karl König The Child with Special Needs: Letters and Essays on Curative Education Publisher: Floris Books 2009 ISBN 0863156932 ISBN 978-0863156939
- Thomas J. Weihs "Children in Need of Special Care" A Condor book Human Horizons series. Editors: Anthea M. Hailey, Michael J. Hailey, N. M. Blitz Souvenir Press Limited, 2000 ISBN 0285635697, ISBN 9780285635692
- Sokolina, Anna, ed., co-author, Architecture and Anthroposophy. (Arkhitektura i Antroposofiia. bilingual ed.) 1st and 2nd edition. 268p. M.: KMK Scientific Press. 2001, ISBN 5-87317-074-6. 2010, ISBN 5-87317-660-4.
- True and False Paths in Spiritual Investigation, first English edition 1927 (online), 2010 edition Kessinger Publishing Company ISBN 9781162592510
- Lorenzo Ravagli, Unter Hammer und Hakenkreuz: Der völkisch-nationalsozialistische Kampf gegen die Anthroposophie, Verlag Freies Geistesleben, ISBN 3-7725-1915-6
- Storr, Anthony (1997) [1996]. "IV. Rudolf Steiner". Feet of Clay: Saints, Sinners, and Madmen: A Study of Gurus. New York: Free Press Paperbacks, Simon & Schuster. pp. 69–70. ISBN 0-684-83495-2.
- Dugan, Dan. Michael Shermer, ed. Anthroposophy and Anthroposophical Medicine. The Skeptic Encyclopedia of Pseudoscience. ABC-CLIO. pp. 31–32. ISBN 978-1-57607-653-8.
- Carlo Willmann, Waldorfpädogogik: Theologische und religionspädagogische Befunde, Böhlau Verlag, 2001. ISBN 3-412-16700-2, pp. 25-8.
- Johannes Hemleben, Rudolf Steiner: A documentary biography, Henry Goulden Ltd, ISBN 0-904822-02-8, pp. 87-91. (German edition Rowohlt Taschenbuch Verlag ISBN 3-499-50079-5)

4

Homeopathy: An Overview

Homeopathy is a form of alternative medicine. They are scientifically not considered effective for treating any condition. Some of the aspects of homeopathy that have been discussed are homeopathic dilutions, electrohomeopathy, arsenicum album and regulation and prevalence of homeopathy. The topics discussed in the section are of great importance to broaden the existing knowledge on homeopathy.

Homeopathy

Homeopathy or homoeopathy is a system of alternative medicine created in 1796 by Samuel Hahnemann, based on his doctrine of *like cures like* (*similia similibus curentur*), a claim that a substance that causes the symptoms of a disease in healthy people would cure similar symptoms in sick people. Homeopathy is a pseudoscience – a belief that is incorrectly presented as scientific. Homeopathic preparations are not effective for treating any condition; large-scale studies have found homeopathy to be no more effective than a placebo, suggesting that any positive feelings that follow treatment are only due to the placebo effect and normal recovery from illness.

Hahnemann believed the underlying causes of disease were phenomena that he termed *miasms*, and that homeopathic preparations addressed these. The preparations are manufactured using a process of homeopathic dilution, in which a chosen substance is repeatedly diluted in alcohol or distilled water, each time with the containing vessel being bashed against an elastic material, (commonly a leather-bound book). Dilution typically continues well past the point where no molecules of the original substance remain. Homeopaths select homeopathics by consulting reference books known as *repertories*, and by considering the totality of the patient's symptoms, personal traits, physical and psychological state, and life history.

Homeopathy is not a plausible system of treatment, as its dogmas about how drugs, illness, the human body, liquids and solutions operate are contradicted by a wide range of discoveries across biology, psychology, physics and chemistry made in the two centuries since its invention. Although some clinical trials produce positive results, multiple systematic reviews have indicated that this is because of chance, flawed research methods, and reporting bias. Continued homeopathic practice, despite the evidence that it does not work, has been criticized as unethical because it discourages the use of effective treatments, with the World Health Organization warning against using homeopathy to try to treat severe diseases such as HIV and malaria. The continued practice of homeopathy, despite a lack of evidence of efficacy, has led to it being characterized within the scientific and medical communities as nonsense, quackery, and a sham.

Assessments by the Australian National Health and Medical Research Council, the United Kingdom's House of Commons Science and Technology Committee and the Swiss Federal Health Office have each concluded that homeopathy is ineffective, and recommended against the practice receiving any further funding.

History

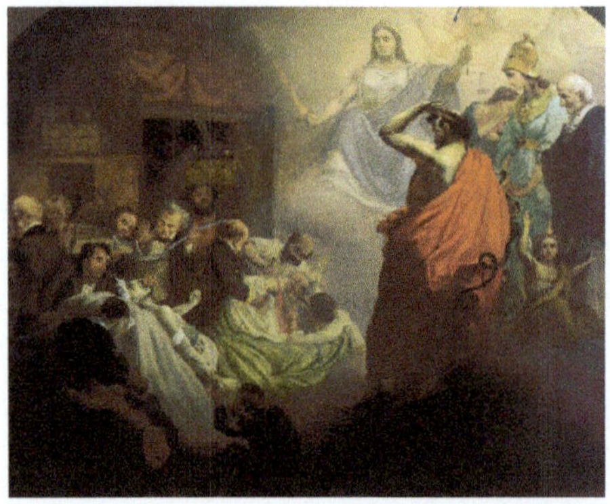

1857 painting by Alexander Beydeman, showing historical figures and personifications of homeopathy observing the brutality of medicine of the 19th century

Historical Context

Homeopaths claim that Hippocrates may have originated homeopathy around 400 BC, when he prescribed a small dose of mandrake root to treat mania, knowing it produces mania in much larger doses. In the 16th century, the pioneer of pharmacology Paracelsus declared that small doses of "what makes a man ill also cures him". Samuel Hahnemann (1755–1843) gave homeopathy its name and expanded its principles in the late 18th century.

In the late 18th and 19th centuries, mainstream medicine used methods like bloodletting and purging, and administered complex mixtures, such as Venice treacle, which was made from 64 substances including opium, myrrh, and viper's flesh. These treatments often worsened symptoms and sometimes proved fatal. Hahnemann rejected these practices – which had been extolled for centuries – as irrational and inadvisable; instead, he advocated the use of single drugs at lower doses and promoted an immaterial, vitalistic view of how living organisms function, believing that diseases have spiritual, as well as physical causes.

Hahnemann's Concept

The term "homeopathy" was coined by Hahnemann and first appeared in print in 1807.

Hahnemann conceived of homeopathy while translating a medical treatise by the Scottish physician and chemist William Cullen into German. Being sceptical of Cullen's theory concerning cinchona's use for curing malaria, Hahnemann ingested some bark specifically to investigate what would happen. He experienced fever, shivering and joint pain: symptoms similar to those of malaria itself. From this, Hahnemann came to believe that all effective drugs produce symptoms in healthy individuals similar to those of the diseases that they treat, in accord with the "law of similars" that had been proposed by ancient physicians. An account of the effects of eating cinchona bark noted by Oliver Wendell Holmes, and published in 1861, failed to reproduce the symptoms Hahnemann reported. Hahnemann's law of similars is a postulate rather than a scientific law.

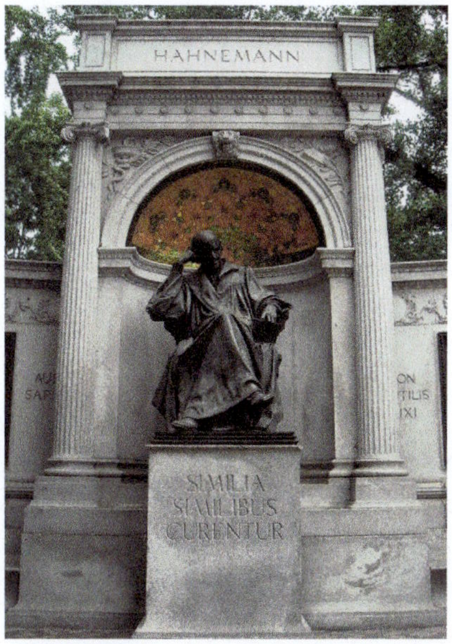

Samuel Hahnemann Monument, Washington D.C. with "Similia Similibus Curentur" - Like cures Like.

Subsequent scientific work showed that cinchona cures malaria because it contains quinine, which kills the *Plasmodium falciparum* parasite that causes the disease; the mechanism of action is unrelated to Hahnemann's ideas.

"Provings"

Hahnemann began to test what effects substances produced in humans, a procedure that would later become known as "homeopathic proving". These tests required subjects to test the effects of ingesting substances by clearly recording all of their symptoms as well as the ancillary conditions under which they appeared. He published a collection of provings in 1805, and a second collection of 65 preparations appeared in his book, *Materia Medica Pura*, in 1810.

Because Hahnemann believed that large doses of drugs that caused similar symptoms would only aggravate illness, he advocated extreme dilutions of the substances; he devised a technique for making dilutions that he believed would preserve a substance's therapeutic properties while removing its harmful effects. Hahnemann believed that this process aroused and enhanced "the spirit-like medicinal powers of the crude substances". He gathered and published a complete overview of his new medical system in his 1810 book, *The Organon of the Healing Art*, whose 6th edition, published in 1921, is still used by homeopaths today.

Miasms and Disease

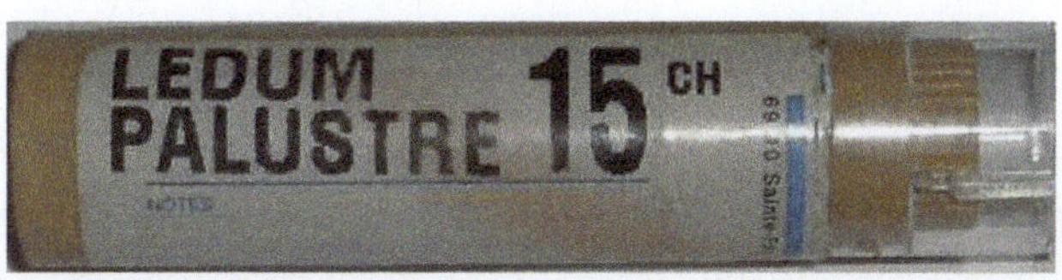

A homeopathic preparation made from marsh tea: the "15C" dilution shown here means the original solution was diluted to $1/10^{30}$ of its original strength. Given that there are many orders of magnitude fewer than 10^{30} molecules in the small sample, the likelihood that it contains even one molecule of the original herb is extremely low.

In the *Organon*, Hahnemann introduced the concept of "miasms" as "infectious principles" underlying chronic disease. Hahnemann associated each miasm with specific diseases, and thought that initial exposure to miasms causes local symptoms, such as skin or venereal diseases. If, however, these symptoms were suppressed by medication, the cause went deeper and began to manifest itself as diseases of the internal organs. Homeopathy maintains that treating diseases by directly alleviating their symptoms, as is sometimes done in conventional medicine, is ineffective because all "disease can generally be traced to some latent, deep-seated, underlying chronic, or inherited tendency". The underlying imputed miasm still remains, and deep-seated ailments can be corrected only by removing the deeper disturbance of the vital force.

Hahnemann's hypotheses for the direct or remote cause of all chronic diseases (miasms) originally presented only three, psora (the itch), syphilis (venereal disease) or sycosis (fig-wart disease). Of these three the most important was *psora* (Greek for "itch"), described as being related to any itching diseases of the skin, supposed to be derived from suppressed scabies, and claimed to be the foundation of many further disease conditions. Hahnemann believed psora to be the cause of such diseases as epilepsy, cancer, jaundice, deafness, and cataracts. Since Hahnemann's time, other miasms have been proposed, some replacing one or more of psora's proposed functions, including tuberculosis and cancer miasms.

The law of susceptibility implies that a negative state of mind can attract hypothetical disease entities called "miasms" to invade the body and produce symptoms of diseases. Hahnemann rejected the notion of a disease as a separate thing or invading entity, and insisted it was always part of the "living whole". Hahnemann coined the expression "allopathic medicine", which was used to pejoratively refer to traditional Western medicine.

Hahnemann's miasm theory remains disputed and controversial within homeopathy even in modern times. The theory of miasms has been criticized as an explanation developed by Hahnemann to preserve the system of homeopathy in the face of treatment failures, and for being inadequate to cover the many hundreds of sorts of diseases, as well as for failing to explain disease predispositions, as well as genetics, environmental factors, and the unique disease history of each patient.

19th Century: Rise to Popularity and Early Criticism

Homeopathy achieved its greatest popularity in the 19th century. It was introduced to the United States in 1825 by Hans Birch Gram, a student of Hahnemann. The first homeopathic school in the US opened in 1835, and in 1844, the first US national medical association, the American Institute of Homeopathy, was established. Throughout the 19th century, dozens of homeopathic institutions appeared in Europe and the United States, and by 1900, there were 22 homeopathic colleges and 15,000 practitioners in the United States. Because medical practice of the time relied on ineffective and often dangerous treatments, patients of homeopaths often had better outcomes than those of the doctors of the time. Homeopathic preparations, even if ineffective, would almost surely cause no harm, making the users of homeopathic preparations less likely to be killed by the treatment that was supposed to be helping them. The relative success of homeopathy in the 19th century may have led to the abandonment of the ineffective and harmful treatments of bloodletting and purging and to have begun the move towards more effective, science-based medicine. One reason for the growing popularity of homeopathy was its apparent success in treating people suffering from infectious disease epidemics. During 19th-century epidemics of diseases such as cholera, death rates in homeopathic hospitals were often lower than in conventional hospitals, where the treatments used at the time were often harmful and did little or nothing to combat the diseases.

From its inception, however, homeopathy was criticized by mainstream science. Sir John Forbes, physician to Queen Victoria, said in 1843 that the extremely small doses of homeopathy were regularly derided as useless, "an outrage to human reason". James Young Simpson said in 1853 of the highly diluted drugs: "No poison, however strong or powerful, the billionth or decillionth of which would in the least degree affect a man or harm a fly." 19th-century American physician and author Oliver Wendell Holmes, Sr. was also a vocal critic of homeopathy and published an essay in 1842 entitled *Homœopathy and Its Kindred Delusions*. The members of the French Homeopathic Society observed in 1867 that some leading homeopathists of Europe not only were abandoning the practice of administering infinitesimal doses but were also no longer defending it. The last school in the US exclusively teaching homeopathy closed in 1920.

Revival in The 20th Century

According to Paul Ulrich Unschuld, the Nazi regime in Germany was fascinated by homeopathy, and spent large sums of money on researching its mechanisms, but without gaining a positive result. Unschuld further argues that homeopathy never subsequently took root in the United States, but remained more deeply established in European thinking.

In the United States, the *Food, Drug, and Cosmetic Act* of 1938 (sponsored by Royal Copeland, a Senator from New York and homeopathic physician) recognized homeopathic preparations as drugs. In the 1950s, there were only 75 pure homeopaths practising in the U.S. However, by the mid to late 1970s, homeopathy made a significant comeback and sales of some homeopathic companies increased tenfold. Some homeopaths give credit for the revival to Greek homeopath George Vithoulkas, who performed a "great deal of research to update the scenarios and refine the theories and practice of homeopathy", beginning in the 1970s, but Ernst and Singh consider it to be linked to the rise of the New Age movement. Whichever is correct, mainstream pharmacy chains recognized the business potential of selling homeopathic preparations. The Food and Drug Administration held a hearing April 20 and 21, 2015, requesting public comment on regulation of homeopathic drugs. The FDA cited the growth of sales of over the counter homeopathic medicines, $2.7 billion as of 2007, many labelled as "natural, safe, and effective".

Bruce Hood has argued that the increased popularity of homeopathy in recent times may be due to the comparatively long consultations practitioners are willing to give their patients, and to an irrational preference for "natural" products which people think are the basis of homeopathic preparations.

Preparations and Treatment

Homeopathic preparations are referred to as "homeopathics" or "remedies". Practitioners rely on two types of reference when prescribing: *materia medica* and repertories. A homeopathic *materia medica* is a collection of "drug pictures", organized alphabetically. These entries describe the symptom patterns associated with individual preparations. A homeopathic repertory is an index of disease symptoms that lists preparations associated with specific symptoms. In both cases different compilers may dispute particular inclusions. The first symptomatic homeopathic *materia medica* was arranged by Hahnemann. The first homeopathic repertory was Georg Jahr's *Symptomenkodex*, published in German in 1835, and translated into English as the *Repertory to the more Characteristic Symptoms of Materia Medica* by Constantine Hering in 1838. This version was less focused on disease categories and would be the forerunner to later works by James Tyler Kent. Repertories, in particular, may be very large.

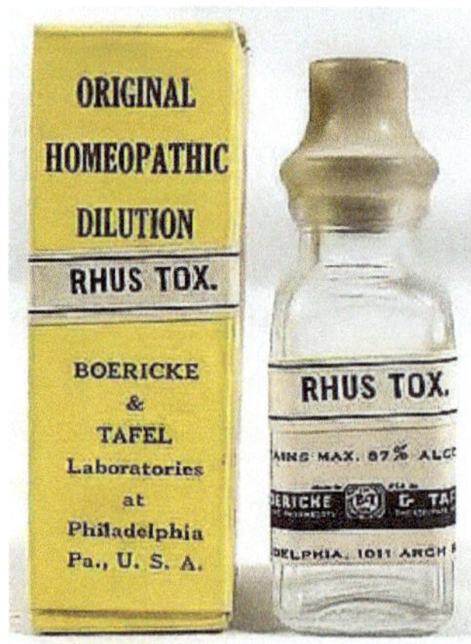

Homeopathic preparation *Rhus toxicodendron*, derived from poison ivy.

Homeopathy uses animal, plant, mineral, and synthetic substances in its preparations, generally referring to them using Latin or faux-Latin names. Examples include *arsenicum album* (arsenic oxide), *natrum muriaticum* (sodium chloride or table salt), *Lachesis muta* (the venom of the bushmaster snake), *opium*, and *thyroidinum* (thyroid hormone).

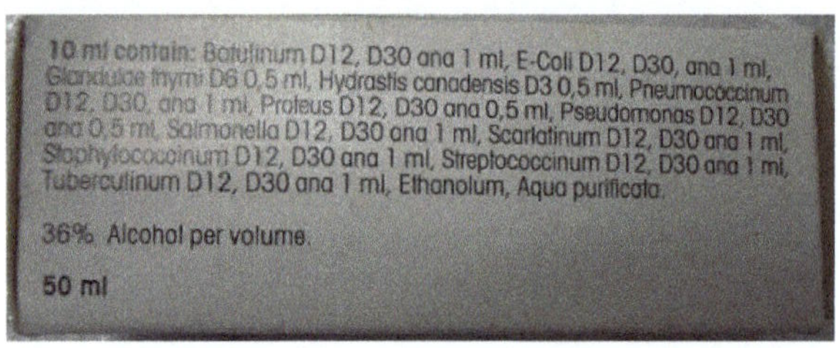

a preparation made from D dilutions of dangerous materials like botulism, E-coli, thymus gland of unspecified origin, pneumonia, pseudomona, proteus, salmonella, scarlet fever, staph, strep and tuberculosis bacteria. Ethanol is listed as being redundantly diluted in alcohol.

Some homeopaths use so-called "nosodes" (from the Greek *nosos*, disease) made from diseased or pathological products such as fecal, urinary, and respiratory discharges, blood, and tissue. Conversely, preparations made from "healthy" specimens are called "sarcodes".

Some modern homeopaths use preparations they call "imponderables" because they do not originate from a substance but some other phenomenon presumed to have been "captured" by alcohol or lactose. Examples include X-rays and sunlight.

Other minority practices include paper preparations, where the substance and dilution are written on pieces of paper and either pinned to the patients' clothing, put in their pockets, or placed under glasses of water that are then given to the patients, and the use of radionics to manufacture preparations. Such practices have been strongly criticized by classical homeopaths as unfounded, speculative, and verging upon magic and superstition.

Preparation

Hahnemann found that undiluted doses caused reactions, sometimes dangerous ones, so specified that preparations be given at the lowest possible dose. He found that this reduced potency as well as side-effects, but formed the view that vigorous shaking and striking on an elastic surface – a process he termed *Schütteln*, translated as *succussion* – nullified this. A common explanation for his settling on this process is said to be that he found preparations subjected to agitation in transit, such as in saddle bags or in a carriage, were more "potent". Hahnemann had a saddle-maker construct a special wooden striking board covered in leather on one side and stuffed with horsehair. Insoluble solids, such as granite, diamond, and platinum, are diluted by grinding them with lactose ("trituration").

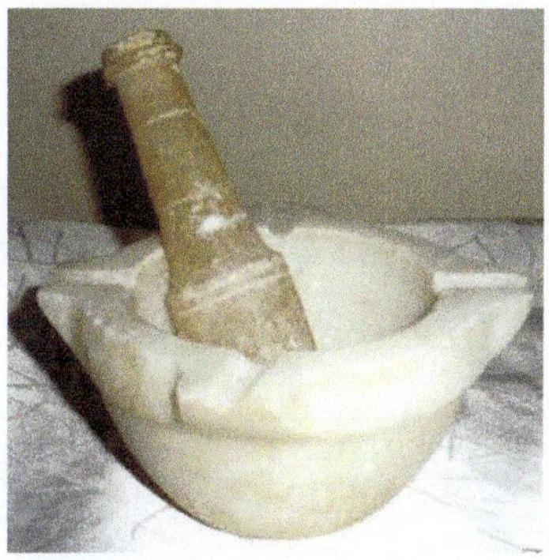

Mortar and pestle used for grinding insoluble solids, such as platinum, into homeopathic preparations

The process of dilution and succussion is termed "dynamization" or "potentization" by homeopaths. In industrial manufacture this may be done by machine.

Serial dilution is achieved by taking an amount of the mixture and adding solvent, but the "Korsakovian" method may also be used, whereby the vessel in which the preparations are manufactured is emptied, refilled with solvent, and the volume of fluid adhering to the walls of the vessel is deemed sufficient for the new batch. The Korsakovian method is sometimes referred to as K on the label of a homeopathic preparation, e.g. 200CK is a 200C preparation made using the Korsakovian method.

Fluxion and radionics methods of preparation do not require succussion. There are differences of opinion on the number and force of strikes, and some practitioners dispute the need for succussion at all while others reject the Korsakovian and other non-classical preparations. There are no laboratory assays and the importance and techniques for succussion cannot be determined with any certainty from the literature.

Dilutions

Three main logarithmic potency scales are in regular use in homeopathy. Hahnemann created the "centesimal" or "C scale", diluting a substance by a factor of 100 at each stage. The centesimal scale was favoured by Hahnemann for most of his life.

A 2C dilution requires a substance to be diluted to one part in 100, and then some of that diluted solution diluted by a further factor of 100.

This works out to one part of the original substance in 10,000 parts of the solution. A 6C dilution repeats this process six times, ending up with the original substance diluted by a factor of $100^{-6}=10^{-12}$ (one part in one trillion or 1/1,000,000,000,000). Higher dilutions follow the same pattern.

In homeopathy, a solution that is more dilute is described as having a higher "potency", and more dilute substances are considered by homeopaths to be stronger and deeper-acting. The end product is often so diluted as to be indistinguishable from the diluent (pure water, sugar or alcohol). There is also a decimal potency scale (notated as "X" or "D") in which the preparation is diluted by a factor of 10 at each stage.

Hahnemann advocated 30C dilutions for most purposes (that is, dilution by a factor of 10^{60}). Hahnemann regularly used potencies up to 300C but opined that "there must be a limit to the matter, it cannot go on indefinitely".

In Hahnemann's time, it was reasonable to assume the preparations could be diluted indefinitely, as the concept of the atom or molecule as the smallest possible unit of a chemical substance was just beginning to be recognized.

The greatest dilution reasonably likely to contain even one molecule of the original substance is 12C.

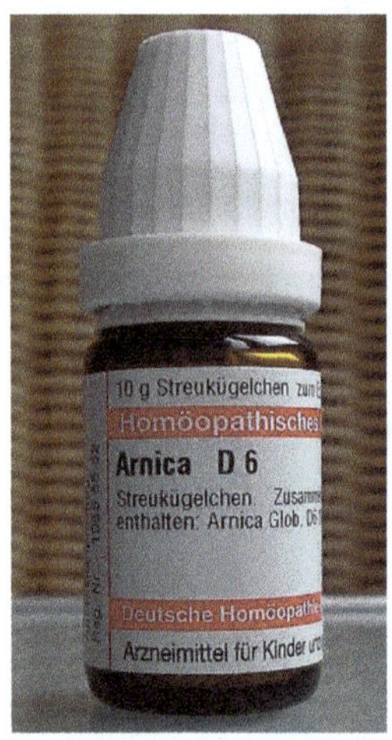

This bottle is labelled *Arnica montana* (wolf's bane) D6, i.e. the nominal dilution is one part in a million (10^{-6}).

Critics and advocates of homeopathy alike commonly attempt to illustrate the dilutions involved in homeopathy with analogies. Hahnemann is reported to have joked that a suitable procedure to deal with an epidemic would be to empty a bottle of poison into Lake Geneva, if it could be succussed 60 times. Another example given by a critic of homeopathy states that a 12C solution is equivalent to a "pinch of salt in both the North and South Atlantic Oceans", which is approximately correct. One-third of a drop of some original substance diluted into all the water on earth would produce a preparation with a concentration of about 13C. A popular homeopathic treatment for the flu is a 200C dilution of duck liver, marketed under the name Oscillococcinum. As there are only about 10^{80} atoms in the entire observable universe, a dilution of one molecule in the observable universe would be about 40C. Oscillococcinum would thus require 10^{320} more universes to simply have one molecule in the final substance. The high dilutions characteristically used are often considered to be the most controversial and implausible aspect of homeopathy.

Not all homeopaths advocate high dilutions. Preparations at concentrations below 4X are considered an important part of homeopathic heritage. Many of the early homeopaths were originally doctors and generally used lower dilutions such as "3X" or "6X", rarely going beyond "12X". The split between lower and higher dilutions followed ideological lines. Those favouring low dilutions stressed pathology and a stronger link to conventional medicine, while those favouring high dilutions emphasized vital force, miasms and a spiritual interpretation of disease. Some products with such relatively lower dilutions continue to be sold, but like their counterparts, they have not been conclusively demonstrated to have any effect beyond that of a placebo.

Provings

A homeopathic "proving" is the method by which the profile of a homeopathic preparation is determined.

At first Hahnemann used undiluted doses for provings, but he later advocated provings with preparations at a 30C dilution, and most modern provings are carried out using ultradilute preparations in which it is highly unlikely that any of the original molecules remain. During the proving process, Hahnemann administered preparations to healthy volunteers, and the resulting symptoms were compiled by observers into a "drug picture".

The volunteers were observed for months at a time and made to keep extensive journals detailing all of their symptoms at specific times throughout the day. They were forbidden from consuming coffee, tea, spices, or wine for the duration of the experiment; playing chess was also prohibited because Hahnemann considered it to be "too exciting", though they were allowed to drink beer and encouraged to exercise in moderation.

After the experiments were over, Hahnemann made the volunteers take an oath swearing that what they reported in their journals was the truth, at which time he would interrogate them extensively concerning their symptoms.

Provings are claimed to have been important in the development of the clinical trial, due to their early use of simple control groups, systematic and quantitative procedures, and some of the first application of statistics in medicine. The lengthy records of self-experimentation by homeopaths have occasionally proven useful in the development of modern drugs: For example, evidence that nitroglycerin might be useful as a treatment for angina was discovered by looking through homeopathic provings, though homeopaths themselves never used it for that purpose at that time. The first recorded provings were published by Hahnemann in his 1796 *Essay on a New Principle*. His *Fragmenta de Viribus* (1805) contained the results of 27 provings, and his 1810 *Materia Medica Pura* contained 65. For James Tyler Kent's 1905 *Lectures on Homoeopathic Materia Medica*, 217 preparations underwent provings and newer substances are continually added to contemporary versions.

Though the proving process has superficial similarities with clinical trials, it is fundamentally different in that the process is subjective, not blinded, and modern provings are unlikely to use pharmacologically active levels of the substance under proving. As early as 1842, Holmes noted the provings were impossibly vague, and the purported effect was not repeatable among different subjects.

Consultation

Homeopaths generally begin with detailed examinations of their patients' histories, including questions regarding their physical, mental and emotional states, their life circumstances and any physical or emotional illnesses. The homeopath then attempts to translate this information into a complex formula of mental and physical symptoms, including likes, dislikes, innate predispositions and even body type.

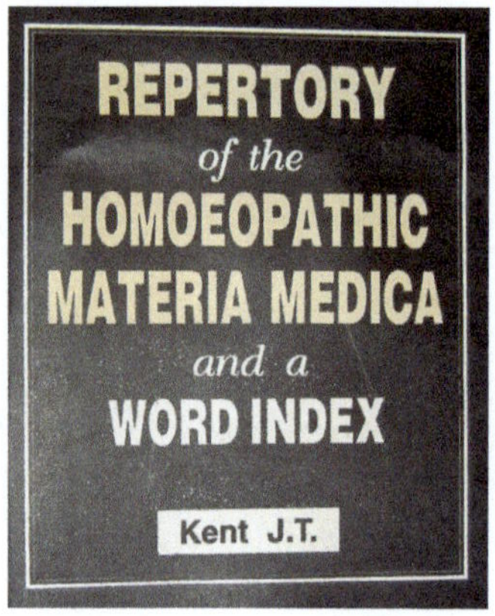

Homeopathic repertory by James Tyler Kent

From these symptoms, the homeopath chooses how to treat the patient using *materia medica* and repertories. In classical homeopathy, the practitioner attempts to match a single preparation to the totality of symptoms (the *simlilum*), while "clinical homeopathy" involves combinations of preparations based on the various symptoms of an illness.

Pills and Active Ingredients

Homeopathic pills are made from an inert substance (often sugars, typically lactose), upon which a drop of liquid homeopathic preparation is placed and allowed to evaporate.

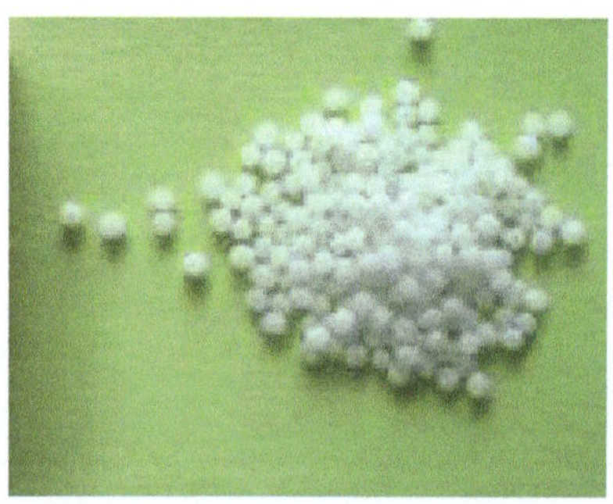

Homeopathic pills, homeopathic preparation *oscillococcinum*

The process of homeopathic dilution results in no objectively detectable active ingredient in most cases, but some preparations (e.g. calendula and arnica creams) do contain pharmacologically active doses. One product, Zicam Cold Remedy, which was marketed as an "unapproved homeopathic" product, contains two ingredients that are only "slightly" diluted: zinc acetate (2X = 1/100 dilution) and zinc gluconate (1X = 1/10 dilution), which means both are present in a biologically active concentration strong enough to have caused some people to lose their sense of smell, a condition termed anosmia. Zicam also listed several normal homeopathic potencies as "inactive ingredients", including *galphimia glauca*, histamine dihydrochloride (homeopathic name, *histaminum hydrochloricum*), *luffa operculata*, and sulfur.

Related and Minority Treatments and Practices

Isopathy

Isopathy is a therapy derived from homeopathy, invented by Johann Joseph Wilhelm Lux in the 1830s. Isopathy differs from homeopathy in general in that the preparations, known as "nosodes", are made up either from things that cause the disease or from products of the disease, such as pus. Many so-called "homeopathic vaccines" are a form of isopathy.

Flower Preparations

Flower preparations can be produced by placing flowers in water and exposing them to sunlight. The most famous of these are the Bach flower remedies, which were developed by the physician and homeopath Edward Bach. Although the proponents of these preparations share homeopathy's vitalist world-view and the preparations are claimed to act through the same hypothetical "vital force" as homeopathy, the method of preparation is different. Bach flower preparations are manufactured in allegedly "gentler" ways such as placing flowers in bowls of sunlit water, and the preparations are not succussed. There is no convincing scientific or clinical evidence for flower preparations being effective.

Veterinary Use

The idea of using homeopathy as a treatment for other animals, termed "veterinary homeopathy", dates back to the inception of homeopathy; Hahnemann himself wrote and spoke of the use of homeopathy in animals other than humans. The FDA has not approved homeopathic products as veterinary medicine in the U.S. In the UK, veterinary surgeons who use homeopathy may belong to the Faculty of Homeopathy and/or to the British Association of Homeopathic Veterinary Surgeons. Animals may be treated only by qualified veterinary surgeons in the UK and some other countries. Internationally, the body that supports and represents homeopathic veterinarians is the International Association for Veterinary Homeopathy.

The use of homeopathy in veterinary medicine is controversial; the little existing research on the subject is not of a high enough scientific standard to provide reliable data on efficacy. Other studies have also found that giving animals placebos can play active roles in influencing pet owners to believe in the effectiveness of the treatment when none exists. The British Veterinary Association's position statement on alternative medicines says that it "cannot endorse" homeopathy, and the Australian Veterinary Association includes it on its list of "ineffective therapies".

The UK's Department for Environment, Food and Rural Affairs (Defra) has adopted a robust position against use of "alternative" pet preparations including homeopathy.

Electrohomeopathy

Electrohomeopathy is a treatment devised by Count Cesare Mattei (1809–1896), who proposed that different "colours" of electricity could be used to treat cancer. Popular in the late nineteenth century, electrohomeopathy has been described as "utter idiocy".

Homeoprophylaxis

The use of homeopathy as a preventive for serious infectious diseases is especially controversial, in the context of ill-founded public alarm over the safety of vaccines stoked by the anti-vaccination movement. Promotion of homeopathic alternatives to vaccines has been characterized as dangerous, inappropriate and irresponsible. In December 2014, Australian homeopathy supplier Homeopathy Plus! were found to have acted deceptively in promoting homeopathic alternatives to vaccines.

Evidence and Efficacy

The low concentration of homeopathic preparations, which often lack even a single molecule of the diluted substance, has been the basis of questions about the effects of the preparations since the 19th century. Modern advocates of homeopathy have proposed a concept of "water memory", according to which water "remembers" the substances mixed in it, and transmits the effect of those substances when consumed. This concept is inconsistent with the current understanding of matter, and water memory has never been demonstrated to have any detectable effect, biological or otherwise. Pharmacological research has found instead that stronger effects of an active ingredient come from higher, not lower doses.

James Randi and the 10:23 campaign groups have highlighted the lack of active ingredients in most homeopathic products by taking large 'overdoses'. None of the hundreds of demonstrators in the UK, Australia, New Zealand, Canada and the US were injured and "no one was cured of anything, either".

Outside of the alternative medicine community, scientists have long considered homeopathy a sham or a pseudoscience, and the mainstream medical community regards it as quackery. There is an overall absence of sound statistical evidence of therapeutic efficacy, which is consistent with the lack of any biologically plausible pharmacological agent or mechanism.

Abstract concepts within theoretical physics have been invoked to suggest explanations of how or why preparations might work, including quantum entanglement, quantum nonlocality, the theory of relativity and chaos theory. Contrariwise, quantum superposition has been invoked to explain why homeopathy does *not* work in double-blind trials. However, the explanations are offered by nonspecialists within the field, and often include speculations that are incorrect in their application of the concepts and not supported by actual experiments. Several of the key concepts of homeopathy conflict with fundamental concepts of physics and chemistry. The use of quantum entanglement to explain homeopathy's purported effects is "patent nonsense", as entanglement is a delicate state which rarely lasts longer than a fraction of a second. While entanglement may result in certain aspects of individual subatomic particles acquiring linked quantum states, this does not mean the particles will mirror or duplicate each other, nor cause health-improving transformations.

Plausibility

The proposed mechanisms for homeopathy are precluded from having any effect by the laws of physics and physical chemistry. The extreme dilutions used in homeopathic preparations usually leave none of the original substance in the final product.

A number of speculative mechanisms have been advanced to counter this, the most widely discussed being water memory, though this is now considered erroneous since short-range order in water only persists for about 1 picosecond. No evidence of stable clusters of water molecules was found when homeopathic preparations were studied using nuclear magnetic resonance, and many other physical experiments in homeopathy have been found to be of low methodological quality, which precludes any meaningful conclusion. Existence of a pharmacological effect in the absence of any true active ingredient is inconsistent with the law of mass action and the observed dose-response relationships characteristic of therapeutic drugs (whereas placebo effects are non-specific and unrelated to pharmacological activity).

Homeopaths contend that their methods produce a therapeutically active preparation, selectively including only the intended substance, though critics note that any water will have been in contact with millions of different substances throughout its history, and homeopaths have not been able to account for a reason why only the selected homeopathic substance would be a special case in their process. For comparison, ISO 3696:1987 defines a standard for water used in laboratory analysis; this allows for a contaminant level of ten parts per billion, 4C in homeopathic notation. This water may not be kept in glass as contaminants will leach out into the water.

Practitioners of homeopathy hold that higher dilutions—described as being of higher *potency*—produce stronger medicinal effects. This idea is also inconsistent with observed dose-response relationships, where effects are dependent on the concentration of the active ingredient in the body. This dose-response relationship has been confirmed in myriad experiments on organisms as diverse as nematodes, rats, and humans. Some homeopaths contend that the phenomenon of hormesis may support the idea of dilution increasing potency, but the dose-response relationship outside the zone of hormesis declines with dilution as normal, and nonlinear pharmacological effects do not provide any credible support for homeopathy.

Physicist Robert L. Park, former executive director of the American Physical Society, is quoted as saying,

"since the least amount of a substance in a solution is one molecule, a 30C solution would have to have at least one molecule of the original substance dissolved in a minimum of 1,000,000,000,000,000,000,000,000,000,000,000,000,000,000,000,000,000,000,000,000 [or 10^{60}] molecules of water. This would require a container more than 30,000,000,000 times the size of the Earth."

Park is also quoted as saying that, "to expect to get even one molecule of the 'medicinal' substance allegedly present in 30X pills, it would be necessary to take some two billion of them, which would total about a thousand tons of lactose plus whatever impurities the lactose contained".

The laws of chemistry state that there is a limit to the dilution that can be made without losing the original substance altogether. This limit, which is related to Avogadro's number, is roughly equal to homeopathic dilutions of 12C or 24X (1 part in 10^{24}).

Scientific tests run by both the BBC's *Horizon* and ABC's *20/20* programmes were unable to differentiate homeopathic dilutions from water, even when using tests suggested by homeopaths themselves.

Efficacy

No individual preparation has been unambiguously shown by research to be different from placebo. The methodological quality of the primary research was generally low, with such problems as weaknesses in study design and reporting, small sample size, and selection bias. Since better quality trials have become available, the evidence for efficacy of homeopathy preparations has diminished; the highest-quality trials indicate that the preparations themselves exert no intrinsic effect. A review conducted in 2010 of all the pertinent studies of "best evidence" produced by the Cochrane Collaboration concluded that "the most reliable evidence – that produced by Cochrane reviews – fails to demonstrate that homeopathic medicines have effects beyond placebo."

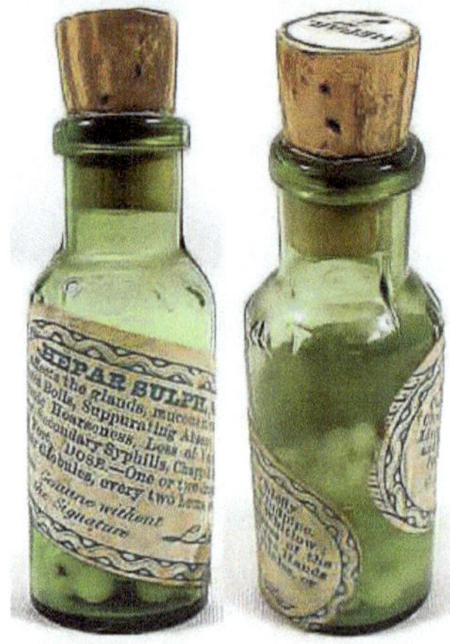

Old bottle of *Hepar sulph* made from calcium sulfide

Government Level Reviews

Government-level reviews have been conducted in recent years by Switzerland (2005), the United Kingdom (2009) and Australia (2015).

The Swiss *programme for the evaluation of complementary medicine* (PEK) resulted in the peer-reviewed Shang publication and a controversial competing analysis by homeopaths and advocates led by Gudrun Bornhöft and Peter Matthiessen, which has misleadingly been presented as a Swiss government report by homeopathy proponents, a claim that has been repudiated by the Swiss Federal Office of Public Health. The Swiss Government terminated reimbursement, though it was subsequently reinstated after a political campaign and referendum for a further six-year trial period.

The United Kingdom's House of Commons Science and Technology Committee sought written evidence and submissions from concerned parties and, following a review of all submissions, concluded that there was no compelling evidence of effect other than placebo and recommended that the Medicines and Healthcare products Regulatory Agency (MHRA) should not allow homeopathic product labels to make medical claims, that homeopathic products should no longer be licensed by the MHRA, as they are not medicines, and that further clinical trials of homeopathy could not be justified. They recommended that funding of homeopathic hospitals should not continue, and NHS doctors should not refer patients to homeopaths. The Secretary of State for Health deferred to local NHS on funding homeopathy, in the name of patient choice. By February 2011 only one third of primary care trusts still funded homeopathy. By 2012, no British universities offered homeopathy courses.

The Australian National Health and Medical Research Council completed a comprehensive review of the effectiveness of homeopathic preparations in 2015, in which it concluded that "there were no health conditions for which there was reliable evidence that homeopathy was effective. No good-quality, well-designed studies with enough participants for a meaningful result reported either that homeopathy caused greater health improvements than placebo, or caused health improvements equal to those of another treatment."

Publication Bias and Other Methodological Issues

The fact that individual randomized controlled trials have given positive results is not in contradiction with an overall lack of statistical evidence of efficacy. A small proportion of randomized controlled trials inevitably provide false-positive outcomes due to the play of chance: a "statistically significant" positive outcome is commonly adjudicated when the probability of it being due to chance rather than a real effect is no more than 5%—a level at which about 1 in 20 tests can be expected to show a positive result in the absence of any therapeutic effect. Furthermore, trials of low methodological quality (i.e. ones which have been inappropriately designed, conducted or reported) are prone to give misleading results. In a systematic review of the methodological quality of randomized trials in three branches of alternative medicine, Linde *et al.* highlighted major weaknesses in the homeopathy sector, including poor randomization. A separate 2001 systematic review that assessed the quality of clinical trials of homeopathy found that such trials were generally of lower quality than trials of conventional medicine.

A related issue is publication bias: researchers are more likely to submit trials that report a positive finding for publication, and journals prefer to publish positive results. Publication bias has been particularly marked in alternative medicine journals, where few of the published articles (just 5% during the year 2000) tend to report null results. Regarding the way in which homeopathy is represented in the medical literature, a systematic review found signs of bias in the publications of clinical trials (towards negative representation in mainstream medical journals, and *vice versa* in alternative medicine journals), but not in reviews.

Positive results are much more likely to be false if the prior probability of the claim under test is low.

Systematic Reviews and Meta-analyses of Efficacy

Both meta-analyses, which statistically combine the results of several randomized controlled trials, and other systematic reviews of the literature are essential tools to summarize evidence of therapeutic efficacy. Early systematic reviews and meta-analyses of trials evaluating the efficacy of homeopathic preparations in comparison with placebo more often tended to generate positive results, but appeared unconvincing overall. In particular, reports of three large meta-analyses warned readers that firm conclusions could not be reached, largely due to methodological flaws in the primary studies and the difficulty in controlling for publication bias. The positive finding of one of the most prominent of the early meta-analyses, published in *The Lancet* in 1997 by Linde et al., was later reframed by the same research team, who wrote:

The evidence of bias [in the primary studies] weakens the findings of our original meta-analysis. Since we completed our literature search in 1995, a considerable number of new homeopathy trials have been published. The fact that a number of the new high-quality trials ... have negative results, and a recent update of our review for the most "original" subtype of homeopathy (classical or individualized homeopathy), seem to confirm the finding that more rigorous trials have less-promising results. It seems, therefore, likely that our meta-analysis at least overestimated the effects of homeopathic treatments.

Subsequent work by John Ioannidis and others has shown that for treatments with no prior plausibility, the chances of a positive result being a false positive are much higher, and that any result not consistent with the null hypothesis should be assumed to be a false positive.

In 2002, a systematic review of the available systematic reviews confirmed that higher-quality trials tended to have less positive results, and found no convincing evidence that any homeopathic preparation exerts clinical effects different from placebo.

In 2005, *The Lancet* medical journal published a meta-analysis of 110 placebo-controlled homeopathy trials and 110 matched medical trials based upon the Swiss government's Programme for Evaluating Complementary Medicine, or PEK. The study concluded that its findings were "compatible with the notion that the clinical effects of homeopathy are placebo effects". This was accompanied by an editorial pronouncing "The end of homoeopathy", which was denounced by the homeopath Peter Fisher.

Other meta-analyses include homeopathic treatments to reduce cancer therapy side-effects following radiotherapy and chemotherapy, allergic rhinitis, attention-deficit hyperactivity disorder and childhood diarrhoea, adenoid vegetation, asthma, upper respiratory tract infection in children, insomnia, fibromyalgia, psychiatric conditions and Cochrane Library reviews of homeopathic treatments for asthma, dementia, attention-deficit hyperactivity disorder, induction of labour, and irritable bowel syndrome. Other reviews covered osteoarthritis, migraines, postoperative ecchymosis and edema, delayed-onset muscle soreness, or eczema and other dermatological conditions.

The results of these reviews are generally negative or only weakly positive, and reviewers consistently report the poor quality of trials. The finding of Linde *et. al.* that more rigorous studies produce less positive results is supported in several and contradicted by none.

Some clinical trials have tested individualized homeopathy, and there have been reviews of this, specifically. A 1998 review found 32 trials that met their inclusion criteria, 19 of which were placebo-controlled and provided enough data for meta-analysis. These 19 studies showed a pooled odds ratio of 1.17 to 2.23 in favour of individualized homeopathy over the placebo, but no difference was seen when the analysis was restricted to the methodologically best trials. The authors concluded that "the results of the available randomized trials suggest that individualized homeopathy has an effect over placebo. The evidence, however, is not convincing because of methodological shortcomings and inconsistencies." Jay Shelton, author of a book on homeopathy, has stated that the claim assumes without evidence that classical, individualized homeopathy works better than nonclassical variations. A systematic review and meta-analysis of trials of individualized homeopathy published in December 2014 concluded that individualized homeopathy may have small effects, but that caution was needed in interpreting the results because of study quality issues – no study included was assessed as being at low risk of bias.

Statements by Major Medical Organizations

Health organizations such as the UK's National Health Service, the American Medical Association, the FASEB, and the National Health and Medical Research Council of Australia, have issued statements of their conclusion that there is "no good-quality evidence that homeopathy is effective as a treatment for any health condition". In 2009, World Health Organization official Mario Raviglione cricitized the use of homeopathy to treat tuberculosis; similarly, another WHO spokesperson argued there was no evidence homeopathy would be an effective treatment for diarrhoea.

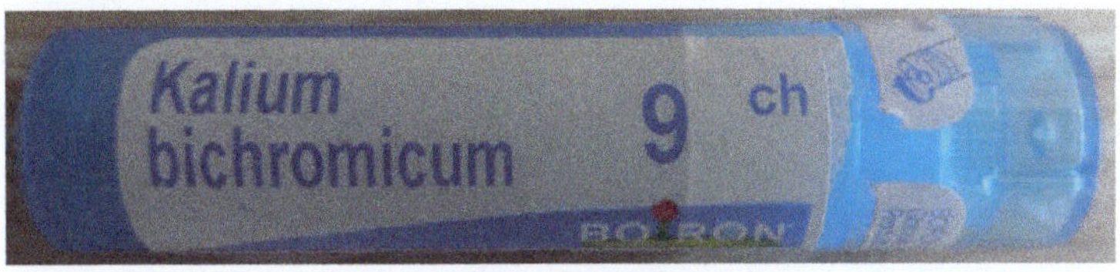

A homeopathic preparation made from potassium dichromate, the chemical compound well known for its toxic and carcinogenic properties

The American College of Medical Toxicology and the American Academy of Clinical Toxicology recommend that no one use homeopathic treatment for disease or as a preventive health measure. These organizations report that no evidence exists that homeopathic treatment is effective, but that there is evidence that using these treatments produces harm and can bring indirect health risks by delaying conventional treatment.

Explanations of Perceived Effects

Science offers a variety of explanations for how homeopathy may appear to cure diseases or alleviate symptoms even though the preparations themselves are inert:

- The placebo effect – the intensive consultation process and expectations for the homeopathic preparations may cause the effect.
- Therapeutic effect of the consultation – the care, concern, and reassurance a patient experiences when opening up to a compassionate caregiver can have a positive effect on the patient's well-being.
- Unassisted natural healing – time and the body's ability to heal without assistance can eliminate many diseases of their own accord.
- Unrecognized treatments – an unrelated food, exercise, environmental agent, or treatment for a different ailment, may have occurred.
- Regression towards the mean – since many diseases or conditions are cyclical, symptoms vary over time and patients tend to seek care when discomfort is greatest; they may feel better anyway but because of the timing of the visit to the homeopath they attribute improvement to the preparation taken.

- Non-homeopathic treatment – patients may also receive standard medical care at the same time as homeopathic treatment, and the former is responsible for improvement.
- Cessation of unpleasant treatment – often homeopaths recommend patients stop getting medical treatment such as surgery or drugs, which can cause unpleasant side-effects; improvements are attributed to homeopathy when the actual cause is the cessation of the treatment causing side-effects in the first place, but the underlying disease remains untreated and still dangerous to the patient.

Purported Effects in Other Biological Systems

While some articles have suggested that homeopathic solutions of high dilution can have statistically significant effects on organic processes including the growth of grain, histamine release by leukocytes, and enzyme reactions, such evidence is disputed since attempts to replicate them have failed. A 2007 systematic review of high-dilution experiments found that none of the experiments with positive results could be reproduced by all investigators.

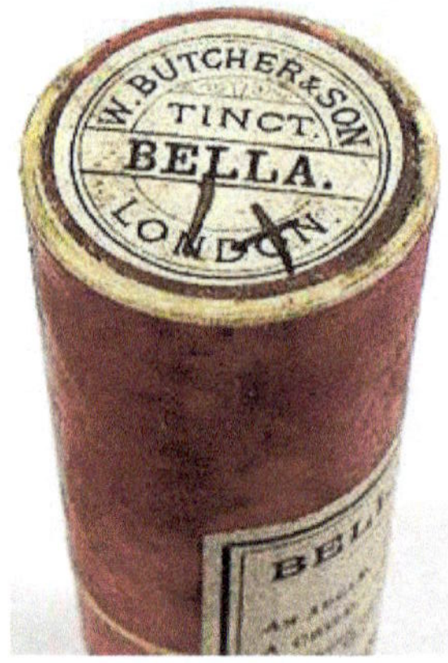

Old homeopathic belladonna preparation.

In 1987, French immunologist Jacques Benveniste submitted a paper to the journal *Nature* while working at INSERM. The paper purported to have discovered that basophils, a type of white blood cell, released histamine when exposed to a homeopathic dilution of anti-immunoglobulin E antibody. The journal editors, sceptical of the results, requested that the study be replicated in a separate laboratory. Upon replication in four separate laboratories the study was published. Still sceptical of the findings, *Nature* assembled an independent investigative team to determine the accuracy of the research, consisting of *Nature* editor and physicist Sir John Maddox, American scientific fraud investigator and chemist Walter Stewart, and sceptic James Randi. After investigating the findings and methodology of the experiment, the team found that the experiments were "statistically ill-controlled", "interpretation has been clouded by the exclusion of measurements in conflict with the claim", and concluded, "We believe that experimental data have been uncritically assessed and their imperfections inadequately reported." James Randi stated that he doubted that there had been any conscious fraud, but that the researchers had allowed "wishful thinking" to influence their interpretation of the data.

In 2001 and 2004, Madeleine Ennis published a number of studies which reported that homeopathic dilutions of histamine exerted an effect on the activity of basophils. In response to the first of these studies, *Horizon* aired a programme in which British scientists attempted to replicate Ennis' results; they were unable to do so.

Ethics and Safety

The provision of homeopathic preparations has been described as unethical. Michael Baum, Professor Emeritus of Surgery and visiting Professor of Medical Humanities at University College London (UCL), has described homoeopathy as a "cruel deception".

Edzard Ernst, the first *Professor of Complementary Medicine* in the United Kingdom and a former homeopathic practitioner, has expressed his concerns about pharmacists who violate their ethical code by failing to provide customers with "necessary and relevant information" about the true nature of the homeopathic products they advertise and sell:

> "My plea is simply for honesty. Let people buy what they want, but tell them the truth about what they are buying. These treatments are biologically implausible and the clinical tests have shown they don't do anything at all in human beings. The argument that this information is not relevant or important for customers is quite simply ridiculous."

Patients who choose to use homeopathy rather than evidence-based medicine risk missing timely diagnosis and effective treatment of serious conditions such as cancer.

In 2013 the UK Advertising Standards Authority concluded that the Society of Homeopaths were targeting vulnerable ill people and discouraging the use of essential medical treatment while making misleading claims of efficacy for homeopathic products.

In 2015 the Federal Court of Australia imposed penalties on a homeopathic company, Homeopathy Plus! Pty Ltd and its director, for making false or misleading statements about the efficacy of the whooping cough vaccine and homeopathic remedies as an alternative to the whooping cough vaccine, in breach of the Australian Consumer Law.

Adverse Effects

Some homeopathic preparations involve poisons such as Belladonna, arsenic, and poison ivy, which are highly diluted in the homeopathic preparation. In rare cases the original ingredients are present at detectable levels. This may be due to improper preparation or intentional low dilution. Serious adverse effects such as seizures and death have been reported or associated with some homeopathic preparations.

On 30 September 2016 the FDA issued a safety alert to consumers warning against the use of homeopathic teething gels and tablets following reports of adverse events after their use. The agency recommended that parents discard these products and "seek advice from their health care professional for safe alternatives" to homeopathy for teething. The pharmacy CVS announced, also on 30 September, that it was voluntarily withdrawing the products from sale and on 11 October Hyland's (the manufacturer) announced that it was discontinuing their teething medicine in the United States though the products remain on sale in Canada. On 12 October Buzzfeed reported that the regulator had "examined more than 400 reports of seizures, fever and vomiting, as well as 10 deaths" over a six year period. The investigation (including analyses of the products) is still ongoing and the FDA does not know yet if the deaths and illnesses were caused by the products. However a previous FDA investigation in 2010, following adverse effects reported then, found that these same products were improperly diluted and contained "unsafe levels of belladonna, also known as deadly nightshade" and that the reports of serious adverse events in children using this product were "consistent with belladonna toxicity".

Instances of arsenic poisoning have occurred after use of arsenic-containing homeopathic preparations. Zicam Cold remedy Nasal Gel, which contains 2X (1:100) zinc gluconate, reportedly caused a small percentage of users to lose their sense of smell; 340 cases were settled out of court in 2006 for 12 million U.S. dollars. In 2009, the FDA advised consumers to stop using three discontinued cold remedy Zicam products because it could cause permanent damage to users' sense of smell. Zicam was launched without a New Drug Application (NDA) under a provision in the FDA's Compliance Policy Guide called "Conditions under which homeopathic drugs may be marketed" (CPG 7132.15), but the FDA warned Matrixx Initiatives, its manufacturer, via a Warning Letter that this policy does not apply when there is a health risk to consumers.

A 2000 review by homeopaths reported that homeopathic preparations are "unlikely to provoke severe adverse reactions". In 2012, a systematic review evaluating evidence of homeopathy's possible adverse effects concluded that "homeopathy has the potential to harm patients and consumers in both direct and indirect ways". One of the reviewers, Edzard Ernst, supplemented the article on his blog, writing: "I have said it often and I say it again: if used as an alternative to an effective cure, even the most 'harmless' treatment can become life-threatening." A 2016 systematic review and meta-analysis found that, in homeopathic clinical trials, adverse effects were reported among the patients who received homeopathy about as often as they were reported among patients who received placebo or conventional medicine.

Lack of Efficacy

The lack of convincing scientific evidence supporting its efficacy and its use of preparations without active ingredients have led to characterizations as pseudoscience and quackery, or, in the words of a 1998 medical review, "placebo therapy at best and quackery at worst". The Chief Medical Officer for England, Dame Sally Davies, has stated that homeopathic preparations are "rubbish" and do not serve as anything more than placebos. Jack Killen, acting deputy director of the National Center for Complementary and Alternative Medicine, says homeopathy "goes beyond current understanding of chemistry and physics". He adds: "There is, to my knowledge, no condition for which homeopathy has been proven to be an effective treatment." Ben Goldacre says that homeopaths who misrepresent scientific evidence to a scientifically illiterate public, have "... walled themselves off from academic medicine, and critique has been all too often met with avoidance rather than argument". Homeopaths often prefer to ignore meta-analyses in favour of cherry picked positive results, such as by promoting a particular observational study (one which Goldacre describes as "little more than a customer-satisfaction survey") as if it were more informative than a series of randomized controlled trials.

Referring specifically to homeopathy, the British House of Commons Science and Technology Committee has stated:

In our view, the systematic reviews and meta-analyses conclusively demonstrate that homeopathic products perform no better than placebos. The Government shares our interpretation of the evidence.

In the Committee's view, homeopathy is a placebo treatment and the Government should have a policy on prescribing placebos. The Government is reluctant to address the appropriateness and ethics of prescribing placebos to patients, which usually relies on some degree of patient deception. Prescribing of placebos is not consistent with informed patient choice - which the Government claims is very important - as it means patients do not have all the information needed to make choice meaningful.

Beyond ethical issues and the integrity of the doctor-patient relationship, prescribing pure placebos is bad medicine. Their effect is unreliable and unpredictable and cannot form the sole basis of any treatment on the NHS.

The National Center for Complementary and Alternative Medicine of the United States' National Institutes of Health states:

Homeopathy is a controversial topic in complementary medicine research. A number of the key concepts of homeopathy are not consistent with fundamental concepts of chemistry and physics. For example, it is not possible to explain in scientific terms how a preparation containing little or no active ingredient can have any effect. This, in turn, creates major challenges to rigorous clinical investigation of homeopathic preparations. For example, one cannot confirm that an extremely dilute preparation contains what is listed on the label, or develop objective measures that show effects of extremely dilute preparations in the human body.

Ben Goldacre noted that in the early days of homeopathy, when medicine was dogmatic and frequently worse than doing nothing, homeopathy at least failed to make matters worse:

During the 19th-century cholera epidemic, death rates at the London Homeopathic Hospital were three times lower than at the Middlesex Hospital. Homeopathic sugar pills won't do anything against cholera, of course, but the reason for homeopathy's success in this epidemic is even more interesting than the placebo effect: at the time, nobody could treat cholera. So, while hideous medical treatments such as blood-letting were actively harmful, the homeopaths' treatments at least did nothing either way.

In Lieu of Standard Medical Treatment

On clinical grounds, patients who choose to use homeopathy in preference to normal medicine risk missing timely diagnosis and effective treatment, thereby worsening the outcomes of serious conditions. Critics of homeopathy have cited individual cases of patients of homeopathy failing to receive proper treatment for diseases that could have been easily diagnosed and managed with conventional medicine and who have died as a result, and the "marketing practice" of criticizing and downplaying the effectiveness of mainstream medicine. Homeopaths claim that use of conventional medicines will "push the disease deeper" and cause more serious conditions, a process referred to as "suppression". Some homeopaths (particularly those who are non-physicians) advise their patients against immunization. Some homeopaths suggest that vaccines be replaced with homeopathic "nosodes", created from biological materials such as pus, diseased tissue, bacilli from sputum or (in the case of "bowel nosodes") faeces. While Hahnemann was opposed to such preparations, modern homeopaths often use them although there is no evidence to indicate they have any beneficial effects. Cases of homeopaths advising against the use of anti-malarial drugs have been identified. This puts visitors to the tropics who take this advice in severe danger, since homeopathic preparations are completely ineffective against the malaria parasite. Also, in one case in 2004, a homeopath instructed one of her patients to stop taking conventional medication for a heart condition, advising her on 22 June 2004 to "Stop ALL medications including homeopathic", advising her on or around 20 August that she no longer needed to take her heart medication, and adding on 23 August, "She just cannot take ANY drugs – I have suggested some homeopathic remedies ... I feel confident that if she follows the advice she will regain her health." The patient was admitted to hospital the next day, and died eight days later, the final diagnosis being "acute heart failure due to treatment discontinuation".

In 1978, Anthony Campbell, then a consultant physician at the Royal London Homeopathic Hospital, criticized statements by George Vithoulkas claiming that syphilis, when treated with antibiotics, would develop into secondary and tertiary syphilis with involvement of the central nervous system, saying that "The unfortunate layman might well be misled by Vithoulkas' rhetoric into refusing orthodox treatment". Vithoulkas' claims echo the idea that treating a disease with external medication used to treat the symptoms would only drive it deeper into the body and conflict with scientific studies, which indicate that penicillin treatment produces a complete cure of syphilis in more than 90% of cases.

A 2006 review by W. Steven Pray of the College of Pharmacy at Southwestern Oklahoma State University recommends that pharmacy colleges include a required course in unproven medications and therapies, that ethical dilemmas inherent in recommending products lacking proven safety and efficacy data be discussed, and that students should be taught where unproven systems such as homeopathy depart from evidence-based medicine.

In an article entitled "Should We Maintain an Open Mind about Homeopathy?" published in the *American Journal of Medicine*, Michael Baum and Edzard Ernst – writing to other physicians – wrote that "Homeopathy is among the worst examples of faith-based medicine... These axioms [of homeopathy] are not only out of line with scientific facts but also directly opposed to them. If homeopathy is correct, much of physics, chemistry, and pharmacology must be incorrect...".

In 2013, Mark Walport, the UK Government Chief Scientific Adviser and head of the Government Office for Science, had this to say: "My view scientifically is absolutely clear: homoeopathy is nonsense, it is non-science. My advice to ministers is clear: that there is no science in homoeopathy. The most it can have is a placebo effect – it is then a political decision whether they spend money on it or not." His predecessor, John Beddington, referring to his views on homeopathy being "fundamentally ignored" by the Government, said: "The only one [view being ignored] I could think of was homoeopathy, which is mad. It has no underpinning of scientific basis. In fact all the science points to the fact that it is not at all sensible. The clear evidence is saying this is wrong, but homoeopathy is still used on the NHS."

Regulation and Prevalence

Homeopathy is fairly common in some countries while being uncommon in others; is highly regulated in some countries and mostly unregulated in others. It is practised worldwide and professional qualifications and licences are needed in most countries. In some countries, there are no specific legal regulations concerning the use of homeopathy, while in others, licences or degrees in conventional medicine from accredited universities are required. In Germany, to become a homeopathic physician, one must attend a three-year training programme, while France, Austria and Denmark mandate licences to diagnose any illness or dispense of any product whose purpose is to treat any illness.

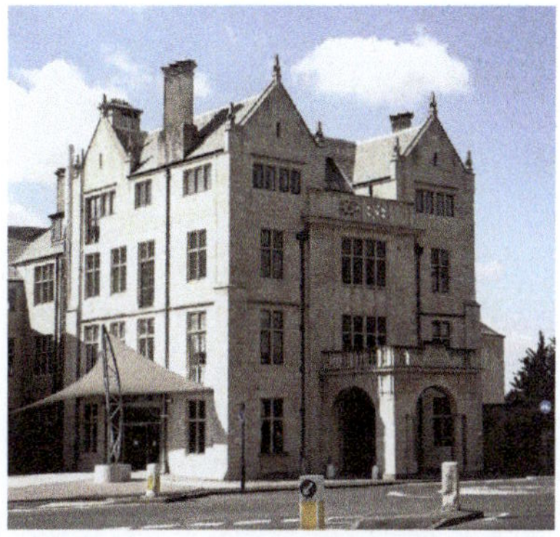

Hampton House, the former site of Bristol Homeopathic Hospital, one of three Homeopathic Hospitals in NHS.

Some homeopathic treatment is covered by the public health service of several European countries, including France, the United Kingdom and Luxembourg. In other countries, such as Belgium, homeopathy is not covered. In Austria, the public health service requires scientific proof of effectiveness in order to reimburse medical treatments and homeopathy is listed as not reimbursable, but exceptions can be made; private health insurance policies sometimes include homeopathic treatment. The Swiss government, after a 5-year trial, withdrew coverage of homeopathy and four other complementary treatments in 2005, stating that they did not meet efficacy and cost-effectiveness criteria, but following a referendum in 2009 the five therapies have been reinstated for a further 6-year trial period from 2012.

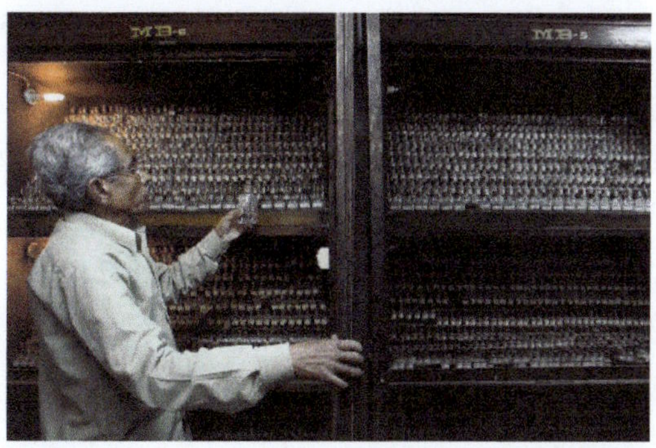

Homeopathics at a homeopathic pharmacy in Varanasi, India.

The Indian government recognizes homeopathy as one of its national systems of medicine; it has established AYUSH or the Department of Ayurveda, Yoga and Naturopathy, Unani, Siddha and Homoeopathy under the Ministry of Health & Family Welfare. The south Indian state of Kerala also gives the final nod for AYUSH department where homeopathy and Ayurveda are the main streams along with Sidha, Unani and Yoga. The Central Council of Homoeopathy was established in 1973 to monitor higher education in homeopathy, and National Institute of Homoeopathy in 1975. A minimum of a recognized diploma in homeopathy and registration on a state register or the Central Register of Homoeopathy is required to practise homeopathy in India.

On 28 September 2016 the UK's Committee of Advertising Practice (CAP) Compliance team wrote to homeopaths in the UK to "remind them of the rules that govern what they can and can't say in their marketing materials." The letter highlights that "homeopaths may not currently make either direct or implied claims to treat medical conditions" and asks them to review their marketing communications "including websites and social media pages" to ensure compliance by 3 November 2016. The letter also includes information on sanctions in the event of non-compliance including, ultimately, "referral by the ASA to Trading Standards under the Consumer Protection from Unfair Trading Regulations 2008."

Public Opposition

In the April 1997 edition of FDA Consumer, William T. Jarvis, the President of the National Council Against Health Fraud, said "Homeopathy is a fraud perpetrated on the public with the government's blessing, thanks to the abuse of political power of Sen. Royal S. Copeland [chief sponsor of the 1938 Food, Drug, and Cosmetic Act]."

Mock "overdosing" on homeopathic preparations by individuals or groups in "mass suicides" have become more popular since James Randi began taking entire bottles of homeopathic sleeping pills before giving lectures. In 2010 The Merseyside Skeptics Society from the United Kingdom launched the 10:23 campaign, encouraging groups to publicly overdose as groups. In 2011 the 10:23 campaign expanded and saw sixty-nine groups participate; fifty-four submitted videos. In April 2012, at the Berkeley SkeptiCal conference, over 100 people participated in a mass overdose, taking *coffea cruda*, which is supposed to treat sleeplessness.

In 2011, the non-profit, educational organizations Center for Inquiry (CFI) and the associated Committee for Skeptical Inquiry (CSI) have petitioned the U.S. Food and Drug Administration (FDA) to initiate 'rulemaking that would require all over-the-counter homeopathic drugs to meet the same standards of effectiveness as non-homeopathic drugs' and 'to place warning labels on homeopathic drugs until such time as they are shown to be effective'. In a separate petition, CFI and CSI request FDA to issue warning letters to Boiron, maker of Oscillococcinum, regarding their marketing tactic and criticize Boiron for misleading labelling and advertising of Oscillococcinum. CFI in Canada is calling for persons that feel they were harmed by homeopathic products to contact them.

In August 2011, a class action lawsuit was filed against Boiron on behalf of "all California residents who purchased Oscillo at any time within the past four years". The lawsuit charged that it "is nothing more than a sugar pill", "despite falsely advertising that it contains an active ingredient known to treat flu symptoms". In March 2012, Boiron agreed to spend up to $12 million to settle the claims of falsely advertising the benefits of its homeopathic preparations.

In July 2012, CBC News reporter Erica Johnson for *Marketplace* conducted an investigation on the homeopathy industry in Canada; her findings were that it is "based on flawed science and some loopy thinking". Center for Inquiry (CFI) Vancouver skeptics participated in a mass overdose outside an emergency room in Vancouver, B.C., taking entire bottles of "medications" that should have made them sleepy, nauseous or dead; after 45 minutes of observation no ill effects were felt. Johnson asked homeopaths and company representatives about cures for cancer and vaccine claims. All reported positive results but none could offer any science backing up their statements, only that "it works". Johnson was unable to find any evidence that homeopathic preparations contain any active ingredient. Analysis performed at the University of Toronto's chemistry department found that the active ingredient is so small "it is equivalent to 5 billion times less than the amount of aspirin ... in a single pellet". Belladonna and ipecac "would be indistinguishable from each other in a blind test".

Following a threat of legal action by the Good Thinking Society campaign group, the British government has stated that the Department of Health will hold a consultation in 2016 regarding whether homeopathic treatments should be added to the NHS treatments blacklist (officially, Schedule 1 of the National Health Service (General Medical Services Contracts) (Prescription of Drugs etc.) Regulations 2004), that specifies a blacklist of medicines not to be prescribed under the NHS.

In March 2016, the University of Barcelona cancelled its Masters degree in Homeopathy citing "lack of scientific basis", after advice from the Spanish Ministry of Health stated that "Homeopathy has not definitely proved its efficacy under any indication or concrete clinical situation". Shortly afterwards, in April 2016, the University of Valencia announced the elimination of its Masters in Homeopathy for 2017.

In June 2016, blogger and sceptic Jithin Mohandas launched a petition through Change.org asking the government of Kerala, India, to stop admitting students to homeopathy medical colleges. Mohandas said that government approval of these colleges makes them appear legitimate, leading thousands of talented students to join them and end up with invalid degrees. The petition asks that homeopathy colleges be converted to regular medical colleges, and that people with homeopathy degrees be provided with training in scientific medicine.

United States Food and Drug Administration (FDA) 2015 Hearing

On April 20–21, 2015, the FDA held a hearing on homeopathic product regulation. Invitees representing the scientific and medical community, and various pro-homeopathy stakeholders, gave testimonials on homeopathic products and the regulatory role played by the FDA. Michael de Dora, a representative from the Center for Inquiry (CFI), on behalf of the organization and dozens of doctors and scientists associated with CFI and the Committee for Skeptical Inquiry (CSI) gave a testimonial which summarized the basis of the organization's objection to homeopathic products, the harm done to the general public and proposed regulatory actions:

The CFI testimonial stated that the principle of homeopathy is at complete odds with the basic principle of modern biology, chemistry and physics and that decades of scientific examination of homeopathic products shows that there is no evidence that it is effective in treating illnesses other than acting as a placebo. Further, it noted a 2012 report by the American Association of Poison Control Centers which listed 10,311 reported cases of poison exposure related to homeopathic agents, among which 8,788 cases were attributed to young children five years of age or younger, as well as examples of harm – including deaths – caused to patients who relied on homeopathics instead of proven medical treatment.

The CFI urged the FDA to announce and implement strict guidelines that "require all homeopathic products meet the same standards as non-homeopathic drugs", arguing that the consumers can only have true freedom of choice (an often used argument from the homeopathy proponents) if they are fully informed on the choices. CFI proposed that the FDA take these three steps:

1. *Testing for homeopathic products* The FDA will mandate that all homeopathic products on the market to perform and pass safety and efficacy tests equivalent to those required of non-homeopathic drugs.
2. *Labelling for homeopathic products* To avert misleading label that the product is regulated by the FDA, all homeopathic products will be required to have prominent labels stating: 1) the products claimed active ingredients in plain English, and 2) the product has not been evaluated by the FDA for either safety or effectiveness.
3. *Regular consumer warnings* Encouraged by the FDA's recent warning of the ineffectiveness of homeopathic products, CFI urged the FDA to issue regular warning to the consumers in addition to warning during public health crises and outbreaks.

Official Conclusions and Recommendations

In March 2015, the National Health and Medical Research Council of Australia issued the following conclusions and recommendations:

- There is no reliable evidence that homeopathy is effective for treating health conditions.
- Homeopathy should not be used to treat health conditions that are chronic, serious, or could become serious.
- People who choose homeopathy may put their health at risk if they reject or delay treatments for which there is good evidence for safety and effectiveness.
- People who are considering whether to use homeopathy should first get advice from a registered health practitioner. Those who use homeopathy should tell their health practitioner, and should keep taking any prescribed treatments.

Homeopathic Dilutions

In homeopathy, homeopathic dilution (known by practitioners as "dynamisation" or "potentisation") is a process in which a substance is diluted with alcohol or distilled water and then vigorously shaken in a process called "succussion". Insoluble solids, such as quartz and oyster shell, are diluted by grinding them with lactose (*trituration*). The founder of homeopathy, Samuel Hahnemann (1755–1843) believed that the process of succussion activated the "vital energy" of the diluted substance, and that successive dilutions increased the "potency" of the preparation, although other strands of homeopathy disagree.

The idea is pseudoscience, because at commonly used dilutions, no molecules of the original material are likely to remain.

Potency Scales

Several potency scales are in use in homeopathy. Hahnemann created the centesimal or "C scale", diluting a substance by a factor of 100 at each stage. The centesimal scale was favored by

Hahnemann for most of his life. A 2C dilution requires a substance to be diluted to one part in one hundred, and then some of that diluted solution diluted by a further factor of one hundred. This works out to one part of the original substance in 10,000 parts of the solution. A 6C dilution repeats this process six times, ending up with the original material diluted by a factor of $100^{-6}=10^{-12}$. Higher dilutions follow the same pattern. In homeopathy, a solution that is more dilute is described as having a higher *potency*, and more dilute substances are considered by homeopaths to be stronger and deeper-acting. The end product is often so diluted that it is indistinguishable from the dilutant (pure water, sugar or alcohol).

There is also the continued flow mode of dilution that is measured on MFC.

Hahnemann advocated 30C dilutions for most purposes (that is, dilution by a factor of 10^{60}). In Hahnemann's time it was reasonable to assume that preparations could be diluted indefinitely, as the concept of the atom or molecule as the smallest possible unit of a chemical substance was just beginning to be recognized. We now know that the greatest dilution that is reasonably likely to contain one molecule of the original substance is 12C, if starting from 1 mole of original substance.

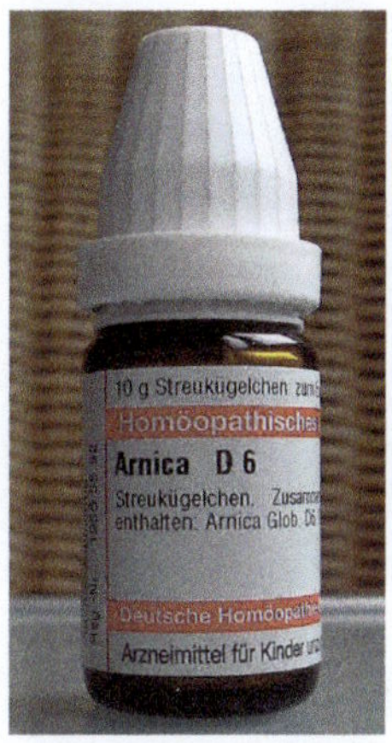

This bottle contains *Arnica montana* (wolf's bane) D6, i.e. the nominal dilution is one part in a million (10^6).

Some homeopaths developed a decimal scale (D or X), diluting the substance to ten times its original volume each stage. The D or X scale dilution is therefore half that of the same value of the C scale; for example, "12X" is the same level of dilution as "6C". Hahnemann never used this scale but it was very popular throughout the 19th century and still is in Europe. This potency scale appears to have been introduced in the 1830s by the American homeopath Constantine Hering. In the last ten years of his life, Hahnemann also developed a quintamillesimal (Q) or LM scale diluting the drug 1 part in 50,000 parts of diluent. A given dilution on the Q scale is roughly 2.35 times its designation on the C scale. For example, a preparation described as "20Q" has about the same concentration as one described with "47C"g.

Potencies of 1000C and above are usually labelled with Roman numeral M and with the centesimal 'C' indicator implied (since all such high potencies are centesimal dilutions): 1M = 1000C; 10M = 10,000C; CM = 100,000C; LM (which would indicate 50,000C) is typically not used because of confusion with the LM potency scale.

The following table is a synopsis comparing the X and C dilution scales and equating them by equivalent dilution. However, the homeopathic understanding of its principles is not explained by dilution but by "potentisation", hence one can not assume that the different potencies can be equated on the basis of equivalence of dilution factors.

X Scale	C Scale	Ratio	Note
1X	–	1:10	described as low potency
2X	1C	1:100	called *higher* potency than 1X by homeopaths
6X	3C	10^{-6}	
8X	4C	10^{-8}	allowable concentration of arsenic in U.S. drinking water
12X	6C	10^{-12}	
24X	12C	10^{-24}	Has a 60% probability of containing one molecule of original material if one mole of the original substance was used.
26X	13C	10^{-26}	If pure water was used as the diluent, no molecules of the original solution remain in the water.
60X	30C	10^{-60}	Dilution advocated by Hahnemann for most purposes: on average, this would require giving two billion doses per second to six billion people for 4 billion years to deliver a single molecule of the original material to any patient.
400X	200C	10^{-400}	Dilution of popular homeopathic flu preparation Oscillococcinum
Note: the "X scale" is also called "D scale". 1X = 1D, 2X = 2D, etc.			

Dilutions

Serial dilution of a solution results, after each dilution step, in fewer molecules of the original substance per litre of solution. Eventually, a solution will be diluted beyond any likelihood of finding a single molecule of the original substance in a litre of the total dilution product.

The Molar Limit

If one begins with a solution of 1 mol/L of a substance, the dilution required to reduce the number of molecules to less than one per litre is 1 part in 1×10^{24} (24X or 12C) since:

$$6.02\times10^{23}/1\times10^{24} = 0.6 \text{ molecules per litre}$$

Homeopathic dilutions beyond this limit (equivalent to approximately 12C) are unlikely to contain a single molecule of the original substance and lower dilutions contain no detectable amount. ISO 3696 (Water for analytical laboratory use) specifies a purity of ten parts per billion, or 10×10^{-9} – this water cannot be kept in glass or plastic containers as they leach impurities into the water, and glassware must be washed with hydrofluoric acid before use. Ten parts per billion is equivalent to a homeopathic dilution of 4C.

Analogies

Critics and advocates of homeopathy alike commonly attempt to illustrate the dilutions involved in homeopathy with analogies. The high dilutions characteristically used are often considered to be the most controversial and implausible aspect of homeopathy.

A popular homeopathic treatment for the flu is a 200C dilution of duck liver, marketed under the name *Oscillococcinum*. As there are only about 10^{80} atoms in the entire observable universe, a dilution of one molecule in the observable universe would be about 40C. Oscillococcinum would thus require 10^{320} more atoms to simply have one molecule in the final substance.

Another illustration of dilutions used in common homeopathic preparations involves comparing a homeopathic dilution to dissolving the therapeutic substance in a swimming pool. There are on the order of 10^{32} molecules of water in an Olympic-size swimming pool and if such a pool were filled with a 15C homeopathic preparation, to have a 63% chance of consuming at least one molecule of the original substance, one would need to swallow 1% of the volume of such a pool, or roughly 25 metric tons of water.

Proposed Explanations

Homeopaths maintain that this water retains some "essential property" of the original material, because the preparation has been shaken after each dilution. Hahnemann believed that the dynamisation or shaking of the solution caused a "spirit-like" healing force to be released from within the substance. Even though the homeopathic preparations are often extremely diluted, homeopaths maintain that a healing force is retained by these homeopathic preparations. Modern advocates of homeopathy have proposed a concept of "water memory", according to which water "remembers" the substances mixed in it, and transmits the effect of those substances when consumed. This concept is inconsistent with the current understanding of matter, and water memory has never been demonstrated to have any detectable effect, biological or otherwise. The claim often given to support "water memory" is that science does not fully understand water. In fact a great deal is known about the structure and properties of liquid water, from both theoretical and experimental studies, because of its importance in biochemistry, its relative molecular simplicity and the quantum mechanical nature of hydrogen bonding which make it a popular substance to study in theoretical chemistry. The actual memory of water can be measured experimentally and is found to be around 50 femtoseconds, which is 0.00000000000005 seconds. Generally considered to be pseudoscience by the scientific community, one disputed study into the so-called memory of water, conducted by Jacques Benveniste, claims to have demonstrated that water can be energetically imprinted upon. Another such study, published in 2003 by Swiss chemist Louis Rey, claims to have found that homeopathically diluted solutions of sodium chloride and lithium chloride have a very different hydrogen bond structure from normal water, as measured by thermoluminescence.

Dilution Debate

Not all homeopaths advocate extremely high dilutions. Many of the early homeopaths were originally doctors and generally used lower dilutions such as "3X" or "6X", rarely going beyond "12X"; these dilution ("trituration") levels were still popular in the late 20th century with advocates of Wilhelm Heinrich Schüßler's 12 biochemic tissue salts, for example. The split between lower and higher dilutions followed ideological lines. Those favoring low dilutions stressed pathology and a strong link to conventional medicine, while those favoring high dilutions emphasised vital force, miasms and a spiritual interpretation of disease. Some products with both low and high dilutions continue to be sold, but like their counterparts, they have not been conclusively demonstrated to have any effect beyond the placebo effect.

Electrohomeopathy

Electrohomoeopathy (or Mattei cancer cure) is a derivative of homeopathy invented in the 19th century by Count Cesare Mattei. The name is derived from a combination of *electro* (referring to an electric bio-energy content supposedly extracted from plants and of therapeutic value, rather than electricity in its conventional sense) and *homeopathy* (referring to an alternative medicinal philosophy developed by Samuel Hahnemann in the 18th century). Electrohomeopathy has been defined as the combination of electrical devices and homeopathy.

Lucrative for its inventor and popular in the late nineteenth century, electrohomoeopathy has been described as "utter idiocy". Like all homeopathy, it is regarded by the medical and scientific communities as pseudoscience and its practice as quackery.

History and Criticism

Electrohomeopathy was devised by Cesare Mattei (1809–1896) in the latter part of the 19th century. Mattei, a nobleman living in a castle in the vicinity of Bologna, studied natural science, anatomy, physiology, pathology, chemistry and botany. He ultimately focused on the supposed therapeutic power of "electricity" in botanical extracts. Mattei made bold, unsupported claims for the efficacy of his treatments, including the claim that his treatments offered a nonsurgical alternative to cancer. His treatment regimens were met with scepticism by mainstream medicine:

The electrohomeopathic system is an invention of Count Mattei who prates of "red", "blue", and "green" electricity, a theory that, in spite of its utter idiocy, has attracted a considerable following and earned a large fortune for its chief promoter.

Notwithstanding criticisms, including a challenge by the British medical establishment to the claimed success of his cancer treatments, electrohomeopathy (or Matteism, as it was sometimes known at the time) had adherents in Germany, France, the USA and the UK by the beginning of the 20th century; electrohomeopathy had been the subject of approximately 100 publications and there were three journals dedicated to it.

Philosophy

Remedies are derived from what are said to be the active micro nutrients or mineral salts of certain plants. One contemporary account of the process of producing electrohomeopathic remedies was as follows:

As to the nature of his remedies we learn ... that ... they are manufactured from certain herbs, and that the directions for the preparation of the necessary dilutions are given in the ordinary jargon of homeopathy. The globules and liquids, however, are "instinct with a potent, vital, electrical force, which enables them to work wonders". This process of "fixing the electrical principle" is carried on in the secret central chamber of a Neo-Moorish castle which Count Mattei has built for himself in the Bolognese Apennines ... The "red electricity" and "white electricity" supposed to be "fixed" in these "vegetable compounds" are in their very nomenclature and suggestion poor and miserable fictions.

According to Mattei's own ideas however, every disease originates in the change of blood or of the lymphatic system or both, and remedies can therefore be mainly divided into two broad categories to be used in response to the dominant affected system. Mattei wrote that having obtained plant extracts, he was "able to determine in the liquid vegetable electricity". Allied to his theories and therapies were elements of Chinese medicine, of medical humours, of apparent Brownianism, as well as modified versions of Samuel Hahnemann's homeopathic principles. Electrohomeopathy has some associations with Spagyric medicine, a holistic medical philosophy claimed to be the practical application of alchemy in medical treatment, so that the principle of modern electrohomeopathy is that disease is typically multi-organic in cause or effect and therefore requires holistic treatment that is at once both complex and natural.

Modern usage

A symposium took place in Bologna in 2008 to mark the 200th anniversary of the birth of Cesare Mattei, with attendees from India, Pakistan, Germany, UK, and the USA. Electrohomeopathy is practised predominantly in India and Pakistan (RAJYA SABHA Parliamentary Bulletin- The Recognition of Electro Homoeopathy System of Medicine Bill, 2015 by Dr. E. M. Sudarsana Natchiappan, M. P), but there are also a number of electrohomeopathy organizations and institutions worldwide.

Arsenicum Album

In homeopathy, arsenicum album (Arsen. alb.) is a solution prepared by diluting aqueous arsenic trioxide generally until there is little or no arsenic remaining in the solution. It is used by homeopaths to treat a range of symptoms that include digestive disorders and, as an application of the homeopathic Law of Similars has been suggested by homeopaths as a treatment for arsenic poisoning. Since the arsenic oxide in a homeopathic preparation is normally non-existent, it is considered generally safe, although cases of arsenic poisoning from poorly prepared homeopathic treatments sold in India have been reported. When properly prepared, however, the extreme dilutions, typically to at least 1 in 10^{24}, or 12C in homeopathic notation, mean that statistically it is extremely unlikely that any pill contains even a molecule of the original arsenic used. While some small, unblinded studies have claimed an effect on reducing arsenic toxicity, they do not recommend its large-scale use, and studies of homeopathic remedies have been shown to generally have problems that prevent them from being considered unambiguous evidence. There is no known mechanism for how arsenicum album could remove arsenic from a body, and there is insufficient evidence for it to be considered effective medicine (for any condition) by the scientific community.

Use in Homeopathy

According to a popular homeopathy guide, arsenicum album is one of the fifteen most important remedies in homeopathy. In classical homeopathy, people are grouped by "constitutional type" named after the homeopathic remedy applied, on the argument that people with similar "body shapes and personalities" suffer from the same type of diseases. "*Arsen. alb.*" types are "tense, restless ambitious individuals" with a tendency toward hypochondriasis, pessimism, need for reassurance, and a meticulous attention to neatness and detail.

For homeopathic use, arsenicum album is prepared by separating arsenic from iron (as in arsenopyrite), cobalt, or nickel by baking at high temperatures. The powder is then ground and diluted with lactose. In the final dilution, statistically most pills will contain zero molecules of the original arsenic used, some might contain a single molecule. The final product is sold as tinctures (liquid), tablets, pellets, or powder.

Key homeopathic uses include treating anxiety and "fear caused by insecurity", digestive disorders and mucosal inflammation, and ailments characterized symptomatically by burning pain. It was also used once for treatment of syphilis.

Research Studies

Several studies have been done into Arsenicum album; however, homeopathic studies are known to have problems, such as evidence of bias, lack of rigour, and failure to blind the experimenters or subjects to which group is being analysed that prevent them from being considered definitive evidence for any effect. In addition, the ideas behind homeopathy are scientifically implausible and directly opposed to fundamental principles of natural science and modern medicine, which means that poorly conducted, small, or unblinded studies are not considered scientific proof of efficacy.

The authors of one unblinded study of mice poisoned with arsenic and then given Arsenicum album, led by Anisur Khuda-Bukhsh, claimed statistically significant reductions were reported in biochemical markers of liver damage. However, other scientists remain doubtful: Andreas Gescher, a biochemical toxicologist interviewed by *New Scientist*, said "This kind of study uses a dilution so high there is hardly anything there... Is it really possible?" and went on to say that he was "extremely sceptical".

Regulation and Prevalence of Homeopathy

Homeopathy is fairly common in some countries while being uncommon in others. In some countries, there are no specific legal regulations concerning the use of homeopathy, while in others, licenses or degrees in conventional medicine from accredited universities are required.

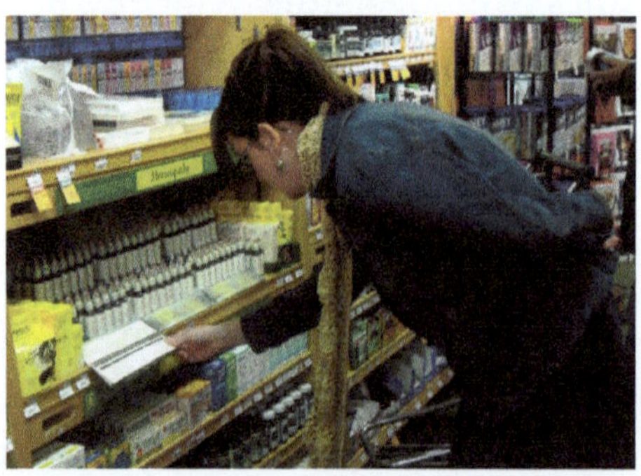

Woman looking at homeopathic remedies

Homeopathy is a pseudoscience and its remedies have been found to be no more effective than placebo.

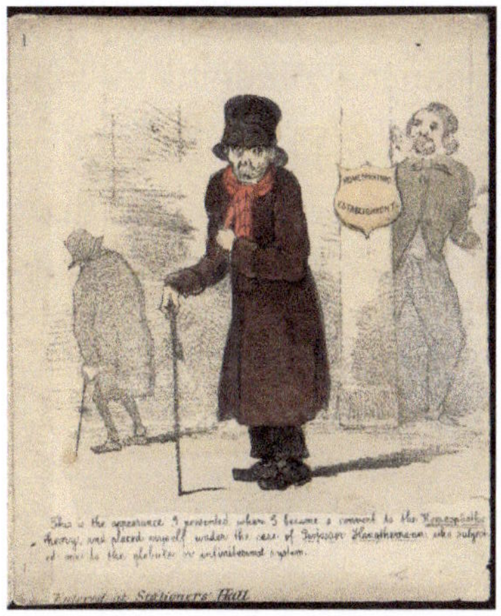

A patient suffering from the effects of homoeopathic treatment (Wellcome Trust).

Europe

Regulations vary in Europe depending on the country. In Austria and Germany, no specific regulations exist, while France and Denmark mandate licenses to diagnose any illness or dispense of any product whose purpose is to treat any illness. Some homeopathic treatment is covered by the national insurance of several European countries, including France, some parts of the United Kingdom, Denmark, and Luxembourg. In other countries, such as Belgium and the Czech Republic, homeopathy is not covered. In Austria, public insurance requires scientific proof of effectiveness in order to reimburse medical treatments, but exceptions are made for homeopathy. In 2004, Germany, which formerly offered homeopathy under its public health insurance scheme withdrew this privilege, with a few exceptions. In June 2005, the Swiss Government, after a 5-year trial, withdrew insurance coverage for homeopathy and four other alternative treatments, stating that they did not meet efficacy and cost-effectiveness criteria. However, following the result of a referendum in 2009 the five therapies were reinstated for a further 6-year trial period from 2012.

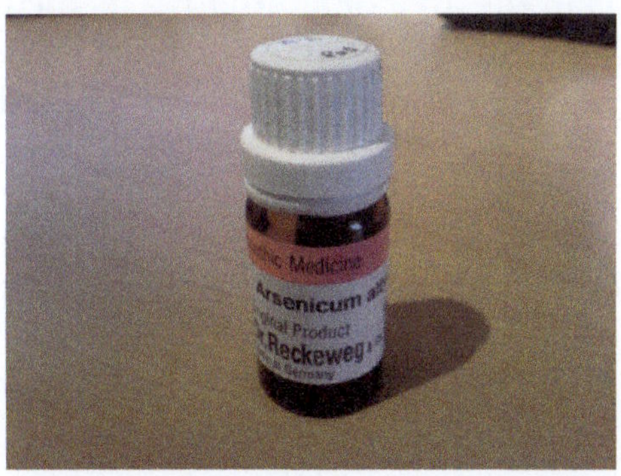

The homeopathic remedy arsenicum album derived from arsenic.

European Union

In 1992, the Council of the European Communities stated in the preamble to its directive that homeopathy was officially recognized in certain member states but only tolerated in others. In any case it was prescribed and used in all member states. To harmonize the market of homeopathic products, the council, by Directive 92/73/EEC directed the member states to implement certain changes in their national legislation. Directive 92/73/EEC was replaced by Directive 2001/83/EC on the Community code relating to medicinal products for human use.

Member states are required to ensure that homeopathic products (for oral or external use) can be registered without proof of therapeutic efficacy, provided that there is a sufficient degree of dilution to guarantee the safety of the product; in particular, the product may not contain either more than one part per 10,000 of the mother tincture or more than 1/100th of the smallest dose used in mainstream medicine, with regard to active principles whose presence in a medicinal product results in the obligation to submit a doctor's prescription. In other words, the dilution must be at least D4/4X/C2, and even higher in special cases. Other homeopathic products can still be registered under the normal rules, and products such as Arnica D1 are legally available.

The labels of homeopathic products registered without proof of efficacy must include the words "homeopathic medicinal product without approved therapeutic indications" as well as "a warning advising the user to consult a doctor if the symptoms persist during the use of the medicinal product".

Belgium

As of 12 May 2014, the exercise of homeopathy is in Belgium is reserved by law to only doctors, dentists and midwives, and should only be used for those indications for which the exercise is shown to be effective according to evidence-based medicine. The Belgian Council of Ministers agreed on July 12, 2013, with the draft royal decree as proposed by the Minister of Social Affairs and Public Health Laurette Onkelinx. The law follows the recommendations of the Belgian Health Care Knowledge Centre (nl). who concluded on the basis of a systematic review of the scientific literature that there is no evidence that homeopathic treatments work better than a placebo. She advised against reimbursement by the compulsory health insurance and advised that only doctors would be allowed to practice homeopathy.

In Belgium, 81% of consultations in the area of alternative medicine involve homeopathy, either alone or in combination with other forms of alternative medicine. Belgium has three homeopathic organizations for medical doctors and pharmacists and two for patients.

France

Homeopathy is the most popular form of alternative medicine in France. Its use rose from 16% of the population in 1982 to 29% in 1987 and 36% in 1992.

Germany

In Germany, the legislation for homeopathic remedies follows European Union (EU) regulations. Homeopathic remedies are subject to registration, but they need not be tested. However, homeopathic remedies that are less diluted than D4, or for which a danger of adverse effects exists, cannot be registered under this rule. They can be sold over-the-counter in pharmacies. Germany is the only member state of the EU in which homeopathic remedies based on minerals or plants, and produced only in very low quantities, do not need to be registered. In other member states only remedies individually prepared in a pharmacy are exempt.

In 2006, homeopathic remedies accounted for 3.16% of sold units in the pharmaceutical sector (1.08% of business volume); 0.48% of prescriptions covered by public health insurance were for homeopathic remedies. A 2008 telephone survey of German adults found that 11.5% had used homeopathy. Homeopathy accounts for 27.4% of patient contacts in the area of alternative medicine.

Italy

A survey of more than 70,000 citizens showed that approximately 4.7 million people in Italy (8.2% of the population) used homeopathy from 1997 to 1999, including being given to 7.7% children under 14 years. Homeopathy use rose from 2.5% in 1991 to 8.2% in 1999, but, despite the increase these numbers are still considered to represent comparatively light use compared to other countries.

Netherlands

In 1991, 40% of general practitioners used homeopathy.

Romania

Romania follows the general practices of EU regarding homeopathy. It is regulated by the National Agency of Drugs and Medical Devices (ANMDM) and is not permitted without a license. Most homeopathic drugs are sold over the counter. Approval of homeopathic drugs was simplified, considering there is no need for excessive testing for most of them.

Sweden

In September 2011, after the National Board of Health and Welfare put a doctor on probation for recommending homeopathy to a patient, Sweden's Supreme Administrative Court ruled that "doctors can recommend homeopathy". In October 2013 a legal review conducted by the National Board of Health and Welfare on behalf of the government concluded that the use of homeopathy by licensed medical professionals is limited to patient-initiated last-resort treatments.

United Kingdom

While the practice of homeopathy in the United Kingdom (UK) is not regulated by law, homeopathic products sold as remedies or medicines are regulated by the Medicines and Healthcare products Regulatory Agency.

In Britain, homeopathy has been in a state of steady decline over recent years. The number of National Health Service (NHS) prescriptions for homeopathic remedies dropped by over 85% between 2000 and 2010 (from 134,000 to 16,359), with homeopathy accounting for only 0.001% of the total 2010 prescribing budget. The Tunbridge Wells Homeopathic Hospital, formerly one of four homeopathic hospitals operated by the NHS, was closed in 2009 following a drop in referrals and a review by the West Kent Primary Care Trust of funding of homeopathy. In September 2010, one of the three remaining NHS-funded homeopathic hospitals, the Royal London Homeopathic Hospital, was renamed as the Royal London Hospital for Integrated Medicine to more accurately reflect the nature of its work. A fifth homeopathic hospital run by the NHS, the Hahnemann Hospital in Liverpool, had been closed in 1976.

In 1991 up to 37% of general practitioners (GPs) used homeopathy, but a review carried out by West Kent NHS Primary Care Trust in 2007 found that less than 1% of registered patients were referred for homeopathic treatment, and that this was almost always at the patient's request rather than as the result of a clinical decision. In 2011 the British Homeopathic Association said that 400 GPs used homeopathy in their everyday practice. The British Homeopathic Dental Association (BHDA) claimed to have 69 dentists, while the British Association of Homeopathic Veterinary Surgeons had 36 vets listed as members. There are over 41,000 GPs and around 24,000 registered veterinary surgeons in the UK, and almost 23,000 dentists doing NHS work in England.

In 2009 there were approximately 2,000 homeopaths, who are not GPs, registered with various organisations. A systematic review of surveys, published in April 2013, concluded that homeopathy is used by UK medical professionals to a minor degree, and that on average referral rates are low.

Around 2009, a few UK universities started closing or reviewing their courses on homeopathy and alternative medicine, after accusations that they were teaching pseudoscience. These courses had been attracting bad publicity and criticism for the universities teaching them. In May 2010 the NHS announced that junior doctors' training would no longer include placements at the Glasgow Homeopathic Hospital. In 2012 and 2013 there were only two universities left in the United Kingdom offering homeopathy degrees.

In February 2010 the Science and Technology Select Committee concluded that: "the NHS should cease funding homeopathy. It also concludes that the Medicines and Healthcare products Regulatory Agency (MHRA) should not allow homeopathic product labels to make medical claims without evidence of efficacy. As they are not medicines, homeopathic products should no longer be licensed by the MHRA." Part of the conclusions state that "When the NHS funds homeopathy, it endorses it. Since the NHS Constitution explicitly gives people the right to expect that decisions on the funding of drugs and treatments are made 'following a proper consideration of the evidence', patients may reasonably form the [misleading] view [inferred from the fact of any NHS financial support] that homeopathy is an evidence-based treatment." Since no evidence of benefit was found – other than the placebo effect – the report's recommendation was that "The Government should stop allowing the funding of homeopathy on the NHS." The government stated that this decision would be left open to the Primary Care Trusts (PCTs), the smaller bodies in charge of regional NHS management, instead of being done by the government itself.

In June 2010, the British Medical Association voted three to one in favour of a motion that homeopathy should be banned from the NHS, and kept from being sold as medicine in pharmacies. In February 2011, out of 104 PCTs who responded to queries, 72 said they did not fund homeopathy, with 10 of these having stopped funding homeopathy in the last four years. By the 2011-2012 financial year the percentage of PCTs funding homeopathy had fallen to 15%.

In July 2013 the Advertising Standards Authority concluded that homeopathy sellers were engaging in false advertising regarding their claims of efficacy of homeopathic products and that at the same time they discouraged users from seeking essential treatments for conditions for which they were needed.

Switzerland

State insurance funding of homeopathy and four other alternative therapies had been withdrawn after a review in 2005, and a 2009 referendum vote called for state backed health insurance to once more pay for these therapies. In 2012 the government reinstated them for a trial period until 2017, pending an independent investigation of the efficacy and cost-effectiveness of the therapies.

The rules for the registration of homeopathic remedies without a concrete field of application are more liberal in Switzerland than they are in member countries of the EU. For homeopathic medicines based on well-known low-risk substances, Swissmedic, the regulatory authority, offers inexpensive registration by means of a simplified electronic registration procedure.

Australia

According to one 1996 study, approximately 4.4% of Australian adults have used homeopathic remedies at least once in their lives, including 1.2% that sought treatment exclusively from homeopathic practitioners.

North America

Canada

In Canada, a study detailing the use of alternative medicines by children in Quebec found that 11% of the sampled 1,911 children used alternative medicines, and 25% of those who did use alternative medicines (less than 3% of all children sampled) used homeopathy. The study also pointed out that homeopathy is more commonly used in children in Canada than in adults, of whom only 19% of alternative medicine users used homeopathy. Physicians who choose to use alternative medicines such as homeopathy must follow guidelines set by their province's College of Physicians and Surgeons. Provincial health care generally does not cover homeopathy.

United States

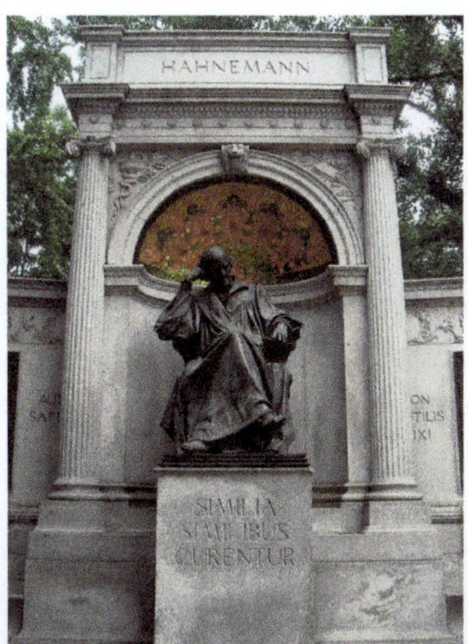

Samuel Hahnemann Monument, Washington D.C. with "Similia Similibus Curentur" - Like cures Like.

The Federal Food, Drug, and Cosmetic Act (FD&C Act) of 1938 recognized homeopathic preparations as drugs, but with significant exceptions. A principal sponsor of the Act was New York Senator and homeopathic physician Royal Copeland, who ensured that homeopathy's own *Homœopathic Pharmacopœia of the United States* (HPUS) be included, as it expressed the "self-professed quality standards" of the homeopathic profession. The finished Act thus created loopholes for the regulation of homeopathic drugs, and they are thus exempted from many of the rules regulating other drugs. The inclusion of HPUS in the Act has since been questioned by "lawyers, doctors, homeopaths, historians, and Food and Drug Administration (FDA) officials."

Homeopathic remedies are regulated by the Food and Drug Administration (FDA), which regulates manufacturing and other standards that are appropriate for homeopathic drugs, mainly through *The Homœopathic Pharmacopœia of the United States* (HPUS) as administered by the Homœopathic Pharmacopœia Convention of the United States and section 400.400 of the FDA *Compliance Policy Guidance Manual*. Homeopathic drugs must be tested for scope of effect, and manufactured and labeled according to the Federal FD&C Act and the HPUS before they are considered official homeopathic drugs. The last bound paper edition of HPUS was published in 1979. It has been replaced by an online database available to subscribers. Official homeopathic drugs can be marketed according to their classification in the HPUS. They are not regulated under the Dietary Supplement Health and Education Act of 1994. Many homeopathic drugs can be sold "over-the-counter"; however, some are classified as prescription-only under all circumstances, and some are classified as prescription-only in various low dilutions. As with all drugs, the labeling requirements are important, as that is one of the primary ways the FDA can regulate drugs. Homeopathic pharmaceutical techniques are not technologically complicated, and the drugs are generally considered to be biologically safe because they are so diluted to the point where there are no molecules from the original solution left in a dose of the final remedy.

The FDA makes significant exemptions for homeopathic *remedies* as compared to other drugs. Here are a few:

1. They are not required to submit new drug applications to the FDA.
2. They are "exempt from good manufacturing practice requirements related to expiration dating".
3. They are exempt from "finished product testing for identity and strength".
4. They may "contain much higher amounts" of alcohol than other drugs, which may contain "no more than 10 percent ... and ... even less for children's medications".

By 2007, in the United States, $3.1 billion were spent on homeopathic medicine and 2.3% of the persons age 18 or over had consulted a practitioner that year. Homeopathy was first established in the United States by Hans Birch Gram in 1825 and rapidly gained popularity. The height of its influence was the end of the 19th century where hardly any city with over 50,000 people was without a homeopathic hospital. In 1890, there were 93 regular schools, 14 of them were fully homeopathic and 8 of them were eclectic. In 1900, there were 121 regular schools, with 22 of them being homeopathic and 10 eclectic. Teaching of homeopathy in the USA declined rapidly in the 20th century. The last purely homeopathic medical school closed in 1920, although homeopathic electives continued to be offered by the Hahnemann Medical School in Philadelphia until the 1940s.

According to one study, in 1990, 0.7% of individuals used homeopathy in the year prior to being questioned; in 1997, 3.4% had used homeopathy at least once in the previous year. According to the same study, of those who used homeopathy, 31.7% had seen a homeopathic practitioner in the past year in 1990 and the number dropped to 16.5% by 1997.

The FDA held a hearing April 20 and 21, 2015, requesting public comment on regulation of homeopathic drugs. Citing the growth of sales of over-the-counter homeopathic medicines, $2.7 billion as of 2007, many labeled as "natural, safe, and effective", the FDA asked:

1. What are consumer and health care provider attitudes towards human drug and biological products labeled as homeopathic?
2. What data sources can be identified or shared with FDA so that the Agency can better assess the risks and benefits of drug and biological products labeled as homeopathic?
3. Are the current enforcement policies under the CPG appropriate to protect and promote public health in light of the tremendous growth in the homeopathic drug market? Are there alternatives to the current enforcement policies of the CPG that would inform FDA's regulatory oversight of drugs labeled as homeopathic? If so, please explain.
4. Are there areas of the current CPG that could benefit from additional clarity? If so, please explain.
5. Is there information regarding the regulation of homeopathic products in other countries that could inform FDA's thinking in this area?
6. A large majority of human drug products labeled as homeopathic are marketed as OTC drugs.These products are available for a wide variety of indications, and many of these indications have never been considered for OTC use under a formal regulatory process. What would be an appropriate regulatory process for evaluating such indications for OTC use?
7. Given the wide range of indications on drug products labeled as homeopathic and available OTC, what processes do companies currently use to evaluate whether such products, including their indications for use, are appropriate for marketing as an OTC drug?
8. Do consumers and health care providers have adequate information to make informed decisions about drug products labeled as homeopathic? If not, what information, including, for example, information in labeling, would allow consumers and health care providers to be better informed about products labeled as homeopathic?

Mexico

In Mexico, homeopathy is currently integrated into the national healthcare system. In 1895, a presidential decree by Gral. Porfirio Díaz established the first homeopathic school and hospital as well as regulations specifying training requirements for homeopathic doctors. Of those individuals who use alternative medicines, over 26% use homeopathy.

South America

Some countries in South America, such as Argentina or Colombia, allow only professional doctors who are qualified and have graduated from a recognised medical school to practice homeopathy. Homeopathy has been regulated in other South American countries, such as Colombia, since the beginning of the 20th century. In Brazil, homeopathy is included in the national health system, and since 1991, physicians who want to practice homeopathy must complete 2,300 hours of education prior to receiving the proper licenses.

Middle East and Asia

India has the largest homeopathic infrastructure in the world, with low estimates at about 64,000, but going as high as 300,000 practising homeopaths. In addition, there are 180 colleges teaching courses, and 7500 government clinics and 307 hospitals which dispense homeopathic remedies. In China and Japan, homeopathy appears to be almost unknown.

Asiatic countries many times were exposed to both homeopathic and non-homeopathic ideas about medicine through invading armies that had ties to Europe. In Malaysia, homeopathy was introduced during World War II by Indian military personnel that formed the bulk of the British army in Asia. The French army brought early modern medicine to Laos during their 1893 invasion. In China, Shanghai had one homeopathic hospital in 1911, and had four later in 1934. In this region, the European models of medicine complemented, but did not replace, the local traditional medicines.

Middle East

Homeopathy is becoming popular in the United Arab Emirates (UAE) and in Iran. The UAE Ministry of Health (MOH) recognizes and regulates the practice of homeopathy in a systematic way. Both medical doctors and lay practitioners can practise homeopathy but they all should pass MOH exams which cover both medical science and homeopathy. The Ministry of Health of Iran recognizes homeopathy as a legal alternative treatment. The Iranian Homeopathic Association, formed with the permission of the Ministry of the Interior and the Ministry of Health, is the reference association for providing standards of homeopathy. In Iran only medical doctors can practice homeopathy.

India

Homoeopathy came to India in early 1810, with travelers, missionaries and military personnel from the West.

Homeopathy research and education is looked after by the Ministry of Ayurveda, Yoga & Naturopathy, Unani, Siddha and Homoeopathy (AYUSH) formed on 9 November 2014, which also takes care of educational standards in the Indian Systems of Medicines and Homoeopathy colleges and promotes research in respective fields. Central Council for Research in Homoeopathy (CCRH) was established as an autonomous organization at New Delhi in 1978 by Govt. of India.

Homeopathic education is regulated by Central Council of Homoeopathy (CCH), a statutory body under the Ministry of Health & Family Welfare, formed in 1973 through Act of Parliament is one of Professional Councils of University Grants Commission (UGC), which monitors all higher education across India.

In 2007 in the state of Uttar Pradesh (population 166 million in 2001) there were 27,548 registered homeopathic practitioners compared with 38,950 medical doctors (referred to as allopaths by those practicing alternative medicine), and 59,783 ayurvedic and 14,905 unani practitioners.

The number of homeopathic doctors in India increased from 105,000 in 1980 to 246,000 in 2010, and the number of homeopathic hospitals/dispensaries increased fourfold – from 1,686 in 1980 to about 7,000 in 2010.

Africa

South Africa

In South Africa, homeopathy is currently regulated by the Allied Health Professions Act, 1982 (Act 63 of 1982) together with the Regulations to the said Act which was set up to provide for the establishment of a statutory body, the Allied Health Professions Council of South Africa (AHPCSA) to regulate the homeopathic profession, amongst ten others. The AHPCSA is one of five Statutory Health Professional Councils regulating health professions in South Africa. Any person wishing to practice Homeopathy in any way whatsover within the borders of South Africa must be registered with the AHPCSA. Registration is a legal requirement and under South African Law it is a criminal offense to practice homeopathy without registration. Homoeopathic registration in South Africa enjoys a standing, rights and privileges similar to that of conventional medical practitioners. This means that the legal scope of practice of a homeopathic practitioner is very similar to that of a conventional medical practitioner. The scope of practice includes also what would generally be applicable to Naturopathic practitioners in countries like the USA.

A Homeopathic Practitioner may diagnose, in fact being a diagnostic primary health care profession, a Homeopathic Practitioner is legally compelled to make a diagnosis and provide the appropriate ICD-10 diagnostic codes. Homeopathic Practitioners also have to be licensed to compound Homeopathic medicine and to dispense any medicine falling within their scope of practice. Both conventional pharmacology and Homoeopharmaceutics are a legal training requirement.

Training therefore is based upon the medical curriculum with Homoeopathy as the primary therapeutic focus. From this perspective it is understandable that (as for Medical Practitioners where the requirement for registration is a MBChB or equivalent) in the case of Homeopathy the requirement for registration is a master's degree in Homeopathy MTech(Hom) or equivalent.

Homoeopathic practitioners are trained diagnosticians, recognised as primary contact practitioners. It should be noted that, whereas the vast majority of international Homoeopathic schools offer skills-oriented Homoeopathic training, South Africa offers professional training at a level required for the practising of Homoeopathy as a primary contact health profession in accordance with the scope of practice of such a profession.

All private Homeopathic colleges were closed during the late 1970s by the South African Department of Health (read the History and Development of Homeopathic Education in South Africa). Existing practitioners were put into a closed register and in terms of the new legislation, and medical doctors were allowed to keep practicing homeopathy regardless of their knowledge of the subject. Nowadays, the only training recognised by the AHPCSA is a five-year full-time master's degree in Homoeopathy offered at the University of Johannesburg and Durban University of Technology.

The M.Tech(Hom) consists of a five-year full-time medico-scientific course based on the medical curriculum with the core focus on classical, clinical, modern and conventional Homoeopathy, Homoeopharmaceutics and ending with a masters research dissertation. Graduates are registered as Homoeopathic practitioners only after having completed their post-graduate internship.

The practice of Homeopathy in South Africa requires medical training as prerequisite. Two routes thus exist for entrance into Homeopathy, either via the medically based homeopathic master's degree course (MTech-Hom) or once a medical practitioner is registered for independent practice, by way of the Post Graduate Diploma in Homeopathy offered by the South African Faculty of Homoeopathy (SAFH). Medical practitioners may register as Homoeopathic practitioners only after successful completion of the post graduate diploma. Once registered, homeopathic practitioners may do the prescribed Compounding and Dispensing course through the University of Pretoria and thereafter apply for a License to Compound and Dispense Homeopathic Medicine from the National Department of Health.

22C. Licensing

(1) Subject to the provisions of this section-

(a) the Director-General may on application in the prescribed manner and on payment of the prescribed fee issue to a medical practitioner, dentist, practitioner, nurse or other person registered under the Health Professions Act, 1974, a licence to compound and dispense medicines, on the prescribed conditions;

(5) No person shall compound or dispense a medicine unless he or she is authorised thereto in terms of the Pharmacy Act, 1974, is a veterinarian or is the holder of a licence as contemplated in subsection(1)(a).

The Medicines Control Council was set up in 1965, and it put all types of medicine under the same standards. It was replaced in 1998 by the South African Medicines and Medical Devices Regulatory Authority, which placed separate procedures for registering regular and alternative medicines, in order to regulate them better.

Nigeria

Both medically qualified practitioners and lay persons can practice homeopathy, with the Congress of Homoeopathic Medicine Practitioners having 30 medical doctors on its register in 2005. The All-Nigeria Homeopathic Medical Organization was founded in 1961, and the first homeopathic practitioner, I. Okogeri, began practice the following year. The Nigerian College of Homoeopathic Medicine, founded in 1972, is recognised by the government of the East Central State. The Nigerian Institute of Homeopathy has special consultative status with the United Nations Department of Economic and Social Affairs.

References

- Kaufman M (1971), Homeopathy in America: The rise and fall of a medical heresy, The Johns Hopkins University Press, ISBN 978-0-8018-1238-5.
- Edzard Ernst; Singh, Simon (2008), Trick or Treatment: The Undeniable Facts about Alternative Medicine,

New York: W. W. Norton, ISBN 0-393-06661-4

- W. Steven Pray (1 August 2003). a History of Nonprescription Product Regulation. Psychology Press. p. 192. ISBN 978-0-7890-1538-9. Retrieved 21 January 2013.
- Robert W. Ullman; Judyth Reichenberg-Ullman (1 October 1994). The patient's guide to homeopathic medicine. Picnic Point Press. pp. 1–2. ISBN 978-0-9640654-2-0. Retrieved 24 January 2013.
- Richard Haehl (1922). Samuel Hahnemann: His Life and Work : Based on Recently Discovered State Papers, Documents, Letters, Etc. B. Jain Publishers. p. 101. ISBN 978-81-7021-693-3. Retrieved 24 January 2013.
- Anne Taylor Kirschmann (2004). A vital force: women in American homeopathy. Rutgers University Press. p. 11. ISBN 978-0-8135-3320-9. Retrieved 28 January 2013.
- Hahnemann S (1833), The organon of the healing art (5th ed.), aphorism 269, ISBN 0-87983-228-2. Hahnemann S (1842), The organon of the healing art (6th ed.) (published 1921), aphorism 270, ISBN 0-87983-228-2
- Whorton JC (2004), Nature Cures: The History of Alternative Medicine in America, New York: Oxford University Press US, pp. 18, 52, ISBN 0-19-517162-4
- Miller, Timothy (1995). America's alternative religions. State University of New York Press, Albany. p. 80. ISBN 978-0-7914-2397-4.
- Winston J (2006), "Homeopathy Timeline", The Faces of Homoeopathy, Whole Health Now, ISBN 0-473-05607-0, retrieved 2007-07-23
- Paul Ulrich Unschuld (9 August 2009). What Is Medicine?: Western and Eastern Approaches to Healing. University of California Press. p. 171. ISBN 978-0-520-94470-1. Retrieved 7 September 2013.
- Lockie, Andrew (2000). Encyclopedia of Homeopathy (1st ed.). New York City, NY: Dorling Kindersley. p. 19. ISBN 978-0-7566-1871-1.
- Mathur KN (2003), Prinzipien der homöopathischen Verschreibung: Synopsis weltweiter klinischer Erfahrungen (in German), Georg Thieme Verlag, pp. 122–123, ISBN 3-8304-9021-6, OCLC 76518035
- Kayne SB (2006), Homeopathic pharmacy: theory and practice (2 ed.), Elsevier Health Sciences, p. 53, ISBN 978-0-443-10160-1
- The volume of all water on earth is about 1.36×10^9 km^3: "Earth's water distribution", Water Science for Schools, United States Geological Survey, 28 August 2006, ISBN 0-07-825402-7
- Bradford, Thomas Lindsley (1895). The Life and Letters of Dr. Samuel Hahnemann. Philadelphia: Boericke & Tafel. pp. 103–104. ISBN 978-1330001509. Retrieved 27 August 2015.
- Rose Shapiro (30 September 2010). Suckers: How Alternative Medicine Makes Fools of Us All. Random House. pp. 97–. ISBN 978-1-4090-5916-5.
- Secretary of State for Health Government Response to the Science and Technology Committee report 'Evidence Check 2: Homeopathy', July 2010 ISBN 978-0-10-179142-7
- Legal status of traditional medicine and complementary/alternative medicine: a worldwide review, World Health Organization, 2001, ISBN 978-92-4-154548-8
- Kayne SB (2006), Homeopathic pharmacy: theory and practice (2 ed.), Elsevier Health Sciences, p. 53, ISBN 978-0-443-10160-1
- Robert ED (1853), Lectures on the theory & practice of homeopathy (PDF), London: B. Jain, pp. 526–7, ISBN 81-7021-311-8

5

Understanding Ayurveda

Ayurveda medicine has its roots in the Indian history. The plants used in Ayurveda are Azadirachta indica, Cedrus deodara, Terminalia arjuna and Phyllanthus emblica. This text has been carefully written to provide an easy understanding of the varied facets of Ayurveda.

Ayurveda

Ayurveda, or Ayurveda medicine, is a system of medicine with historical roots in the Indian subcontinent. Globalized and modernized practices derived from Ayurveda traditions are a type of complementary or alternative medicine. In the Western world, Ayurveda therapies and practices (which are manifold) have been integrated in general wellness applications and as well in some cases in medical use.

The main classical Ayurveda treatises begin with legendary accounts of the transmission of medical knowledge from the Gods to sages, and thence to human physicians. Thus, the Sushruta Samhita narrates how Dhanvantari, "greatest of the mighty celestial," incarnated himself as Divodāsa, a mythical king of Varanasi, who then taught medicine to a group of wise physicians, including Sushruta himself. Ayurveda therapies have varied and evolved over more than two millennia. Therapies are typically based on complex herbal compounds, while treatises introduced mineral and metal substances (perhaps under the influence of early Indian alchemy or *rasaśāstra*). Ancient Ayurveda treatises also taught surgical techniques, including rhinoplasty, perineal lithotomy, the suturing of wounds, and the extraction of foreign objects.

Although laboratory experiments suggest it is possible that some substances in Ayurveda might be developed into effective treatments, there is no evidence that any are effective as currently proffered. Ayurveda medicine is considered pseudoscientific. Other researchers consider it a protoscience, or trans-science system instead. Close to 21% of Ayurveda U.S. and Indian-manufactured patent medicines sold through the Internet were found to contain toxic levels of heavy metals, specifically lead, mercury, and arsenic. The public health implications of such metallic contaminants in India are unknown.

Some scholars assert that Ayurveda originated in prehistoric times, and that some of the concepts of Ayurveda have existed from the time of the Indus Valley Civilization or even earlier. Ayurveda developed significantly during the Vedic period and later some of the non-Vedic systems such as Buddhism and Jainism also developed medical concepts and practices that appear in the classical Ayurveda treatises. Humoral balance is emphasized, and the suppressing of natural urges is considered unhealthy and claimed to lead to illness. Ayurveda names three elemental substances, the *doshas* (called Vata, Pitta and Kapha), and states that a balance of the doshas results in health, while imbalance results in disease. Ayurveda has eight canonical components, which are derived from classical Sanskrit literature. Some of the oldest known Ayurvedic texts include the *Suśrutha Sachitā* and *Charaka Sachitā*, which are written in Sanskrit. Ayurveda practitioners had developed various medicinal preparations and surgical procedures by the medieval period.

Eight Components

The earliest classical Sanskrit works on Ayurveda describe medical science as being divided into eight components. This characterization of the physicians' art as the teaching found in "the medicine that has eight components" is first found in the Sanskrit epic, the *Mahābhārata*. The components are:

- *Kāyacikitsā*: general medicine, medicine of the body
- *Kaumāra-bhṛtya*: the treatment of children, paediatrics
- *Śalyatantra*: surgical techniques and the extraction of foreign objects
- *Śālākyatantra:* treatment of ailments affecting ears, eyes, nose, mouth, etc. ("ENT")
- *Bhūtavidyā*: pacification of possessing spirits, and the people whose minds are affected by such possession
- *Agadatantra*: toxicology
- *Rasāyanatantra*: rejuvenation and tonics for increasing lifespan, intellect and strength
- *Vājīkaraṇatantra*: aphrodisiacs and treatments for increasing the volume and viability of semen and sexual pleasure.

Principles and Terminology

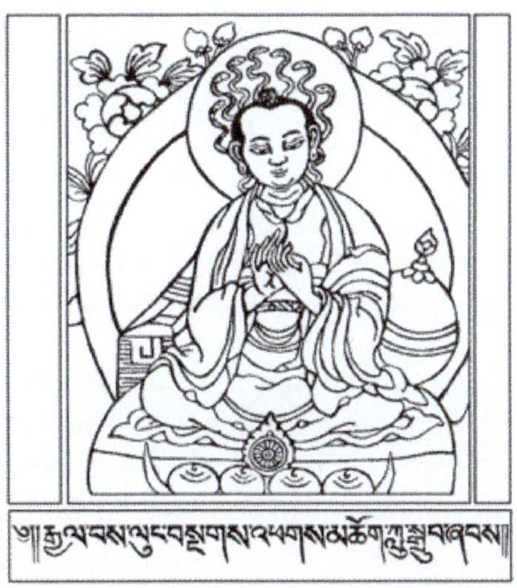

Several philosophers in India combined religion and traditional medicine—notable examples being that of Hinduism and Ayurveda. Shown in the image is the philosopher Nagarjuna—known chiefly for his doctrine of the *Madhyamaka* (middle path)—who wrote medical works *The Hundred Prescriptions* and *The Precious Collection*, among others.

The central theoretical ideas of Ayurveda developed in the mid-first millennium BCE, and show parallels with Sāṅkhya and Vaiśeṣika philosophies and with Buddhism and Jainism. Balance is emphasized, and suppressing natural urges is considered unhealthy and claimed to lead to illness. For example, to suppress sneezing is said to potentially give rise to shoulder pain. However, people are also cautioned to stay within the limits of reasonable balance and measure when following nature's urges. For example, emphasis is placed on moderation of food intake, sleep, and sexual intercourse.

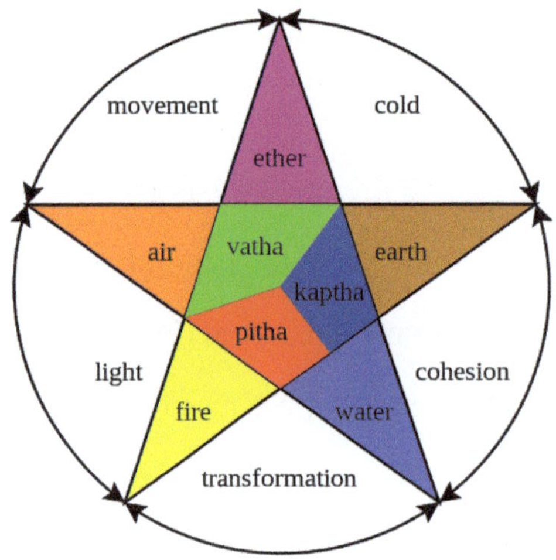

The three do-has and the five elements from which they are composed.

Ayurveda names seven basic tissues (dhatu), which are plasma (*rasa*), blood (*rakta*), muscles (*māmsa*), fat (*meda*), bone (*asthi*), marrow (*majja*), and semen (*shukra*). Like the medicine of classical antiquity, Ayurveda has historically divided bodily substances into five classical elements (Sanskrit *[maha]panchabhuta*, viz. earth, water, fire, air and ether. There are also twenty gunas (qualities or characteristics) which are considered to be inherent in all substances. These are organized in ten pairs of antonyms: heavy/light, cold/hot, unctuous/dry, dull/sharp, stable/mobile, soft/hard, non-slimy/slimy, smooth/coarse, minute/gross, and viscous/liquid.

Ayurveda also names three elemental substances, the *doshas* (called Vata, Pitta and Kapha), and states that a balance of the doshas results in health, while imbalance results in disease. One Ayurvedic view is that the doshas are balanced when they are equal to each other, while another view is that each human possesses a unique combination of the doshas which define this person's temperament and characteristics. In either case, it says that each person should modulate their behavior or environment to increase or decrease the doshas and maintain their natural state.

In medieval taxonomies of the Sanskrit knowledge systems, Ayurveda is assigned a place as a subsidiary Veda (upaveda). Some medicinal plant names from the *Atharvaveda* and other Vedas can be found in subsequent Ayurveda literature. The earliest recorded theoretical statements about the canonical models of disease in Ayurveda occur in the earliest Buddhist Canon.

Practice

Ayurvedic doctors regard physical existence, mental existence, and personality as a unit, with each element being able to influence the others. This is a holistic approach used during diagnosis and therapy, and is a fundamental aspect of Ayurveda. Another part of Ayurvedic treatment says that there are channels (*srotas*) which transport fluids, and that the channels can be opened up by massage treatment using oils and Swedana (fomentation). Unhealthy channels are thought to cause disease.

Diagnosis

Ayurveda has eight ways to diagnose illness, called Nadi (pulse), Mootra (urine), Mala (stool), Jihva (tongue), Shabda (speech), Sparsha (touch), Druk (vision), and Aakruti (appearance). Ayurvedic practitioners approach diagnosis by using the five senses. For example, hearing is used to observe the condition of breathing and speech. The study of the lethal points or *marman marma* is of special importance.

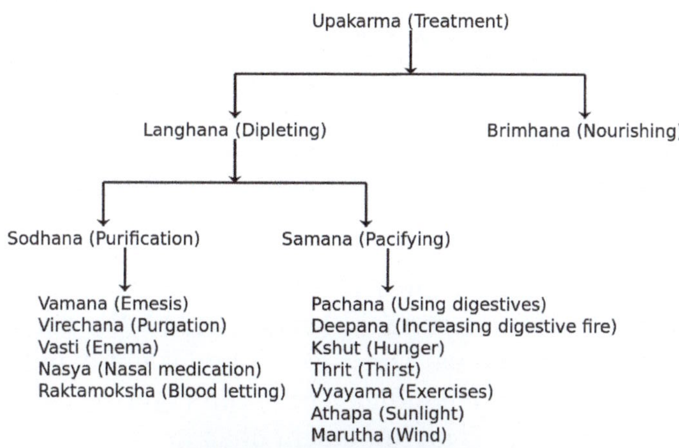

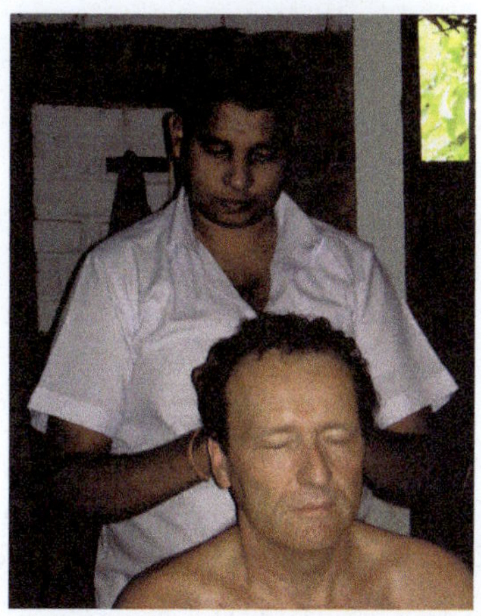

An Ayurvedic practitioner applying oils using head massage.

Treatment and Prevention

Two of the eight branches of classical Ayurveda deal with surgery, but contemporary Ayurveda tends to stress attaining vitality by building a healthy metabolic system and maintaining good digestion and excretion. Ayurveda also focuses on exercise, yoga, and meditation. One type of prescription is a Sattvic diet.

Ayurveda follows the concept of Dinacharya, which says that natural cycles (waking, sleeping, working, meditation etc.) are important for health. Hygiene, including regular bathing, cleaning of teeth, skin care, and eye washing, is also a central practice.

Substances Used

Plant-based treatments in Ayurveda may be derived from roots, leaves, fruits, bark, or seeds such as cardamom and cinnamon. In the 19th century, William Dymock and co-authors summarized hundreds of plant-derived medicines along with the uses, microscopic structure, chemical composition, toxicology, prevalent myths and stories, and relation to commerce in British India. Animal products used in Ayurveda include milk, bones, and gallstones. In addition, fats are prescribed both for consumption and for external use. Consumption of minerals, including sulphur, arsenic, lead, copper sulfate and gold, are also prescribed. The addition of minerals to herbal medicine is called *rasa shastra*.

Ayurveda uses alcoholic beverages called *Madya*, which are said to adjust the doshas by increasing Pitta and reducing Vatta and Kapha. Madya are classified by the raw material and fermentation process, and the categories include: sugar-based, fruit-based, cereal-based, cereal-based with herbs, fermentated with vinegar, and tonic wines. The intended outcomes can include causing purgation, improving digestion or taste, creating dryness, or loosening joints. Ayurvedic texts describe Madya as non-viscid and fast-acting, and say that it enters and cleans minute pores in the body.

Purified opium is used in eight Ayurvedic preparations and is said to balance the Vata and Kapha doshas and increase the Pitta dosha. It is prescribed for diarrhea and dysentery, for increasing the sexual and muscular ability, and for affecting the brain. The sedative and pain-relieving properties of opium are not considered in Ayurveda. The use of opium is not found in the ancient Ayurvedic texts, and is first mentioned in the *Sarngadhara Samhita* (1300-1400 CE), a book on pharmacy used in Rajasthan in Western India, as an ingredient of an aphrodisiac to delay male ejaculation. It is possible that opium was brought to India along with or before the Mohammedan conquest. The book *Yoga Ratnakara* (1700-1800 CE, unknown author), which is popular in Maharashtra, uses opium in a herbal-mineral composition prescribed for diarrhea. In the *Bhaisajya Ratnavali*, opium and camphor are used for acute gastroenteritis. In this drug, the respiratory depressant action of opium is counteracted by the respiratory stimulant property of Camphor. Later books have included the narcotic property for use as analgesic pain reliever.

Cannabis indica is also absent from the ancient Ayurveda books, and is first mentioned in the *Sarngadhara Samhita* as a treatment for diarrhea. In the *Bhaisajya Ratnavali* it is named as an ingredient in an aphrodisiac.

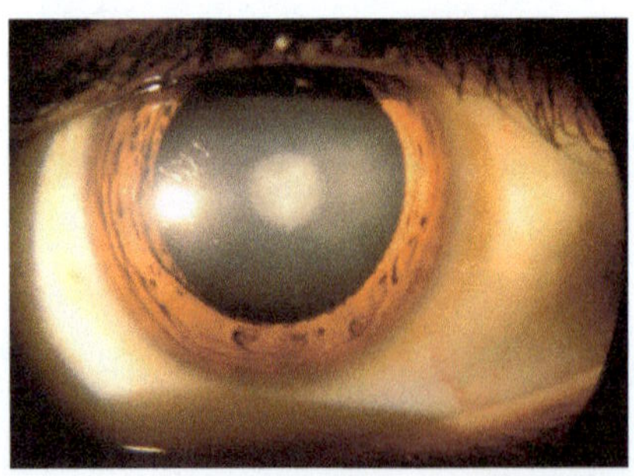

Cataract in human eye – magnified view seen on examination with a slit lamp. Cataract surgery is mentioned in the *Sushruta Samhita*, as a procedure to be performed with a *jabamukhi salaka*, a curved needle used to loosen the obstructing phlegm and push it out of the field of vision. The eye would later be soaked with warm butter and then bandaged.

Ayurveda says that both oil and tar can be used to stop bleeding, and that traumatic bleeding can be stopped by four different methods: ligation of the blood vessel, cauterisation by heat, use of preparations to facilitate clotting, and use of preparations to constrict the blood vessels. Oils are also used in a number of ways, including regular consumption, anointing, smearing, head massage, application to affected areas, and oil pulling. Liquids may also be poured on the patient's forehead, a technique called shirodhara.

Panchakarma

According to Ayurveda, the technique of panchakarma eliminates toxic elements from the body. Panchakarma includes Vamana, Virechana, Basti, Nasya and Raktamokshana. It is preceded by Poorvakarma as a preparatory step, and is followed by Paschatkarma and Peyadikarma.

Current Status

Based on the World Health Assembly resolution on traditional medicine (WHA62.13, compare as well the 2008 Beijing declaration on traditional medicine), the WHO has established a traditional medicine strategy, which involves, among other complementary health systems, Ayurveda. The first previous global strategy was published in 2002 and dealt especially with herbal medicines. The current version (2014-2023) is beginning to consider aspects of T&CM practices and practitioners and whether and how they should be integrated into overall health service delivery. It is as well part of the 2013 WHO, WIPO, WTO TRIPS study on health innovation and access to medicines.

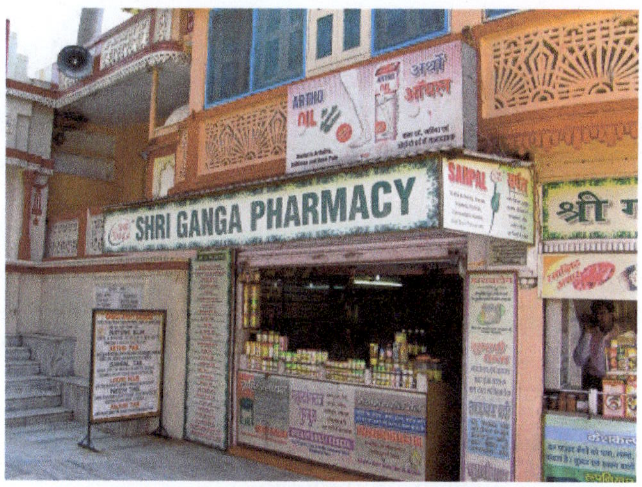

A typical Ayurvedic pharmacy, Rishikesh.

As well the WTO mentions Ayurveda in its intellectual property strategy. Traditional medicine, including Ayurveda, contributes significantly to the health status of many communities, and is increasingly used within certain communities in developed countries. Along that, traditional medicine has a long history of use in health maintenance and in disease prevention and treatment, particularly for chronic diseases. Suitable recognition of traditional medicine is an important element of national health policies and has as well important basis for new products with significant export potential. WTO, WIPO and WHO ask for respect for both the economic value and the social and cultural significance of traditional knowledge and supports documentation of traditional medical knowledge and enhanced regulation of quality, safety and efficacy of such products. The WHO paper asks to integrate traditional and complementary medicine services, where appropriate, into health care service delivery and self-health care and to promote an improved universal health coverage by doing so.

India

Kandamkulathy Ayurveda Hospital, Mala, Kerala

According to some sources, up to 80 percent of people in India use some form of traditional medicine, a category which includes Ayurveda.

In 1970, the Indian Medical Central Council Act which aimed to standardise qualifications for Ayurveda practitioners and provide accredited institutions for its study and research was passed by the Parliament of India. In 1971, the Central Council of Indian Medicine (CCIM) was established under the Department of Ayurveda, Yoga and Naturopathy, Unani, Siddha and Homoeopathy (AYUSH), Ministry of Health and Family Welfare, to monitor higher education in Ayurveda in India. The Indian government supports research and teaching in Ayurveda through many channels at both the national and state levels, and helps institutionalise traditional medicine so that it can be studied in major towns and cities. The state-sponsored Central Council for Research in Ayurvedic Sciences (CCRAS) is designed to do research on Ayurveda. Many clinics in urban and rural areas are run by professionals who qualify from these institutes. As of 2013, India has over 180 training centers offer degrees in traditional Ayurvedic medicine.

To fight biopiracy and unethical patents, in 2001 the government of India set up the Traditional Knowledge Digital Library as a repository for formulations of various systems of Indian medicine, such as Ayurveda, Unani and Siddha. The formulations come from over 100 traditional Ayurveda books. An Indian Academy of Sciences document quoting a 2003-04 report informs that India had 4,32,625 (equivalent to 432,625 in Western numbering) registered medical practitioners, 13,925 dispensaries, 2,253 hospitals and a bed strength of 43,803. 209 under-graduate teaching institutions and 16 post-graduate institutions. Insurance companies cover expenses for Ayurvedic treatments in case of conditions such as spinal cord disorders, bone disorder, arthritis and cancer. Such claims comprise 5-10 percent of the country's health insurance claims.

Maharashtra Andhashraddha Nirmoolan Samiti, an organisation dedicated to fighting superstition in India, considers Ayurveda to be pseudoscience.

Other Countries in The Indian Subcontinent

About 75%-80% of the population of Nepal use Ayurveda, and it is the most practiced form of medicine in the country.

The Sri Lankan tradition of Ayurveda is similar to the Indian tradition. Practitioners of Ayurveda in Sri Lanka refer to Sanskrit texts which are common to both countries. However, they do differ in some aspects, particularly in the herbs used.

In 1980, the Sri Lankan government established a Ministry of Indigenous Medicine to revive and regulate Ayurveda. The Institute of Indigenous Medicine (affiliated to the University of Colombo) offers undergraduate, postgraduate, and MD degrees in Ayurveda Medicine and Surgery, and similar degrees in unani medicine. In the public system, there are currently 62 Ayurvedic hospitals and 208 central dispensaries, which served about 3 million people (about 11% of Sri Lanka's population) in 2010. In total, there are about 20,000 registered practitioners of Ayurveda in the country.

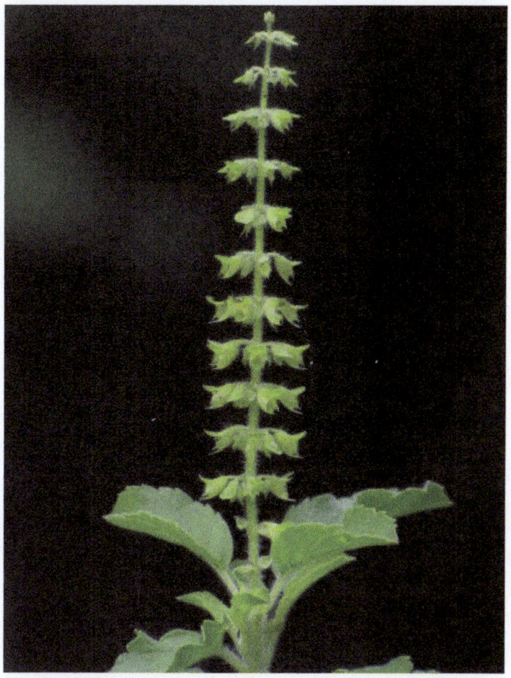

Tulsi-flower (holy basil), an Ayurvedic herb

According to the Mahavamsa, an ancient chronicle of Sinhalese royalty from the sixth century C.E., King Pandukabhaya of Sri Lanka (reigned 437 BCE to 367 BCE) had lying-in-homes and Ayurvedic hospitals (Sivikasotthi-Sala) built in various parts of the country. This is the earliest documented evidence available of institutions dedicated specifically to the care of the sick anywhere in the world. Mihintale Hospital is the oldest in the world.

Outside The Indian Subcontinent

Ayurveda is a system of traditional medicine developed during antiquity and the medieval period, and as such is comparable to pre-modern Chinese and European systems of medicine. However, beginning in the 1960s, Ayurveda has been advertised as alternative medicine in the Western world. Due to different laws and medical regulations in the rest of the world, the unregulated practice and commercialisation of Ayurveda has raised ethical and legal issues. In some instances, Ayurvedic practices or terminology have also been adapted specifically for Western consumption, notably in the case of "Maharishi Ayurveda" in the 1980s. In some cases, this involved active fraud on the part of proponents of Ayurveda in an attempt to falsely represent the system as equal to the standards of modern medical research.

Baba Hari Dass was an early proponent who helped bring Ayurveda to the US in the early 1970s. He taught classes derived from the *Suśrutha Sa⍰hitā* and the *Charaka Sa⍰hitha*, leading to the establishment of the Mount Madonna Institute, College of Ayurveda, Ayurveda World, and Ayurvedic pharmacy. He invited several notable Ayurvedic teachers, including Vasant Lad, Sarita Shrestha, and Ram Harsh Singh. The Ayurvedic practitioner Michael Tierra wrote that "[t]he history of Ayurveda in North America will always owe a debt to the selfless contributions of Baba Hari Dass."

In the United States, the practice of Ayurveda is not licensed or regulated by any state. Practitioners of Ayurveda can be licensed in other healthcare fields such as massage therapy or midwifery, and a few states have approved schools teaching Ayurveda.

Classification and Efficacy

Although laboratory experiments suggest it is possible that some substances in Ayurveda might be developed into effective treatments, there is no evidence that any are effective in themselves. According to Cancer Research UK, no significant scientific evidence has shown effectiveness of Ayurvedic medicine for the treatment of any disease, although massage and relaxation are often beneficial for some cancer patients and there are indications from animal studies that some herbal products used in Ayurveda might be explored further.

Today, ayurvedic medicine is considered pseudoscientific on account of its confusion between reality and metaphysical concepts. Other researchers debate whether it should be considered a proto-science, an unscientific, or trans-science system instead.

A review of the use of Ayurveda for cardiovascular disease concluded that the evidence is not convincing for the use of any Ayurvedic herbal treatment for heart disease or hypertension, but that many herbs used by Ayurvedic practitioners could be appropriate for further research.

Research

In India, research in Ayurveda is undertaken by the Central Council for Research in Ayurveda and Siddha (CCRAS), through a national network of research institutes.

In Nepal, the National Ayurvedic Training and Research Centre (NATRC) researches medicinal herbs in the country.

Research into ayurveda has been characterized as pseudoscience. Both the lack of scientific soundness in the theoretical foundations of ayurveda and the quality of research have been criticized.

Use of Toxic Metals

Rasa shastra, the practice of adding metals, minerals or gems to herbal preparations, may include toxic heavy metals such as lead, mercury and arsenic. The public health implications of metals in rasa shastra in India is unknown. Adverse reactions to herbs are described in traditional Ayurvedic texts, but practitioners are reluctant to admit that herbs could be toxic and that reliable information on herbal toxicity is not readily available. There is a communication gap between practitioners of modern medicine and Ayurveda.

Some traditional Indian herbal medicinal products contain harmful levels of heavy metals, including lead. A 1990 study on Ayurvedic medicines in India found that 41% of the products tested contained arsenic, and that 64% contained lead and mercury. A 2004 study found toxic levels of heavy metals in 20% of Ayurvedic preparations made in South Asia and sold in the Boston area, and concluded that Ayurvedic products posed serious health risks and should be tested for heavy-metal contamination. A 2008 study of more than 230 products found that approximately 20% of remedies (and 40% of *rasa shastra* medicines) purchased over the Internet from U.S. and Indian suppliers contained lead, mercury or arsenic.

Heavy metals are thought of as active ingredients by advocates of Indian herbal medicinal products. Ayurvedic proponents believe that the toxicity of these materials is reduced through purification processes such as *samskaras* or *shodhanas* (for metals). These are similar to the Chinese *pao zhi*, although the Ayurvedic techniques are more complex and may involve prayers as well as physical pharmacy techniques. However, these products have nonetheless caused severe lead poisoning and other toxic effects. Between 1978 and 2008, "more than 80 cases of lead poisoning associated with Ayurvedic medicine use [were] reported worldwide". In 2012, the U.S. Centers for Disease Control and Prevention (CDC) linked Ayurvedic drugs to lead poisoning, based on cases where toxic materials were found in the blood of pregnant women who had taken Ayurvedic drugs.

In India, the government ruled that Ayurvedic products must be labelled with their metallic content. However, in *Current Science*, a publication of the Indian Academy of Sciences, M. S. Valiathan said that "the absence of post-market surveillance and the paucity of test laboratory facilities [in India] make the quality control of Ayurvedic medicines exceedingly difficult at this time". In the United States, most Ayurvedic products are marketed without having been reviewed or approved by the FDA. Since 2007, the FDA has placed an import alert on some Ayurvedic products in order to prevent them from entering the United States.

History

The origins of Ayurveda have been traced back to around 5,000 BCE, when they originated as an oral tradition. Some of the concepts of Ayurveda have been discovered since the times of Indus Valley Civilization. The first recorded forms of Ayurveda as medical texts evolved from the Vedas. Ayurveda is a discipline of the upaveda or "auxiliary knowledge" in Vedic tradition. The origins of Ayurveda are also found in Atharvaveda, which contains 114 hymns and incantations described as magical cures for disease. There are various legendary accounts of the origin of Ayurveda, e.g. that it was received by Dhanvantari (or Divodasa) from Brahma. Tradition also holds that the writings of Ayurveda were influenced by a lost text by the sage Agnivesa.

Ayurveda is one of the few systems of medicine developed in ancient times that is still widely practiced in modern times. As such, it is open to the criticism that its conceptual basis is obsolete and that its contemporary practitioners have not taken account of the developments of Modern Establishment Medicine. Responses to this situation led to an impassioned debate in India during the early decades of the twentieth century, between proponents of unchanging tradition (*śuddha* "pure" ayurveda) and those who thought ayurveda should modernise and syncretize (*aśuddha* "impure, tainted" ayurveda). The political debate about the place of ayurveda in contemporary India has continued to the present (2015), both in the public arena and in government. Debate about the place of Ayurvedic medicine in the contemporary internationalized world also continues today (2015).

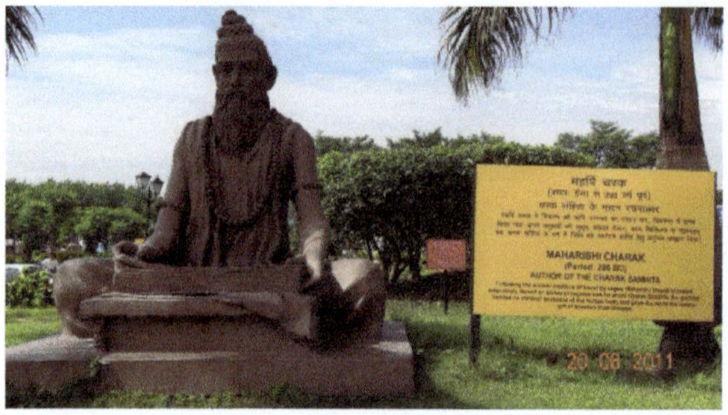

Charaka

Main Texts

There are three principal early texts on Ayurveda include the Charaka Samhita, the Sushruta Samhita and the Bhela Samhita. The Sushruta Samhita is based on an original from the 6th century BCE, and was updated by the Buddhist scholar Nagarjuna in the 2nd century CE. The Charaka Samhita, written by Charaka, and the Bhela Samhita, attributed to Atreya Punarvasu, are also dated to the 6th century BCE. The Charaka Samhita was also updated by Dridhabala during the early centuries of the Common Era.

The Bower Manuscript is also of special interest to historians due to its inclusion of excerpts from the Bheda Samhita and its description of concepts in Central Asian Buddhism. In 1987, A. F. R. Hoernle identified the scribe of the medical portions of the manuscript to be a native of India using a northern variant of the Gupta script, who had migrated and become a Buddhist monk in a monastery in Kucha. The Chinese pilgrim Fa Hsien (c. 337–422 AD) wrote about the healthcare system of the Gupta empire (320–550) and described the institutional approach of Indian medicine. This is also visible in the works of Charaka, who describes about hospital and how it should be equipped.

Other early texts are the Agnivesha Samhita, Kasyapa Samhita and Harita Samhita. The original edition of the Agnivesha Samhita, by Agnivesa, is dated to 1500 BCE, and it was later modified by Charaka. Kasyapa Samhita includes the treatise of Jivaka Kumar Bhaccha and is dated to the 6th century BCE. While Harita Samhita is dated to an earlier period, it is attributed to Harita, who was a disciple of Punarvasu Atreya. Some later texts are *Astanga nighantu* (8th Century) by Vagbhata, *Paryaya ratnamala* (9th century) by Madhava, *Siddhasara nighantu* (9th century) by Ravi Gupta, *Dravyavali* (10th Century), and *Dravyaguna sangraha* (11th century) by Cakrapanidatta, among others.

Illnesses Portrayed

Underwood and Rhodes state that the early forms of traditional Indian medicine identified fever, cough, consumption, diarrhea, dropsy, abscesses, seizures, tumours, and leprosy, and that treatments included plastic surgery, couching (a form of cataract surgery), puncturing to release fluids in the abdomen, extraction of foreign bodies, treatment of anal fistulas, treating fractures, amputations, cesarean sections, and stitching of wounds. The use of herbs and surgical instruments became widespread. During this period, treatments were also prescribed for complex ailments, including angina pectoris, diabetes, hypertension, and stones.

Further Development and Spread

Ayurveda flourished throughout the Indian Middle Ages. Dalhana (fl. 1200), Sarngadhara (fl. 1300) and Bhavamisra (fl. 1500) compiled works on Indian medicine. The medical works of both Sushruta and Charaka were also translated into the Chinese language in the 5th century, and during the 8th century, they were translated into the Arabic and Persian language. The 9th-century Persian physician Muhammad ibn Zakariya al-Razi was familiar with the text. The Arabic works derived from the Ayurvedic texts eventually also reached Europe by the 12th century. In Renaissance Italy, the Branca family of Sicily and Gaspare Tagliacozzi (Bologna) were influenced by the Arabic reception of the Sushruta's surgical techniques.

British physicians traveled to India to observe rhinoplasty being performed using native methods, and reports on Indian rhinoplasty were published in the *Gentleman's Magazine* in 1794. Instruments described in the *Sushruta Samhita* were further modified in Europe. Joseph Constantine Carpue studied plastic surgery methods in India for 20 years and, in 1815, was able to perform the first major rhinoplasty surgery in the western world, using the "Indian" method of nose reconstruction. In 1840 Brett published an article about this technique.

During the period of colonial British rule of India, the practice of Ayurveda was neglected by the British Indian Government, in favor of modern medicine. After Indian independence, there was more focus on Ayurveda and other traditional medical systems. Ayurveda became a part of the Indian National health care system, with state hospitals for Ayurveda established across the country. However, the treatments of traditional medicines were not always integrated with others.

Plants Used in Ayurveda

Azadirachta Indica

Azadirachta indica, also known as Neem, Nimtree, and Indian Lilac is a tree in the mahogany family Meliaceae. It is one of two species in the genus *Azadirachta*, and is native to India and the Indian subcontinent including Nepal, Pakistan, Bangladesh, and Sri Lanka. It typically is grown in tropical and semi-tropical regions. Neem trees now also grow in islands located in the southern part of Iran. Its fruits and seeds are the source of neem oil.

Description

Neem is a fast-growing tree that can reach a height of 15–20 metres (49–66 ft), and rarely 35–40 metres (115–131 ft). It is evergreen, but in severe drought it may shed most or nearly all of its leaves. The branches are wide and spreading. The fairly dense crown is roundish and may reach a diameter of 15–20 metres (49–66 ft) in old, free-standing specimens. The neem tree is very similar in appearance to its relative, the Chinaberry (*Melia azedarach*).

The opposite, pinnate leaves are 20–40 centimetres (7.9–15.7 in) long, with 20 to 31 medium to dark green leaflets about 3–8 centimetres (1.2–3.1 in) long. The terminal leaflet often is missing. The petioles are short.

The (white and fragrant) flowers are arranged in more-or-less drooping axillary panicles which are up to 25 centimetres (9.8 in) long. The inflorescences, which branch up to the third degree, bear from 150 to 250 flowers. An individual flower is 5–6 millimetres (0.20–0.24 in) long and 8–11 millimetres (0.31–0.43 in) wide. Protandrous, bisexual flowers and male flowers exist on the same individual tree.

The fruit is a smooth (glabrous), olive-like drupe which varies in shape from elongate oval to nearly roundish, and when ripe is 1.4–2.8 centimetres (0.55–1.10 in) by 1.0–1.5 centimetres (0.39–0.59 in). The fruit skin (exocarp) is thin and the bitter-sweet pulp (mesocarp) is yellowish-white and very fibrous. The mesocarp is 0.3–0.5 centimetres (0.12–0.20 in) thick. The white, hard inner shell (endocarp) of the fruit encloses one, rarely two, or three, elongated seeds (kernels) having a brown seed coat.

Etymology

Neem is a Hindi noun derived from Sanskrit Nimba.

Vernacular Names

Names for this plant in various languages include;

- Arabic - Neeb, Azad-darakhul-hind, Shajarat Alnnim
- Assamese - Neem (নীম)
- Bengali - Nim (নিম)
- English - Margosa, Neem Tree
- French - Azadirac de l'Inde, margosier, margousier
- German - Indischer zedrach, Grossblaettiger zedrach
- Gujarati - Dhanujhada, Limbda
- Hausa - Darbejiya, Dogonyaro, Bedi
- Hindi - Neem
- Kannada - Bevu
- Kiswahili - Muarubaini
- Khmer - Sdau (ស្ដៅ)
- Malay - Mambu (وبمم)
- Malayalam - Aryaveppu (ആര്യവേപ്പ്)
- Manipuri - Neem (নীম)
- Marathi - Kadunimba
- Myanmar - Burma- Tamar

- Nepal - Neem
- Nigerian - Dongoyaro
- Odiya - Neem (ନିମ)
- Persian - Azad Darakth e hind, neeb, nib
- Portuguese - Nimbo, Margosa, Amargoseira
- Punjabi - Nimmh (ਨਿੰਮ੍ਹ)
- Sanskrit - Arishta, Pakvakrita, Nimbaka
- Sinhala - Kohomba (කොහොඹ)
- Sindhi - Nimm (نم)
- Somali - Geed Hindi
- Tamil - Veppai, Sengumaru
- Telugu - Vepa
- Thai - Sadao
- tulu-besappu
- Urdu - Neem (نیم)

Ecology

The neem tree is noted for its drought resistance. Normally it thrives in areas with sub-arid to sub-humid conditions, with an annual rainfall of 400–1,200 millimetres (16–47 in). It can grow in regions with an annual rainfall below 400 mm, but in such cases it depends largely on ground water levels. Neem can grow in many different types of soil, but it thrives best on well drained deep and sandy soils. It is a typical tropical to subtropical tree and exists at annual mean temperatures of 21–32 °C (70–90 °F). It can tolerate high to very high temperatures and does not tolerate temperature below 4 °C (39 °F). Neem is one of a very few shade-giving trees that thrive in drought-prone areas e.g. the dry coastal, southern districts of India, and Pakistan. The trees are not at all delicate about water quality and thrive on the merest trickle of water, whatever the quality. In India and tropical countries where the Indian diaspora has reached, it is very common to see neem trees used for shade lining streets, around temples, schools and other such public buildings or in most people's back yards. In very dry areas the trees are planted on large tracts of land.

Weed Status

Neem is considered a weed in many areas, including some parts of the Middle East, most of Sub-Saharan Africa including West Africa and Indian Ocean states, and some parts of Australia. Ecologically, it survives well in similar environments to its own, but its weed potential has not been fully assessed.

In April 2015, *A. indica* was declared a class B and C weed in the Northern Territory, Australia, meaning its growth and spread must be controlled and plants or propagules are not allowed to be brought into the NT. It is illegal to buy, sell, or transport the plants or seeds. Its declaration as a weed came in response to its invasion of waterways in the "Top End" of the territory.

After being introduced into Australia, possibly in the 1940s, *A. indica* was originally planted in the Northern Territory to provide shade for cattle. Trial plantations were established between the 1960s and 1980s in Darwin, Queensland, and Western Australia, but the Australian neem industry did not prove viable. The tree has now spread into the savanna, particularly around waterways, and naturalised populations exist in several areas.

Uses

Neem leaves are dried in India and placed in cupboards to prevent insects eating the clothes, and also in tins where rice is stored. Neem leaves are dried and burnt in the tropical regions to keep away mosquitoes. These flowers are also used in many Indian festivals like Ugadi. As an ayurvedic herb, neem is also used in baths.

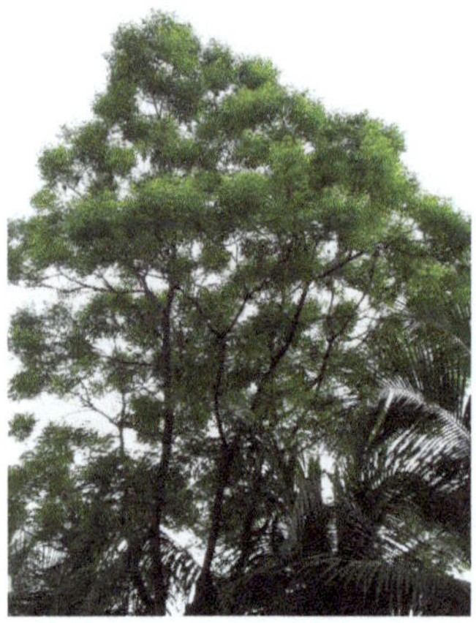

Neem tree

As A Vegetable

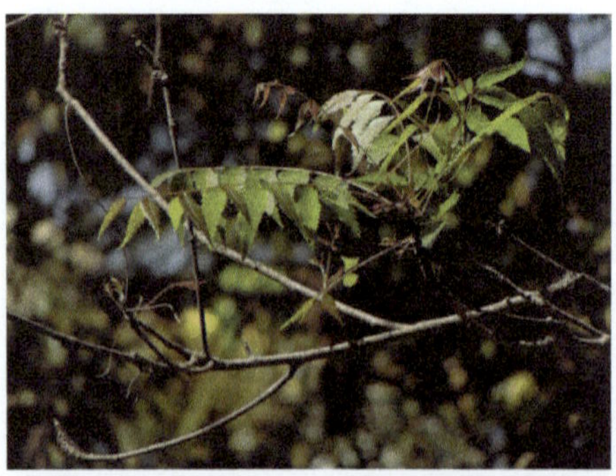

Tender neem leaves used as medicine, Karnataka, India

The tender shoots and flowers of the neem tree are eaten as a vegetable in India. A souplike dish called *Veppampoo charu* (Tamil) (translated as "neem flower rasam") made of the flower of neem is prepared in Tamil Nadu. In West Bengal, young neem leaves are fried in oil with tiny pieces of eggplant (brinjal). The dish is called *nim begun* and is the first item during a Bengali meal that acts as an appetizer. It is eaten with rice.

Neem is used in parts of mainland Southeast Asia, particularly in Cambodia aka sdov—ស្ដៅ, Laos (where it is called *kadao*), Thailand (where it is known as *sadao* or *sdao*), Myanmar (where it is known as *tamar*) and Vietnam (where it is known as *sầu đâu* and is used to cook the salad *gỏi sầu đâu*). Even lightly cooked, the flavour is quite bitter and the food is not enjoyed by all inhabitants of these nations, though it is believed to be good for one's health. Neem gum is a rich source of protein. In Myanmar, young neem leaves and flower buds are boiled with tamarind fruit to soften its bitterness and eaten as a vegetable. Pickled neem leaves are also eaten with tomato and fish paste sauce in Myanmar.

Traditional Medicinal Use

Products made from neem trees have been used in India for over two millennia for their medicinal properties. Neem products are believed by Siddha and Ayurvedic practitioners to be Anthelmintic, antifungal, antidiabetic, antibacterial, antiviral, contraceptive, and sedative. It is considered a major component in siddha medicine and Ayurvedic and Unani medicine and is particularly prescribed for skin diseases. Neem oil is also used for healthy hair, to improve liver function, detoxify the blood, and balance blood sugar levels. Neem leaves have also been used to treat skin diseases like eczema, psoriasis, etc.

Insufficient research has been done to assess the purported benefits of neem, however. In adults, short-term use of neem is safe, while long-term use may harm the kidneys or liver; in small children, neem oil is toxic and can lead to death. Neem may also cause miscarriages, infertility, and low blood sugar.

Safety Issues

Neem oil can cause some forms of toxic encephalopathy and ophthalmopathy if consumed in large quantities.

Pest and Disease Control

Neem is a key ingredient in non-pesticidal management (NPM), providing a natural alternative to synthetic pesticides. Neem seeds are ground into a powder that is soaked overnight in water and sprayed onto the crop. To be effective, it must be applied repeatedly, at least every ten days. Neem does not directly kill insects on the crop. It acts as an anti-feedant, repellent, and egg-laying deterrent, protecting the crop from damage. The insects starve and die within a few days. Neem also suppresses the hatching of pest insects from their eggs. Neem cake is often sold as a fertilizer.

Neem oil has been shown to avert termite attack as an ecofriendly and economical agent.

Neem Oil for Polymeric Resins

Applications of neem oil in the preparation of polymeric resins have been documented in the recent reports. The synthesis of various alkyd resins from neem oil is reported using a monoglyceride (MG) route and their utilization for the preparation of PU coatings. The alkyds are prepared from reaction of conventional divalent acid materials like phthalic and maleic anhydrides with MG of neem oil. In other reports, different routes for preparation of polymeric resins from neem oil also are reported.

Construction

The juice of this plant is a potent ingredent for a mixture of wall plaster, according to the Samarā□ga□a Sūtradhāra, which is a Sanskrit treatise dealing with Śilpaśāstra (Hindu science of art and construction).

Other Uses

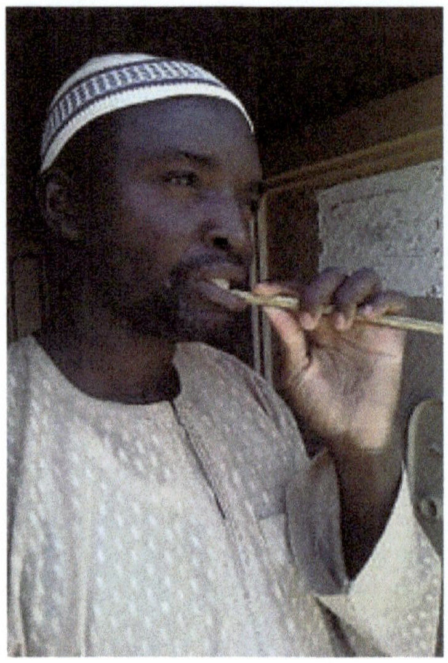

cleaning teeth by chewing stick

- Toiletries: Neem oil is used for preparing cosmetics such as soap, shampoo, balms, and creams as well as toothpaste
- Animal Treatment: Used to treat sweet itch and mud fever in horses
- Toothbrush: Traditionally, slender neem twigs (called datun) are first chewed as a toothbrush and then split as a tongue cleaner. This practice has been in use in India, Africa, and the Middle East for centuries. Many of India's 80% rural population still start their day with the chewing stick, while in urban areas neem toothpaste is preferred. Neem twigs are still collected and sold in markets for this use, and in rural India one often sees youngsters in the streets chewing on neem twigs. It has been found to be as effective as a toothbrush in reducing plaque and gingival inflammation.
- Tree: Besides its use in traditional Indian medicine, the neem tree is of great importance for its anti-desertification properties and possibly as a good carbon dioxide sink.
- Neem gum is used as a bulking agent and for the preparation of special purpose foods.
- Neem blossoms are used in Andhra Pradesh, Tamil Nadu, and Karnataka to prepare Ugadi pachhadi. A mixture of neem flowers and jaggery (or unrefined brown sugar) is prepared and

offered to friends and relatives, symbolic of sweet and bitter events in the upcoming new year, Ugadi. "*Bevina hoovina gojju*" (a type of curry prepared with neem blossoms) is common in Karnataka throughout the year. Dried blossoms are used when fresh blossoms are not available. In Tamil Nadu, a rasam (veppam poo rasam) made with neem blossoms is a culinary specialty.

- Cosmetics : Neem is perceived in India as a beauty aid. Powdered leaves are a major component of at least one widely used facial cream. Purified neem oil is also used in nail polish and other cosmetics.
- Bird repellent: Neem leaf boiled in water can be used as a very cost-effective bird repellent, especially for sparrows.
- Lubricant : Neem oil is non-drying and it resists degradation better than most vegetable oils. In rural India, it is commonly used to grease cart wheels.
- Fertilizer : Neem has demonstrated considerable potential as a fertilizer. Neem cake is widely used to fertilize cash crops, particularly sugarcane and vegetables.
- Plant protectant : Ploughed into the soil, it protects plant roots from nematodes and white ants, probably as it contains the residual limonoids. In Karnataka, people grow the tree mainly for its green leaves and twigs, which they puddle into flooded rice fields before the rice seedlings are transplanted.
- Resin : An exudate can be tapped from the trunk by wounding the bark. This high protein material is not a substitute for polysaccharide gum, such as gum arabic. It may, however, have a potential as a food additive, and it is widely used in South Asia as "Neem glue".
- Bark : Neem bark contains 14% tannin, an amount similar to that in conventional tannin-yielding trees (such as Acacia decurrens). Moreover, it yields a strong, coarse fibre commonly woven into ropes in the villages of India.
- Honey : In parts of Asia neem honey commands premium prices, and people promote apiculture by planting neem trees.
- Soap : 80% of India›s supply of neem oil now is used by neem oil soap manufacturers. Although much of it goes to small-scale speciality soaps, often using cold-pressed oil, large-scale producers also use it, mainly because it is cheap. Additionally it is antibacterial and antifungal, soothing, and moisturising. It can be made with up to 40% neem oil.]]. Generally, the crude oil is used to produce coarse laundry soaps.
- Against pox viruses : In India, people who are affected with pox viruses are generally made to lie in bed made of neem leaves and branches. The belief is that it prevents the spreading of pox virus to others and has been in practice since early centuries.

Association with Hindu Festivals in India

Neem leaf or bark is considered an effective pitta pacifier because of its bitter taste. Hence, it is traditionally recommended during early summer in Ayurveda (that is, the month of Chaitra as per the Hindu Calendar which usually falls in the month of March – April).

In the Indian states of Telangana, Andhra Pradesh and Karnataka, Neem flowers are very popular for their use in 'Ugadi Pachhadi' (soup-like pickle), which is made on Ugadi day. In Telangana, Andhra Pradesh, and Karnataka, a small amount of Neem and Jaggery (Bevu-Bella) is consumed on Ugadi day, the Telugu and Kannada new year, indicating that one should take both bitter and sweet things in life, joy and sorrow.

During Gudi Padva, which is the New Year in the state of Maharashtra, the ancient practice of drinking a small quantity of neem juice or paste on that day, before starting festivities, is found. As in many Hindu festivals and their association with some food to avoid negative side-effects of the season or change of seasons, neem juice is associated with Gudi Padva to remind people to use it during that particular month or season to pacify summer pitta.

In Tamil Nadu during the summer months of April to June, the Mariamman temple festival is a thousand-year-old tradition. The Neem leaves and flowers are the most important part of the Mariamman festival. The statue of the goddess Mariamman will be garlanded with Neem leaves and flowers. During most occasions of celebrations and weddings the people of Tamil Nadu adorn their surroundings with the Neem leaves and flowers as a form of decoration and also to ward off evil spirits and infections.

In the eastern coastal state of Odisha the famous Jagannath temple deities are made up of Neem heart wood along with some other essential oils and powders.

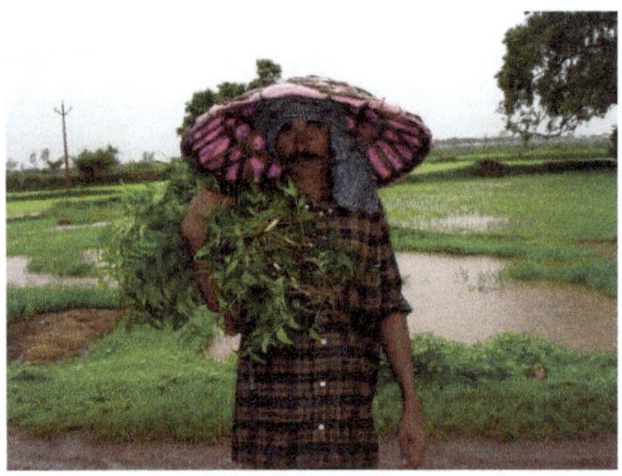

Native of Chhattisgarh with Neem branches and leaves for Hareli Festival

Chemical Compounds

Ayurveda was the first to bring the anthelmintic, antifungal, antibacterial, and antiviral constituents of the Neem tree to the attention of natural products chemists. The process of extracting neem oil involves extracting the water-insoluble components with ether, petrol ether, ethyl acetate, and dilute alcohol. The provisional naming was *nimbin* (sulphur-free crystalline product with melting point at 205 °C, empirical composition $C_7H_{10}O_2$), *nimbinin* (with similar principle, melting at 192 °C), and *nimbidin* (cream-coloured containing amorphous sulphur, melting at 90–100 °C). Siddiqui identified *nimbidin* as the main active antibacterial ingredient, and the highest yielding bitter component in the neem oil. These compounds are stable and found in substantial quantities in the Neem. They also serve as natural insecticides.

Neem-coated urea is being used an alternate to plain urea fertilizer in India. It reduces pollution, improves fertilizer's efficacy and soil health.

Genome and Transcriptomes

Neem genome and transcriptomes from various organs have been sequenced, analyzed, and published by Ganit Labs in Bangalore, India.

ESTs were identify by generation of subtractive hybridization libraries of neem fruit, leaf, fruit mesocarp, and fruit endocarp by CSIR-CIMAP Lucknow.

Cultural and Social Impact

In Theravada Buddhism, the neem tree is said to have been used to achieve enlightenment (*bodhi*) by Tissa, the twentieth reincarnation of Lord Buddha. Some sources claim, however, that *Terminalia tomentosa* was the Bodhi tree used.

In 1995, the European Patent Office (EPO) granted a patent on an anti-fungal product derived from neem to the United States Department of Agriculture and W. R. Grace and Company. The Indian government challenged the patent when it was granted, claiming that the process for which the patent had been granted had been in use in India for more than 2,000 years. In 2000, the EPO ruled in India's favour, but W. R. Grace appealed, claiming that prior art about the product had never been published in a scientific journal. On 8 March 2005, that appeal was lost and the EPO revoked the Neem patent.

Symbolism

Previously, neem had been declared as the national tree of the former Hyderabad State, now defunct.

Biotechnology

The biopesticide produced by extraction from the tree seeds contains limonoids. Currently, the extraction process has disadvantages such as contamination with fungi and heterogeneity in the content of limonoids due to genetic, climatic, and geographical variations. To overcome these problems, production of limonoids from plant cell suspension and hairy root cultures in bioreactors has been studied, including the development of a two-stage bioreactor process that enhances growth and production of limonoids with cell suspension cultures of *A. indica*.

Cedrus Deodara

Cedrus deodara (deodar cedar, Himalayan cedar, or deodar/devdar/devadar/devadaru; Sanskrit devadāru, Hindi: *devadār*, *dāruk*; Urdu: رادويد/ رای‌د *deodār*; Kannada:Chinese: 雪松 *xuě sōng*) is a species of cedar native to the western Himalayas in eastern Afghanistan, northern Pakistan (especially in Khyber Pakhtunkhwa) and India (Jammu and Kashmir, Himachal Pradesh, Sikkim, Darjeeling and Uttarakhand states), southwesternmost Tibet in (China) and western Nepal, occurring at 1,500–3,200 m (4,921–10,499 ft) altitude. It is a large evergreen coniferous tree reaching 40–50 m (131–164 ft) tall, exceptionally 60 m (197 ft) with a trunk up to 3 m (10 ft) in diameter. It has a conic crown with level branches and drooping branchlets.

The leaves are needle-like, mostly 2.5–5 cm (0.98–1.97 in) long, occasionally up to 7 cm (2.8 in) long, slender (1 mm (0.039 in) thick), borne singly on long shoots, and in dense clusters of 20–30 on short shoots; they vary from bright green to glaucous blue-green in colour. The female cones are barrel-shaped, 7–13 cm (2.8–5.1 in) long and 5–9 cm (2.0–3.5 in) broad, and disintegrate when mature (in 12 months) to release the winged seeds. The male cones are 4–6 cm (1.6–2.4 in) long, and shed their pollen in autumn.

Etymology

The botanical name, which is also the English common name, derives from the Sanskrit term *devadāru*, which means "wood of the gods", a compound of *deva* "god" and *dāru* "wood, tree".

Cultural Importance in The Indian Subcontinent

Among Hindus, as the etymology of deodar suggests, it is worshiped as a divine tree. Deva, the first half of the Sanskrit term, means *divine*, *deity*, or *deus*. Dāru, the second part, is cognate with (related to) the words *durum*, *druid*, *tree*, and *true*.

Several Hindu legends refer to this tree. For example, Valmiki Ramayan – Kishkinda khanda-stanza 4-43-13 reads:

lodhra padmaka khaNDeSu devadaaru vaneSu ca |

raavaNaH saha vaidehyaa maargitavyaa tataH tataH || || 4-43-13

That means "In the stands of Lodhra trees, Padmaka trees and in the woods of Devadaru, or Deodar trees, Ravana is to be searched there and there, together with Sita. [4-43-13]"

Forests full of Deodar or Devadāru trees were the favorite living place of ancient Indian sages and their families who were devoted to the Hindu god Shiva. To please Lord Shiva, the sages used to perform very difficult tapasya (meditation) practices in deodar forests. Also the ancient Hindu epics and Shaivite texts regularly mention *Darukavana*, meaning a forest of deodars, as a sacred place.

The deodar is the national tree of Pakistan.

Cultivation and Uses

The most cold-tolerant trees originate in the northwest of the species' range in Kashmir and Paktia Province, Afghanistan. Selected cultivars from this region are hardy to USDA zone 7 or even zone 6, tolerating temperatures down to about −30 °C (−22 °F). Named cultivars from this region include 'Eisregen', 'Eiswinter', 'Karl Fuchs', 'Kashmir', 'Polar Winter', and 'Shalimar'. Of these, 'Eisregen', 'Eiswinter', 'Karl Fuchs', and 'Polar Winter' were selected in Germany from seed collected in Paktia; 'Kashmir' was a selection of the nursery trade, whereas 'Shalimar' originated from seeds collected in 1964 from Shalimar Gardens, India (in the Kashmir region) and propagated at the Arnold Arboretum.

This plant has gained the Royal Horticultural Society's Award of Garden Merit.

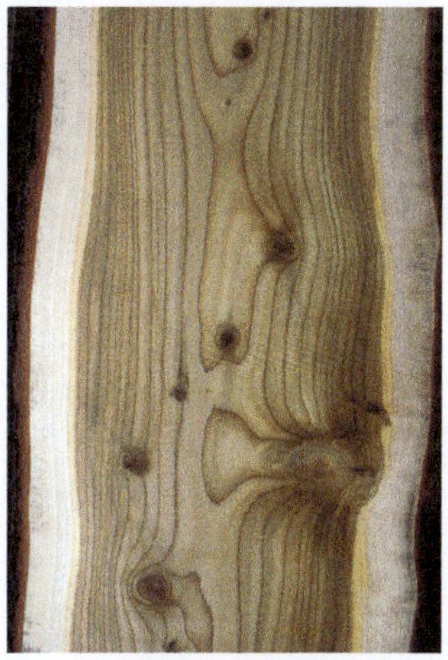

It is widely grown as an ornamental tree, often planted in parks and large gardens for its drooping foliage. General cultivation is limited to areas with mild winters, with trees frequently killed by temperatures below about −25 °C (−13 °F), limiting it to USDA zone 7 and warmer for reliable growth. It can succeed in rather cool-summer climates, as in Stateline, Nevada, and Ushuaia, Argentina.

Construction Material

Deodar is in great demand as building material because of its durability, rot-resistant character and fine, close grain, which is capable of taking a high polish. Its historical use to construct religious temples and in landscaping around temples is well recorded. Its rot-resistant character also makes it an ideal wood for constructing the well-known houseboats of Srinagar, Kashmir. In Pakistan and India, during the British colonial period, deodar wood was used extensively for construction of barracks, public buildings, bridges, canals and railway cars. Despite its durability, it is not a strong timber, and its brittle nature makes it unsuitable for delicate work where strength is required, such as chair-making.

Herbal Ayurveda

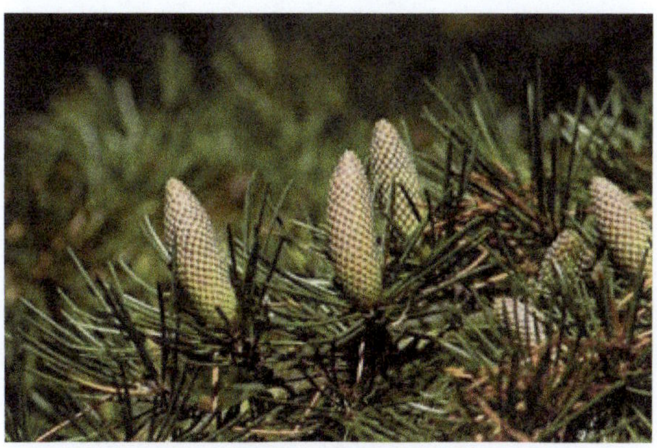

Cones of Deodar

The use of *C. deodara* in Ayurvedic medicines is well recorded.

The inner wood is aromatic and used to make incense. Inner wood is distilled into essential oil. As insects avoid this tree, the essential oil is used as insect repellent on the feet of horses, cattle and camels. It also has antifungal properties and has some potential for control of fungal deterioration of spices during storage. The outer bark and stem are astringent.

Because of its antifungal and insect repellent properties, rooms made of Deodar (Cedrus deodara) wood are used to store meat and food grains like oats and wheat in Shimla, Kullu and Kinnaur district of Himachal Pradesh. In Himachal people suffering from asthma or other respiratory problems are advised to sit under a Deodar tree early in the morning.

Cedar oil is often used for its aromatic properties, especially in aromatherapy. It has a characteristic woody odour which may change somewhat in the course of drying out. The crude oils are often yellowish or darker in colour. Its applications cover soap perfumes, household sprays, floor polishes and insecticides and is also used in microscope work as a clearing oil.

Chemistry

The bark of *Cedrus deodara* contains large amounts of taxifolin. The wood contains cedeodarin (6-methyltaxifolin), dihydromyricetin (ampelopsin), cedrin (6-methyldihydromyricetin), cedrinoside and deodarin (3′,4′,5,6-tetrahydroxy-8-methyl dihydroflavonol). The main components of the needle essential oil include α-terpineol (30.2%), linalool (24.47%), limonene (17.01%), anethole (14.57%), caryophyllene (3.14%) and eugenol (2.14%). The deodar cedar also contains lignans and the phenolic sesquiterpene himasecolone together with isopimaric acid. Other compounds have been identified as (−)-matairesinol, (−)-nortrachelogenin and a dibenzylbutyrolactollignan (4,4',9-trihydroxy-3,3'-dimethoxy-9,9'-epoxylignan).

Terminalia Arjuna

Terminalia arjuna is a tree of the genus *Terminalia*. It is commonly known as arjuna or arjun tree in English, thella maddi in Telugu, kumbuk in Sinhala, marudha maram in Tamil and neer maruthu in Malayalam.

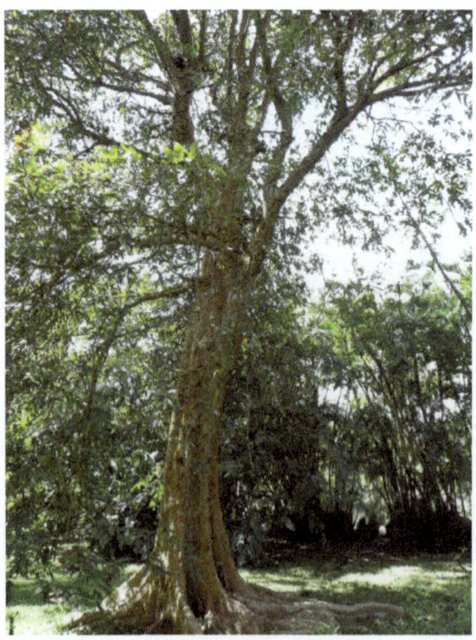

Terminalia arjuna

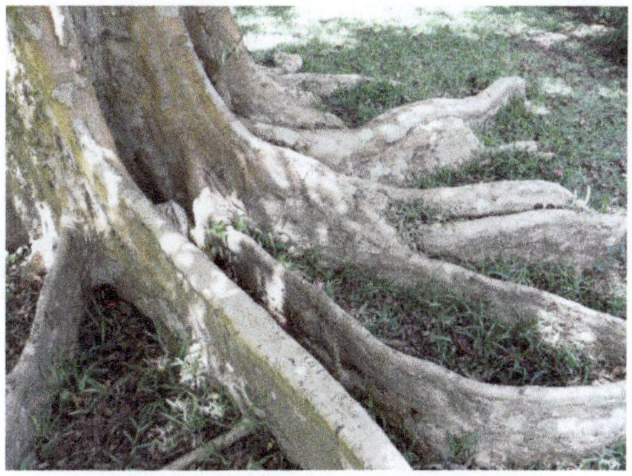

Terminalia arjuna lower trunk

Description

The arjuna is about 20–25 metres tall; usually has a buttressed trunk, and forms a wide canopy at the crown, from which branches drop downwards. It has oblong, conical leaves which are green on the top and brown below; smooth, grey bark; it has pale yellow flowers which appear between March and June; its glabrous, 2.5 to 5 cm fibrous woody fruit, divided into five wings, appears between September and November.

Distribution and Habitat

The arjuna is usually found growing on river banks or near dry river beds in Bangladesh, Uttar Pradesh, Madhya Pradesh, West Bengal and south and central India. It is known as *matthimara* in Kannada, *neer maruthu* in Malayalam 'marutha maram' (marutham pattai) in Tamil, thella maddi in Telugu and *kohda* in Rajasthan.

Importance

Silk Production

The arjuna is one of the species whose leaves are fed on by the *Antheraea paphia* moth which produces the tassar silk, a wild silk of commercial importance.

Alternative Medicine

The arjuna was introduced into Ayurveda as a treatment for heart disease by Vagbhata (c. 7th century CE). It is traditionally prepared as a milk decoction. In the Ashtānga Hridayam, but was also mentioned in many ancient Indian vedas, and was a known practice for thousands of years, passed down by tradition, before vagbhata mentioned it in his writings. Vagbhata mentions arjuna in the treatment of wounds, hemorrhages and ulcers, applied topically as a powder. Arjuna is an excellent medicine for Heart, it has the capability to even reverse heart failure. The Arjuna plant (lat. Terminalia Arjuna) has traditionally been used to treat heart disease for centuries, which is why it got the nickname "Guardian of the heart." It's named after the hero of the famous epic "Mahabharata", because of its protective effects. Arjuna is an evergreen tree of the Combretaceae family, which grows along the rivers of West Bengal in the drained beds of central and southern India. In Ayurveda,it's considered a sacred plant.

Scientific Research

Recent studies in rat model have shown its preventive potential in monocrotaline induced pulmonary artery hypertension. It prevents rise in right ventricular systolic pressure, right ventricular hypertrophy, % medial wall thickness, echo-cardiographic changes through inhibition of reactive oxygen species (ROS)Reactive_oxygen_species mediated pulmonary vascular remodeling. It has also been identified to inhibit NADPH oxidase (NOX1)NADPH_oxidase in lung homogenate.

In Buddhism

In Theravada Buddhism, arjuna is said to have used as the tree for achieved enlightenment, or Bodhi by tenth Lord Buddha called "Anomadassi - අනෝමදස්සී". The plant is known as කුඹුක් (kumbuk) in Sinhala in Sri Lanka.

Phyllanthus Emblica

Phyllanthus emblica, also known as emblic, emblic myrobalan, myrobalan, Indian gooseberry, Malacca tree, or amla from Sanskrit amalika is a deciduous tree of the family Phyllanthaceae. It is known for its edible fruit of the same name.

Plant Morphology and Harvesting

The tree is small to medium in size, reaching 1–8 m (3 ft 3 in–26 ft 3 in) in height. The branchlets aren't glabrous or finely pubescent, 10–20 cm (3.9–7.9 in) long, usually deciduous; the leaves are simple, subsessile and closely set along branchlets, light green, resembling pinnate leaves. The flowers are greenish-yellow. The fruit is nearly spherical, light greenish yellow, quite smooth and hard on appearance, with six vertical stripes or furrows.

Ripening in autumn, the berries are harvested by hand after climbing to upper branches bearing the fruits. The taste of Indian emblic is sour, bitter and astringent, and it is quite fibrous. In India, it is common to eat emblic steeped in salt water and red chilli powder to make the sour fruits palatable.

Cultural and Religious Significance

Fruit with young leaves and flower buds.

The tree is considered sacred by Hindus as God Vishnu is believed to dwell in it. The tree is worshiped on Amalaka Ekadashi.

In other Hindu beliefs, Amla is said to have originated from the drops of Amrit which spilled on earth accidentally, because of the fight of Gods and Demons after ksheera sagar manthan. And hence also this religious belief makes claims that it almost cures every disease and is also good in extending the longevity of life.

In the Sanskrit Buddhist tradition half an amalaka fruit was the final gift to the Buddhist sangha by the great Indian emperor Ashoka. This is illustrated in the Ashokavadana in the following verses:

"A great donor, the lord of men, the eminent Maurya Ashoka, has gone from being lord of Jambudvipa [the continent] to being lord of half a myrobalan." (Strong, 1983, p. 99) This deed became so famous that a stupa was created to mark the place of the event in modern-day Patna and was known as the Amalaka stupa.

According to Hindu tradition, Adi Shankara of Kerala composed and recited the Kanakadhara stotram in praise of Mahalakshmi to make a poor Brahmin lady get wealth, in return for a single amla presented to him as bhiksha on an auspicious dwadashi day. Contemporary poet/philosopher Ravi Teja Yelamanchili wrote a book titled Amalaki. The book is based on Advaita Vedanta of Sri Adi Shankaracharya.

According to a Tamil legend, Avvaiyar, a female poet, ethicist and political activist of the Sangam period was gifted with one amla by King Athiyaman to give her long life.

In Theravada Buddhism, this plant is said to have been used as the tree for achieving enlightenment, or Bodhi by twenty first Lord Buddha called "Pussa - පුස්ස".

Traditional Uses

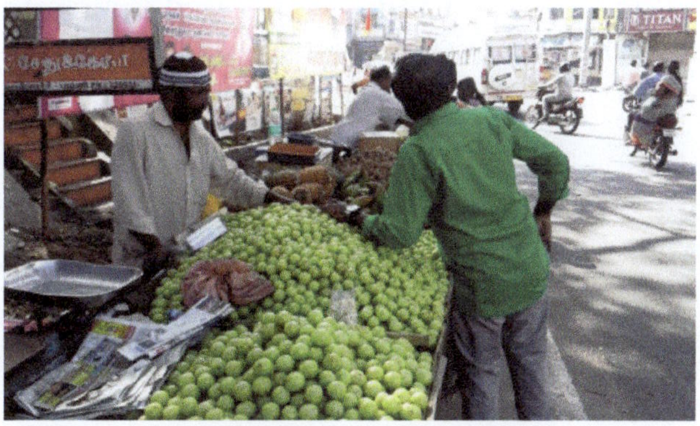

Emblic seller in Pollachi, India

Traditional Medicine

In traditional Indian medicine, dried and fresh fruits of the plant are used. All parts of the plant are used in various Ayurvedic/Unani medicine (*Jawarish amla*) herbal preparations, including the fruit, seed, leaves, root, bark and flowers. According to Ayurveda, amla fruit is sour (*amla*) and astringent (*kashaya*) in taste (*rasa*), with sweet (*madhura*), bitter (*tikta*) and pungent (*katu*) secondary tastes (*anurasas*). Its qualities (*gunas*) are light (*laghu*) and dry (*ruksha*), the postdigestive effect (*vipaka*) is sweet (*madhura*) and its energy (*virya*) is cooling (*shita*).

According to Ayurveda, amla balances all three doshas. While amla is unusual in that it contains five out of the six tastes recognized by Ayurveda, it is most important to recognize the effects of the "virya", or potency, and "vipaka", or post-digestive effect. Considered in this light, amla is particularly helpful in reducing *pitta* because of its cooling energy. It also balances both Pitta and *vata* by virtue of its sweet taste. The *kapha* is balanced primarily due to its drying action. It may be used as a *rasayana* (rejuvenative) to promote longevity, and traditionally to enhance digestion (*dipanapachana*), treat constipation (*anuloma*), reduce fever (*jvaraghna*), purify the blood (*raktaprasadana*), reduce cough (*kasahara*), alleviate asthma (*svasahara*), strengthen the heart (*hrdaya*), benefit the eyes (*chakshushya*), stimulate hair growth (*romasanjana*), enliven the body (*jivaniya*), and enhance intellect (*medhya*).

In Ayurvedic polyherbal formulations, Indian gooseberry is a common constituent, and most notably is the primary ingredient in an ancient herbal *rasayana* called *Chyawanprash*. This formula, which contains 43 herbal ingredients as well as clarified butter, sesame oil, sugar cane juice, and honey, was first mentioned in the Charaka Samhita as a premier rejuvenative compound.

In Chinese traditional therapy, this fruit is called *yuganzi* (余甘子), which is used to treat throat inflammation.

Culinary Use

Maharashtra is one of the largest producers and suppliers of Indian gooseberries. In this region the fruit is commonly pickled with salt, oil, and spices. The amla fruit is eaten raw or cooked into various dishes. In Andhra Pradesh, tender varieties are used to prepare *dal* (a lentil preparation), and *amle ka murabbah*, a sweet dish made by soaking the berries in sugar syrup until they are candied. It is traditionally consumed after meals.

In the Batak area of Sumatra, Indonesia, the inner bark is used to impart an astringent, bitter taste to the broth of a traditional fish soup known as *holat*.

Other Uses

Popularly used in inks, shampoos and hair oils, the high tannin content of Indian gooseberry fruit serves as a mordant for fixing dyes in fabrics. Amla shampoos and hair oil are traditionally believed to nourish the hair and scalp and prevent premature grey hair.

In Kerala, well beds are lined with *Emblica* timber (നെല്ലിപ്പലക) to get clean and sweet water for drinking and cooking.

Pharmacological Research

In Vitro (On Cells)

Indian gooseberry has undergone preliminary research, demonstrating *in vitro* antiviral and antimicrobial properties. There is preliminary evidence *in vitro* that its extracts induce apoptosis and modify gene expression in osteoclasts involved in rheumatoid arthritis and osteoporosis. It may prove to have potential activity against some cancers.

In Vivo (In Animals)

One recent animal study found treatment with *E. officinalis* reduced severity of acute pancreatitis (induced by L-arginine in rats). It also promoted the spontaneous repair and regeneration process of the rat pancreas occurring after an acute attack.

Experimental preparations of leaves, bark or fruit have shown potential efficacy against laboratory models of disease, such as for inflammation, cancer, age-related renal disease, and diabetes.

Emblica officinalis tea may ameliorate diabetic neuropathy due to aldose reductase inhibition.

In rats it significantly reduced blood glucose, food intake, water intake and urine output in diabetic rats compared with the non- diabetic control group.

Another recent study with alloxan-induced diabetic rats given an aqueous amla fruit extract has shown significant decrease of the blood glucose, as well as triglyceridemic levels and an improvement of the liver function caused by a normalization of the liver-specific enzyme alanine transaminase activity.

Clinical Studies

A human pilot study demonstrated a reduction of blood cholesterol levels in both normal and hypercholesterolemic men with treatment.

Chemical Constituents

Although these fruits are reputed to contain high amounts of ascorbic acid (vitamin C), up to 445 mg per 100 g, the specific contents are disputed, and the overall antioxidant strength of amla may derive instead from its high density of ellagitannins such as emblicanin A (37%), emblicanin B (33%), punigluconin (12%) and pedunculagin (14%). It also contains punicafolin and phyllanemblinin A, phyllanemblin other polyphenols: flavonoids, kaempferol, ellagic acid and gallic acid.

Vernacular Names

Names for this plant in various languages include:
Lozü in Ao languages
halïlaj or *ihlïlaj* (هليلج اهليلج) in Arabic
amlakhi in Assamese
balakka in Batak language, an Indonesian language
amloki (আমলকী) in Bengali
Amlai in Bodo language
anmole (庵摩勒) in Chinese
ambare in Garo language
āmla in Gujarati
ānvalā in Hindi
Kantout Prei (កន្ទួតព្រៃ) in Khmer
Bettada nellikaayi in Kannada
sohmylleng in Khasi
āvāo in Konkani
mak kham bom in Lao
melaka (ملاك) in Malay, A state in Malaysia, Malacca was named after this tree.
nelli (നെല്ലി) in Malayalam
heikru in Manipuri
āvaā (or *awla*) in Marathi
sunhlu in Mizo
zee phyu thee in Myanmar
amalā in Nepali
anlaa (ଅଁଳା) in Oriya
Suaklu in Paite

Aula (ਔਲਾ) in Punjabi
amalika in Sanskrit
Dhatric in Sanskrit, Maithili
nelli (නෙල්ලි) in Sinhala
Nelli (Root Word) or Nellikkāy *or Nellikani* in Tamil
aavnlaa (*amla* or *ambla* or *awla*) in Urdu
usiri kaay in Telugu
ma kham pom (มะขามป้อม) in Thai
skyu ru ra (སྐྱུ་རུ་ར་) in Tibetan
Amla (آملہ) in Urdu

Ayurvedic Acupressure

Ayurvedic Acupressure (also known as Marma therapy) is a particular kind of massage or an alternative medical treatment, which integrates the knowledge of ancient Ayurveda and the principles of acupressure, allegedly to completely heal and cure physical, mental, emotional and spiritual illnesses.

According to Charaka Samhitā, an early text on Ayurveda (Indian traditional medicine), the cosmos and its correspondence – the human body, are composed of both physical (Visible) and metaphysical (Invisible) forces.

Ayurvedic acupressure talks about 10 elements – 5 physical and 5 metaphysical.

- 5 physical elements: – Space, Air, Fire, Water and Earth.
- 5 metaphysical elements: – Time, Direction, Mind, Soul and Tam (Origin).

In Ayurveda the pressure points or the meridians are called Marma points. These are considered as energy points, just as Chinese refer them as pressure points, and they help in stimulating not only circulation, but also improve mental and emotional outlook. The Marma points are located throughout the body.

Treatment in Ayurvedic Acupressure can be easily done without needles by:

- Applying pressure with finger
- Seeds
- Magnets
- Colours

The Acupressure shodh prashikshan evam upchar sansthan Allahabad is an non government organization working for the last 20 years in popularizing the Ayurvedic Acupressure

There are many branches of acupressure/acupuncture as we know it today. They are

- Traditional Chinese Medicine (TCM)
- Ayurvedic Acupressure
- Sujok
- Reflexology

These are just some of the forms. The scope and theories of each are a bit different.

Ayurveda in The United States

Ayurveda is an indigenous medical system of India that arose over 2,000 years ago. Despite its long history, this system has a dynamic, continually changing past and present: as Ayurveda spreads form the East to the West and encounters new influences, it has become redefined by cultural and social biases.

History of Ayurveda in The West

Initial Western Encounters with Ayurveda

Ayurvedic doctors and European doctors initially encountered one another through the spice trade that also exchanged botanicals and pharmaceuticals. Some Indian medicinal knowledge had already spread through texts and oral transmission. Later, the export of medicines along with the basic knowledge of their traditional applications became an international, large-scale commercial enterprise. By the nineteenth and twentieth centuries, during the British colonial period, this exchange reached its peak. Colonial Britain and British scholars initially took a keen interest in the ancient medical system and encouraged the study and practice of Ayurveda.

A 1924 article in The Lancet provides interesting insight into Western attitudes toward Ayurveda. The anonymous author, presumably of Western origin and education, writes in reaction to the establishment of a new scientific journal, the *Journal of Ayurveda,* published from Calcutta, India and edited by a Western-educated medical doctor and Sanskrit scholar. The writer notes that in earlier literature, Ayurvedic practitioners denounced Western medicine entirely, alienating the West; he then writes that the new magazine showcases efforts to use empirical scientific methods to test the efficacy of Ayurvedic treatments and consequently allies itself closely with Western biomedicine advances. The brief article thus indicates that a new collaborative relationship was forming based on mutual respect. Even at this early stage, there were well-known Western scholars who encouraged Ayurveda as the primary medical practice of India, although this respect was reserved for "modern Ayurveda," that which was supported with the more "progressive Western medicine" and did not only depend on "charms and incantations."

As the colonial era ended, a nationalistic push to standardize Ayurvedic education was born; the age-old teaching system of passing down knowledge exclusively from master to disciple or through family lines (thereby maintaining educational lineages) began to come to an end. By this time Western biomedicine had earned a name as reputable and even "superior," so when Ayurvedic colleges developed and became established, Ayurveda was recast in Western terms and taught alongside biomedicine in order to seem competent. For the first time, Ayurveda had to directly compete with another medical system, though previously it had coexisted for centuries among various medical traditions.

Ayurveda Arrives in The West

Besides the initial pre-colonial and colonial transfers of Indian medical knowledge, Ayurveda arrived to North America and Europe as Indian immigrants spread across the globe. However, very little information about Indian medicine (homogeneous or otherwise) became accessible to the public (Source12). In the 1970s and 1980s, the political and social environment was largely characterized by an effort and rebellion against the mainstream. During this time, Ayurveda came into public view primarily through the New Age movement that rallied around the work of a few individual spiritual leaders. The New Age movement is centered on the idea that a new epoch of human history is approaching and as a result teaches that humans must strive to achieve spiritual balance and wellness. The recently standardized system of biomedicine of this time began to represent empiricism, commercialism, and impersonal industry, and those who comprised the New Age Movement looked to alternative systems of medicine that would be personalized, ethical/spiritual, less expensive, and holistic. Thus when the New Age movement brought Ayurveda into the American public eye, and the system was introduced in juxtaposition to mainstream medicine. Ayurveda could not and did not become popularized as a legitimate medical system.

"New Age Ayurveda"

Several paradigms of Ayurveda unique to Western practice have emerged over the past few decades, but perhaps the most pervasive paradigm imprinted in the mind of the American public is a form of practice termed "New Age Ayurveda." Although the New Age movement slowly died out in past decades, many of its core ideologies have begun to resurface in recent years, bringing along with it a revival of sorts for a new form of Ayurveda. The earliest successful promoters of Ayurveda in America included individuals like Maharishi Mahesh Yogi, Deepak Chopra, Vasant Lad, David Frawley, etc.; who sought to popularize their particular varieties of Ayurvedic practices to a larger audience. These varieties of Ayurveda all share a common acceptance of New Age beliefs and incorporate many of these beliefs into their practices. Zysk (2001) identifies four particular characteristics unique to New Age Ayurveda in America in particular: linking Ayurveda to Indian spirituality (using yoga in particular), depicting Ayurveda as ancient beyond evidence, calling Ayurveda the foundation of mind-body medicine, and trying to use Western scientific principles to prove that Ayurveda is legitimate and more effective than biomedicine. Such forms also tend to make extensive, broad claims about efficacy and "correctness" that directly contradicts even the writings of classical texts. New Age Ayurveda often claims to be without side effects, that natural remedies can provide great benefit without any detriment to other aspects of health. Classical Ayurveda distinctly refutes this by warning that prescribing inappropriate remedies or misdiagnosing a malady can result in illness. Classical Ayurveda also employs methods such as surgery for various diseases (such as cancer) along with rational therapies for understanding and healing the mind, which are often ignored or even refuted in New Age Ayurveda against the classical opinion

Classical or Traditional Ayurveda in India also has no references to such techniques as Reiki, Pranic Healing and Chakra-balancing that are being practiced as part of modern-day American Ayurveda, either. While techniques such as Pranayama were employed in Yogic healing, these systems dramatically differ from the "faith healing" techniques in New Age Ayurveda circles. While traditional Tantric Ayurveda did employ these practices, they were more in-depth and elaborate systems that required several decades of study and practice by sadhaks or spiritual adepts.

Ayurveda has experienced many historically or academically inconsistent portrayals as a five- to eight-thousand-year-old practice, as a direct descendant of the Vedic medicine, as a Tantric tradition, etc. For any particular version of New Age Ayurveda, one or more of these claims are made as a method to increase authenticity (no matter how misleading), and therefore also popularity and recognition. Even these small controversies have caused a general rift between the scientific or academic communities and Ayurveda practitioners, resulting in a general disgust with and misconceptions about the whole medical system. Modern American practices have appropriated authentic practices so drastically that Western Ayurveda has taken a form of "wellness and self-help culture" which scholars and academics critically view as the commoditization of a deep and complex tradition.

Ayurveda in A Contemporary Lens

Influential Representatives and Writings

In the 1980s and '90's, Ayurveda was brought to the attention of the American public primarily through a few key individuals who found a ready audience in the young middle class white men and women who were dissatisfied with established religions and spiritual organizations of the time. These individuals, with mixed and matched education in Ayurveda returned to America with their own compilation and version of Ayurvedic principles and practices. They established their own schools of Ayurvedic learning and wrote extensively on their brand of Ayurveda, successfully reaching their market and making a lasting impression on the development of current Western Ayurveda.

One of the first non-academic books that introduced Ayurveda to the general public in America was Vasant Lad's *Ayurveda: The Science of Self-Healing*. Lad is a product of the earlier New Age movement, and he learned extensively under several gurus in India through the traditional master-disciple system; he also earned degrees in Ayurvedic Science from Tilak Ayurveda College. His interesting background of traditional educational lineage as well as the nationally standardized schooling is reflected in his unconventional presentation of Ayurveda. Published in 1984, Lad's first book shows a dedication to traditional Ayurveda, but it also mentions many supposedly Ayurvedic practices and tools that are not found in any Ayurvedic texts, ancient or recent. What perhaps more profoundly influenced America's initial perceptions of Ayurveda is his definition of Ayurveda as a way of innovative and empirical thought rather than one of strict adherence to classical texts.

Robert Svoboda, a similar figure whose Ayurvedic education has roots in both formal and traditional Indian systems of schooling, also contributed to the promotion of Ayurveda in the late 1990s. Rather than defining Ayurveda in a Western framework, his written work primarily set Ayurveda within its own concepts. His 1998 work Prakriti: Your Ayurvedic Constitution avoided all discussion of Western or allopathic parallels, unlike predecessors who still used Western terms to juxtapose Ayurveda with biomedicine. However, the Ayurveda he explains is different from the classical Ayurveda; the emphasis is on eating, nutrition, and routine, while disease diagnostics and treatment take a backseat. His particular brand of Ayurveda makes a strong appeal to those seeking a blend of spirituality, mystique, and medicine, a characteristic trait of New Age ideology.

Deepak Chopra began his medical career in strictly biomedical sense, and he earned his medical degree in the US and specialized in endocrinology. Though Chopra is not formally or traditionally trained in Ayurveda, he spent time with vaidyas (Ayurveda practitioners) in the 1980s and eventually studied and worked with Maharishi Mahesh Yogi in the first wave of New Age Ayurvedic promotion. In his early days, Chopra established Maharishi Ayur-Ved Products International Inc., though he later separated from the group in order to pursue further individual growth and success. Chopra has written dozens of best-selling books for American audiences that portray a distinctive brand of Ayurveda, stripped of most of the Sanskrit terms, classical principles, and technical concepts. His work concerns itself primarily with issues of "quality of life" and uses accessible concepts of mind-body medicine to bridge Ayurveda and Western biomedicine. The books make use of a spiritual, optimistic tone and format that appeal to a wide audience. The overarching conceptual connections, often phrased in terms of Western science or biomedicine, are not diagnostic or treatment-based; thus the books essentially ignore a large part of Ayurveda itself: the diagnosis of disease and subsequent treatment. Over the past few decades as his popularity has increased, Deepak Chopra has become the quintessential Ayurveda practitioner in the American public's eye.

David Frawley, founder of the American Institute of Vedic Studies, initially earned a Doctor of Oriental Medicine degree through a New Mexico-based correspondence course. He later studied with Vasant Lad and Ayurveda practitioners in India and decided to become a teacher of Ayurveda himself. His approach to Ayurveda is a conventionally a Traditional approach that relates Ayurveda to Indian astrology, Hinduism, and Vedic studies. For example, he argues the traditional Yogic view of chakras in traditional Yoga and Ayurveda against the New Age views. Frawley is particularly concerned with antiquity and the classical Vedic texts as a justification or proof of authenticity, and in his many books, he often interconnects Vedic and Hindu history with that of Ayurveda and looks back to the ancient Tantric and spiritual traditions of Ayurveda, notably through Vasishtha Ganapati Muni and BL Vashta. He has coauthored books alongside traditional BAMS (Bachelor of Ayurvedic Medicine and Surgery) Physicians from India, notably Dr. Vasant Lad, Dr. Subhash Ranade and Dr. Avinash Lele.

Baba Hari Dass was one of the early proponents who helped bring Ayurveda to the US in the beginning of 1970s. He combined Patanjali's Ashtanga Yoga, Samkhya, and Ayurveda in his teachings. As interest grew, he taught classes in the *three dosha* theory, pulse detection and personal *prakriti* types derived from the classic scriptures of the *Suśrutha Sa⍰hitā* and the *Charaka Sa⍰hitha*, leading to the establishment of the Mount Madonna Institute, College of Ayurveda, Ayurveda World, and Ayurvedic pharmacy. His emphasis was often placed on ayurvedic remedies, *pancha karma*, *svedan* massage and other practices that were helpful in yogic life and in attaining dosha balance. During a period of expansion in the 1980s and 1990s, he invited several notable Ayurveidic teachers, Dr. Vasant Lad, Sarita Shrestha, M.D., Professor Ram Harsh Singh, Ph.D, Dr. Shekhar Annambhotla, BAMS, MD (Ayurveda) and others. Michael Tierra, Ayurvedic medicine practitioner, wrote: "The history of Ayurveda in North America will always owe a debt to the selfless contributions of Baba Hari Dass" (*The way of Ayurvedic Herbs*, Lotus Press, 2008, XIV).

Popular Americanized Practices

In recent years, Western Ayurveda has been drained of most of the details and distinguishing features of the first millennium classical literature, including descriptions of extreme therapies or the use of animal products in treatments. Health in the alternative medicine context has been transformed into a booming industry that propagates a diluted, exoticized and romanticized version of Ayurveda for Western markets.

Today American Ayurveda has specialized its chief market even further to young, white, middle to upper class women. The past couple decades have brought a surge in products, books, and classes that address women, through Ayurvedic versions of beauty care, yoga, aromatherapy, weight loss programs, etc. Interestingly, this trend has reached India as well; even modern Indian Ayurveda is being marketed for both Indian and Western female audiences. Perhaps one of the most obvious examples of the misappropriation of Ayurveda as an attractive marketing label is the burgeoning Ayurvedic spa culture. Aimed primarily at elite and wealthy Western women, Ayurvedic resorts located in remote locations in the US or the most scenic paradises in India provide the most expensive and elaborate commoditization of Ayurveda. Ayurveda Yoga Villa, located in Kerala, India is the archetypical example of spa culture; providing Ayurvedic massages, cosmetic treatments, yoga classes, and spiritual rejuvenation, the resort "assures the effectiveness of the applications of Ayurveda and yoga."

Slightly more accessible to the masses are the herbal medicines, "Ayurvedic yoga classes," books/ DVDs that comprise the general "self-help" market. The chosen market is still by and large well off and female, but these practices are more accessible to a wider socioeconomic group. With celebrity endorsements of various practices and treatments, studios and spas selling "Ayurvedic packages," and dozens companies specializing in Ayurvedic and yoga accessories and products, the transformation from practice to product becomes even more evident. Thus in the West, Ayurveda is rarely associated with science or medicine, and becomes instead another market to be exploited.

American Practitioners

Scott Gerson, who received his M.D. degree from the Mount Sinai School of Medicine and completed his Internal Medicine training in New York, initially studied Ayurvedic medicine at Benaras Hindu University and the Ayurvedic College in Tiruvanathapuram and earned his M.Phil. and Ph.D. in Ayurveda jointly from the University of Pune and Tilak Ayurved Mahavidyalaya (Pune). He is an Adjunct Professor at TAMV in the Department of Kayachikitsa. Dr. Gerson established The National Institute of Ayurvedic Medicine in 1984 (now The Gerson Institute of Ayurvedic Medicine) where his medical practice specializes in the diagnosis and treatment of difficult disease. His brand of Ayurveda differs from others in that he integrates, where appropriate, conventional Western medicine with the full range of Ayurvedic therapeutics including herbal medicines, individualized diets, Vedic meditation and related practices, and comprehensive medical Panchakarma (the subject of his doctoral thesis).

In Pop Culture Media

The realm of popular print and Internet literature is vast and still growing: there are a plethora of articles and books on Ayurveda (in the Western sense) that are successful because they capitalize on the romance and mystique of India and alternative therapies. The majority of these is not written by Ayurvedic doctors, and most articles simply prescribe the "Ayurvedic lifestyle" and provide guidelines for ideal eating, sleeping, and exercise routines. Garden-variety lifestyle magazines such as *Living Green Magazine* that feature pieces like "An Ayurvedic Approach to Staying Cool" are more often than not the American public's only education about Ayurveda. These articles are typically written by authors with no education or training in Ayurveda and providing only vague details that pertain to classical Ayurveda: "Through vedic principals, it's believed that to live optimally in balance your Dosha should be in fact, IN balance." These articles and guidelines focus on lifestyle/beauty routines and philosophy rather than historical or technical concepts.

Ayurveda in Academia

In Western Academic Literature

In the realm of academia, few researchers or doctors have published literature about Ayurveda in technical peer-reviewed journals. Even then, scholastic works on Ayurveda are barely known or read outside of a few relevant but small academic circles. In the past decade however, due to the resurgence of popular Ayurveda in America, those in the field of biomedicine have cautiously begun to reconsider Ayurveda as a legitimate medical science and are trying to glean relevant and useful knowledge using Western methods.

Agni (Ayurveda)

Agni is the "fire," that drives all digestion and metabolism in the Indian medical practice of Ayurveda. The digestive and absorption process is called Pakwagni (digestive fire).

Background

The pachak (stomach and small intestine) has 13 Jatharagni (digestive enzymes or "fire") that occur in four different states: samagni (normal), Visamagni (abnormal), Tikshanagni (increased) and Mandagni (decreased).

Samanagni is the state of complete balance. All three doshas: vata, pitta and kaphha are in total balance. When Agni is disturbed by Vata, the condition is known as Vishamagni. When Pitta affects Agni, the condition is known Tikshagni. When Kapha affects Agni, the condition is known Mandagni.

The composer of Hareet Samhita writes that condition of Samanagni depends upon whether the doshas (Vata, pitta, and kaphha) are all in normal stage. When Vata, Pitta, Kaphha are unequal, the condition is known as Vishamagni. When Pitta is higher than normal, the condition is known as Teekshagni. When Vata and Kaphha are higher than normal, the condition is known as Mandagni.

Samagni

The agni Samagni digests and assimilates food properly thus increasing the quality of dhatus (supportive tissues of the body). Persons having Samanagni always are hale and healthy. The body of

Samanagni is balanced in Dhatus and Indriya. Because they are balanced, neither Mand, Visham or Teekshana is the object of treatments

Vishamagni

This type of Agni alternates between digesting food quickly and slowly. When this agni is affected by the Vata Dosha, it creates cholera, diarrhoea, infective diarrhoea, dysentery, vatadi diseases, spleenomegaly, gulm/abdominal tumour, colic, flatulence, wind formation and accumulation, eructations etc. This is narrated by the Hareet in Hareet Samhita.

In Dhanvantari Samhita, Dhanvantari writes that when the Jatharagni (digestive fire) alternates from digesting food completely and from producing symptoms such as colic, eructations, diarrhoea, heaviness in or rumbling in the abdomen, wind in the intestines, or dysentery, Vishamagni is present.

Tikshnagni

Tikshna means very quick/very sharp/very fast. Agni means digestive power or digestive capacity. Tikshnagni is a state of very quick digestion of food regardless of the type of food. Acharya Sushruta states that when food digests very quickly, this type of agni is known as "Tikshnagni". When the power of digestion is increased from normal to above normal, food digests very quickly and produces hunger or the desire for food. When food digests, the throat, the mouth cavity and the lips become dry with a burning sensation. This condition is known "Bhasmak Roga" according to Ayurveda.

In Hareeta Samhita, food is eaten fully and yet, the person is not satiated by food desiring even more food. If their eyes becomes yellow, there is a burning sensation present and the body's strength is deficient, this indicates Tikshnagni. When Vata and Pitta becomes weak and Pitta becomes strong and acute, the condition is known as Bhasmagni or Bhasmak.

The complications from the Bhasmak Roga are jaundice, anaemia, hepatitis, yellow skin, diarrhoea, tuberculosis, vertigo, hepatomegaly, urine anomalies, colic, unconsciousness, hemophilia, hematomasis, hemorrhage, sour eructations, hyperacidity, burning, pain, inflammation in urination etc. The body is emaciated and weak.

Mandagni

Mandagni is a Sanskrit word. "Manda" means slow and "agni" means digestive fire or digestive capacity. The meaning of the mandagni is slow digestive power or slow digestion capacity. Those who are having Mandagni eat very little and are unable to digest the smallest amount of food. Dhanavantri says that Agni digests the least amount of food in the greatest amount of time. Because food is undigested, this produces heaviness in the abdomen, heaviness in the head, asthma and respiratory problems, bronchitis, cough, excessive salivation from the mouth, nausea and fatigue.

- Sushruta Samhita
- Traditional medicine

References

- Wujastyk, Dominik (2003). "Indian Medicine". In Flood, Gavin. The Blackwell Companion to Hinduism. Oxford: Blackwell. p. 394. ISBN 978-1405132510.
- Clifford, Terry (2003). Tibetan Buddhist Medicine and Psychiatry. 42. Motilal Banarsidass Publications. ISBN 81-208-1784-2.
- Zysk, Kenneth G. (1998). Asceticism and Healing in Ancient {India}: Medicine in the {Buddhist} Monastery. Delhi: Motilal Banarsidass. ISBN 81-208-1507-6.
- Sharma, A. K. (2003). "Panchkarma Therapy in Ayurvedic Medicine". In Mishra, Lakshmi Chandra. Scientific Basis for Ayurvedic Therapies. Boca Raton, FL: CRC Press. p. 43. ISBN 0-8493-1366-X.
- WHO traditional medicine strategy: 2014-2023. 1.Medicine, Traditional. 2.Complementary therapies. 3.Health planning. 4.Delivery of health care. 5.Health policy. I.World Health Organization. ISBN 978 92 4 150609 0
- Quack, Johannes (2011). Disenchanting India: Organized Rationalism and Criticism of Religion in India. Oxford University Press. p. 213. ISBN 9780199812608.
- Guneratne, Arjun (2009). Culture and the Environment in the Himalaya. Routledge contemporary South Asia series, #24. New York: Routledge. pp. 84–85. ISBN 978-0-415-77883-1.
- Bausell, R. Barker (2007). Snake Oil Science: The Truth About Complementary and Alternative Medicine. Oxford University Press. p. 259. ISBN 9780195383423.
- Elizabeth R. Mackenzie; Birgit Rakel (2006). Complementary and Alternative Medicine for Older Adults: A Guide to Holistic Approaches to Healthy Aging. Springer. p. 215. ISBN 9780826138064.
- Frawley, David; Ranade, Subhash (2001). Ayurveda, Nature's Medicine. Lotus Press. p. 11. ISBN 9780914955955. Retrieved 6 January 2015.
- Singh, Rana P. B.; Rana, Pravin S. (2002). Banaras Region: A Spiritual and Cultural Guide. Varanasi, India: Indica Books. p. 31. ISBN 81-86569-24-3.
- Berger, Rachel (2013). Ayurveda made modern : political histories of indigenous medicine in North India, 1900-1955. New York, NY: Palgrave Macmillan. ISBN 9780230284555.
- Mohammad Ali Jazayery; Werner Winter (1988). Samhita Languages and Cultures: Studies in Honor of Edgar C. Polomé Check |url= value (help). Walter de Gruyter. p. 116. ISBN 9783110102048.
- Glucklich, Ariel (2008). The Strides of Vishnu: Hindu Culture in Historical Perspective. Oxford, England: Oxford University Press. p. 141. ISBN 978-0-19-531405-2.
- Upinder Singh (2008). A History of Ancient and Early Medieval India: From the Stone Age to the 12th Century. Pearson. ISBN 9788131711200.
- Anil Kumar Mehta; Naveen K. Gupta; R. N. Sharma (2002). Health & Harmony Through Ayurveda. B. Jain Publishers. p. 41. ISBN 9788170219347.
- Dagmar Wujastyk (2002). Well-Mannered Medicine: Medical Ethics and Etiquette in Classical Ayurveda. Oxford University Press. ISBN 9780199856275.
- Humphrey James, Welch (1993). Haddows, Gordon, ed. The World Checklist of Conifers. Bromyard: Landsman's Bookshop. ISBN 978-0-900513-09-1.
- "Cedarwood Oils". Flavours and fragances of plant origin. Food and Agriculture Organization of the United Nations. 1995. ISBN 92-5-103648-9.
- Pole, Sebastian (2006). Ayurvedic Medicine: The Principles of Traditional Practice. Singing Dragon. pp. 126–127. ISBN 978-1-84819-113-6.

6

Herbalism: Theories and Approaches

The use of plants for the purpose of medicine is termed as herbalism. It also, at times, includes fungal and bee products. This chapter focuses on the history of herbalism and also lists herbs with known adverse effects. In order to completely understand herbalism, it is necessary to understand the theories and approaches related to herbalism.

Herbalism

Herbalism is the use of plants for medicinal purposes, and the study of botany for such use. Plants have been the basis for medical treatments through much of human history, and such traditional medicine is still widely practiced today. Modern medicine recognizes herbalism as a form of alternative medicine, as the practice of herbalism is not strictly based on evidence gathered using the scientific method. Modern medicine, does, however, make use of many plant-derived compounds as the basis for evidence-tested pharmaceutical drugs. Phytotherapy, and phytochemistry work to apply modern standards of effectiveness testing to herbs and medicines that are derived from natural sources. The scope of herbal medicine is sometimes extended to include fungal and bee products, as well as minerals, shells and certain animal parts.

History

Archaeological evidence indicates that the use of medicinal plants dates at least to the Paleolithic age, approximately 60,000 years ago. Written evidence of herbal remedies dates back over 5,000 years, to the Sumerians, who compiled lists of plants. A number of ancient cultures wrote about plants and their medical uses in books called *herbals*. In ancient Egypt, herbs are mentioned in Egyptian medical papyri, depicted in tomb illustrations, or on rare occasions found in medical jars containing trace amounts of herbs. Among the oldest, lengthiest, and most important medical papyri of ancient Egypt, the Ebers Papyrus dates from about 1550 BC, and covers more than 700 drugs, mainly of plant origin. The earliest known Greek herbals come from Theophrastus of Eresos who in the 4th c. B.C. wrote in Greek *Historia Plantarum*, from Diocles of Carystus who wrote during the 3rd century B.C, and from Krateuas who wrote in the 1st century B.C. Only a few fragments of these works have survived intact, but from what remains scholars have noted a large amount of overlap with the Egyptian herbals. Seeds likely used for herbalism have been found in archaeological sites of Bronze Age China dating from the Shang Dynasty (c. 1600 BC–c. 1046 BC). Over a hundred of the 224 drugs mentioned in the *Huangdi Neijing*, an early Chinese medical text, are herbs. Herbs also commonly featured in the medicine of ancient India, where the principal treatment for diseases was diet. *De Materia Medica*, originally written in Greek by Pedanius Dioscorides (c. 40 – 90 AD) of Anazarbus, Cilicia, a Greek physician, pharmacologist and botanist, is a particularly important example of such writings. The documentation of herbs and their uses was a central part of both Western and Eastern medical scholarship through to the 1600s, and these works played an important role in the development of the science of botany.

Modern Herbal Medicine

The World Health Organization (WHO) estimates that 80 percent of the population of some Asian and African countries presently use herbal medicine for some aspect of primary health care. Pharmaceuticals are prohibitively expensive for most of the world's population, half of whom lived on less than $2 U.S. per day in 2002. In comparison, herbal medicines can be grown from seed or gathered from nature for little or no cost.

Many of the pharmaceuticals currently available to physicians have a long history of use as herbal remedies, including opium, aspirin, digitalis, and quinine. According to the World Health Organization, approximately 25% of modern drugs used in the United States have been derived from plants. At least 7,000 medical compounds in the modern pharmacopoeia are derived from plants. Among the 120 active compounds currently isolated from the higher plants and widely used in modern medicine today, 80% show a positive correlation between their modern therapeutic use and the traditional use of the plants from which they are derived.

Clinical Tests

In 2015 the Australian Government's Department of Health published the results of a review of alternative therapies that sought to determine if any were suitable for being covered by health insurance; Herbalism was one of 17 topics evaluated for which no clear evidence of effectiveness was found.

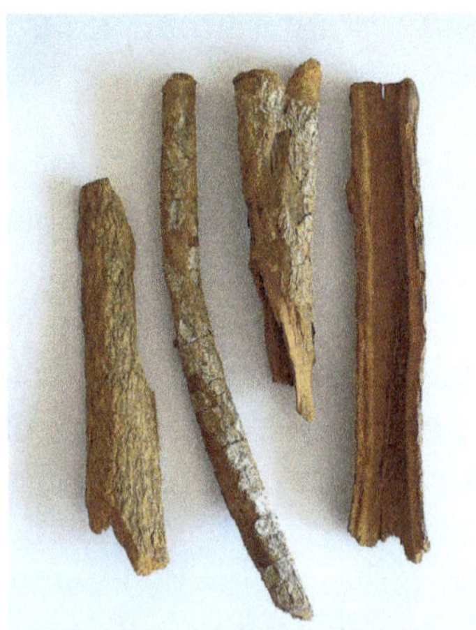

The bark of the cinchona tree contains quinine, which today is a widely prescribed treatment for malaria, especially in countries that cannot afford to purchase the more expensive anti-malarial drugs produced by the pharmaceutical industry.

In a 2010 survey of the most common 1000 plant-derived compounds, only 156 had clinical trials published. Preclinical studies (tissue-culture and animal studies) were reported for about one-half of the plant products, while 12% of the plants, although available in the Western market, had "no substantial studies" of their properties. Strong evidence was found that 5 were toxic or allergenic, so that their use ought to be discouraged or forbidden. Nine plants had considerable evidence of therapeutic effect.

According to Cancer Research UK, "there is currently no strong evidence from studies in people that herbal remedies can treat, prevent or cure cancer".

The U.S. National Center for Complementary and Integrative Health of the National Institutes of Health funds clinical trials of the effectiveness of herbal medicines and provides "fact sheets" summarizing the effectiveness and side effects of many plant-derived preparations.

Prevalence of Use

The use of herbal remedies is more prevalent in patients with chronic diseases such as cancer, diabetes, asthma and end-stage renal disease. Multiple factors such as gender, age, ethnicity, education and social class are also shown to have association with prevalence of herbal remedies use.

A survey released in May 2004 by the National Center for Complementary and Integrative Health focused on who used complementary and alternative medicines (CAM), what was used, and why it was used. The survey was limited to adults, aged 18 years and over during 2002, living in the United States. According to this survey, herbal therapy, or use of natural products other than vitamins and minerals, was the most commonly used CAM therapy (18.9%) when all use of prayer was excluded.

Herbal remedies are very common in Europe. In Germany, herbal medications are dispensed by apothecaries (e.g., Apotheke). Prescription drugs are sold alongside essential oils, herbal extracts, or herbal teas. Herbal remedies are seen by some as a treatment to be preferred to pure medical compounds that have been industrially produced.

In India the herbal remedy is so popular that the government of India has created a separate department—AYUSH—under the Ministry of Health & Family Welfare. The National Medicinal Plants Board was also established in 2000 by the Indian government in order to deal with the herbal medical system.

Herbal Preparations

There are many forms in which herbs can be administered, the most common of which is in the form of a liquid that is drunk by the patient—either an herbal tea or a (possibly diluted) plant extract. Whole herb consumption is also practiced either fresh, in dried form or as fresh juice.

Several methods of standardization may be determining the amount of herbs used. One is the ratio of raw materials to solvent. However different specimens of even the same plant species may vary in chemical content. For this reason, thin layer chromatography is sometimes used by growers to assess the content of their products before use. Another method is standardization on a signal chemical.

Herbal teas, or tisanes, are the resultant liquid of extracting herbs into water, though they are made in a few different ways. Infusions are hot water extracts of herbs, such as chamomile or mint, through steeping. Decoctions are the long-term boiled extracts, usually of harder substances like roots or bark. Maceration is the old infusion of plants with high mucilage-content, such as sage, thyme, etc. To make macerates, plants are chopped and added to cold water. They are then left to stand for 7 to 12 hours (depending on herb used). For most macerates 10 hours is used.

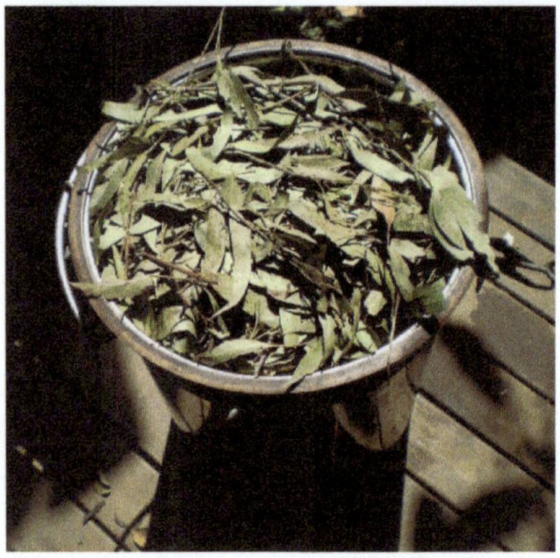

Leaves of *Eucalyptus olida* being packed into a steam distillation unit to gather its essential oil.

Tinctures are alcoholic extracts of herbs, which are generally stronger than herbal teas. Tinctures are usually obtained by combining 100% pure ethanol (or a mixture of 100% ethanol with water) with the herb. A completed tincture has an ethanol percentage of at least 25% (sometimes up to 90%). Herbal wine and elixirs are alcoholic extract of herbs, usually with an ethanol percentage of 12-38%. Herbal wine is a maceration of herbs in wine, while an elixir is a maceration of herbs in spirits (e.g., vodka, grappa, etc.). Extracts include liquid extracts, dry extracts, and nebulisates. Liquid extracts are liquids with a lower ethanol percentage than tinctures. They are usually made by vacuum distilling tinctures. Dry extracts are extracts of plant material that are evaporated into a dry mass. They can then be further refined to a capsule or tablet. A nebulisate is a dry extract created by freeze-drying. Vinegars are prepared in the same way as tinctures, except using a solution of acetic acid as the solvent. Syrups are extracts of herbs made with syrup or honey. Sixty-five parts of sugar are mixed with thirty-five parts of water and herb. The whole is then boiled and macerated for three weeks.

The exact composition of an herbal product is influenced by the method of extraction. A tea will be rich in polar components because water is a polar solvent. Oil on the other hand is a non-polar solvent and it will absorb non-polar compounds. Alcohol lies somewhere in between.

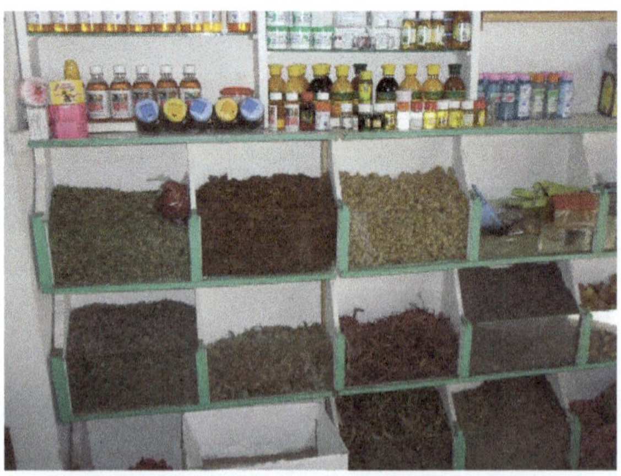

A herb shop in the souk of Marrakesh, Morocco

Many herbs are applied topically to the skin in a variety of forms. Essential oil extracts can be applied to the skin, usually diluted in a carrier oil. Many essential oils can burn the skin or are simply too high dose used straight; diluting them in olive oil or another food grade oil such as almond oil can allow these to be used safely as a topical. Salves, oils, balms, creams and lotions are other forms of topical delivery mechanisms. Most topical applications are oil extractions of herbs. Taking a food grade oil and soaking herbs in it for anywhere from weeks to months allows certain phytochemicals to be extracted into the oil. This oil can then be made into salves, creams, lotions, or simply used as an oil for topical application. Many massage oils, antibacterial salves, and wound healing compounds are made this way. One can also make a poultice or compress using the whole herb or the appropriate part of the plant, which is usually crushed or dried and re-hydrated with a small amount of water and then applied directly in a bandage, cloth, or just as is.

Inhalation, as in aromatherapy, can be used as a mood changing treatment to fight a sinus infection or cough , or to cleanse the skin on a deeper level (steam rather than direct inhalation here)

Safety

A number of herbs are thought to be likely to cause adverse effects. Furthermore, "adulteration, inappropriate formulation, or lack of understanding of plant and drug interactions have led to adverse reactions that are sometimes life threatening or lethal." Proper double-blind clinical trials are needed to determine the safety and efficacy of each plant before they can be recommended for medical use. Although many consumers believe that herbal medicines are safe because they are "natural", herbal medicines and synthetic drugs may interact, causing toxicity to the patient. Herbal remedies can also be dangerously contaminated, and herbal medicines without established efficacy, may unknowingly be used to replace medicines that do have corroborated efficacy.

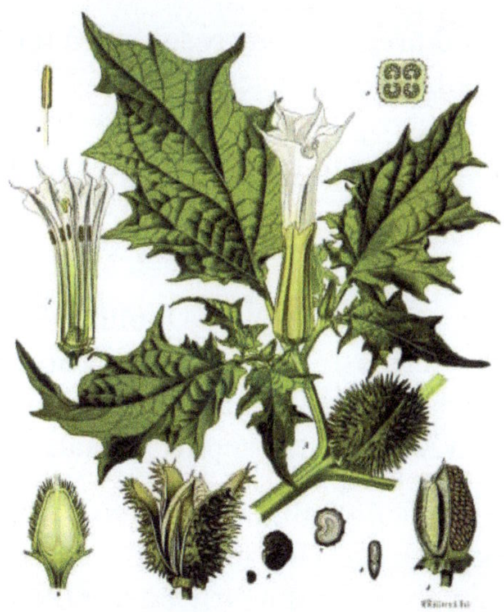

Datura stramonium is a highly effective treatment for asthma symptoms when smoked, because it contains atropine, which acts as an antispasmodic in the lungs. However, datura is also an extremely powerful hallucinogen and overdoses of the tropane alkaloids in it can result in hospitalization or death.

Standardization of purity and dosage is not mandated in the United States, but even products made to the same specification may differ as a result of biochemical variations within a species of plant. Plants have chemical defense mechanisms against predators that can have adverse or lethal effects on humans. Examples of highly toxic herbs include poison hemlock and nightshade. They are not marketed to the public as herbs, because the risks are well known, partly due to a long and colorful history in Europe, associated with "sorcery", "magic" and intrigue. Although not frequent, adverse reactions have been reported for herbs in widespread use. On occasion serious untoward outcomes have been linked to herb consumption. A case of major potassium depletion has been attributed to chronic licorice ingestion., and consequently professional herbalists avoid the use of licorice where they recognize that this may be a risk. Black cohosh has been implicated in a case of liver failure. Few studies are available on the safety of herbs for pregnant women, and one study found that use of complementary and alternative medicines are associated with a 30% lower ongoing pregnancy and live birth rate during fertility treatment. Examples of herbal treatments with likely cause-effect relationships with adverse events include aconite, which is often a legally restricted herb, ayurvedic remedies, broom, chaparral, Chinese herb mixtures, comfrey, herbs containing certain flavonoids, germander, guar gum, liquorice root, and pennyroyal. Examples of herbs where a high degree of confidence of a risk long term adverse effects can be asserted include ginseng, which is unpopular among herbalists for this reason, the endangered herb goldenseal, milk thistle, senna, against which herbalists generally advise and rarely use, aloe vera juice, buckthorn bark and berry, cascara sagrada bark, saw palmetto, valerian, kava, which is banned in the European Union, St. John's wort, Khat, Betel nut, the restricted herb Ephedra, and Guarana.

There is also concern with respect to the numerous well-established interactions of herbs and drugs. In consultation with a physician, usage of herbal remedies should be clarified, as some herbal remedies have the potential to cause adverse drug interactions when used in combination with various prescription and over-the-counter pharmaceuticals, just as a patient should inform a herbalist of their consumption of orthodox prescription and other medication.

For example, dangerously low blood pressure may result from the combination of an herbal remedy that lowers blood pressure together with prescription medicine that has the same effect. Some herbs may amplify the effects of anticoagulants. Certain herbs as well as common fruit interfere with cytochrome P450, an enzyme critical to much drug metabolism.

Labeling Accuracy

A 2013 study published in the journal BMC Medicine found that one-third of herbal supplements sampled contained no trace of the herb listed on the label. The study found products adulterated with filler including allergens such as soy, wheat, and black walnut. One bottle labeled as St. John's Wort was found to actually contain Alexandrian senna, a laxative.

Researchers at the University of Adelaide found in 2014 that almost 20 per cent of herbal remedies surveyed were not registered with the Therapeutic Goods Administration, despite this being a condition for their sale. They also found that nearly 60 per cent of products surveyed had ingredients that did not match what was on the label. Out of 121 products, only 15 had ingredients that matched their TGA listing and packaging.

In 2015 the New York Attorney General issued cease and desist letters to four major U.S. retailers (GNC, Target, Walgreens, and Walmart) who are accused of selling herbal supplements that were mislabeled and potentially dangerous. 24 products were tested by DNA barcoding as part of the investigation, all but five contained DNA that did not match the products' labels. The investigation was prompted by the 2013 BMC study.

Practitioners of Herbalism

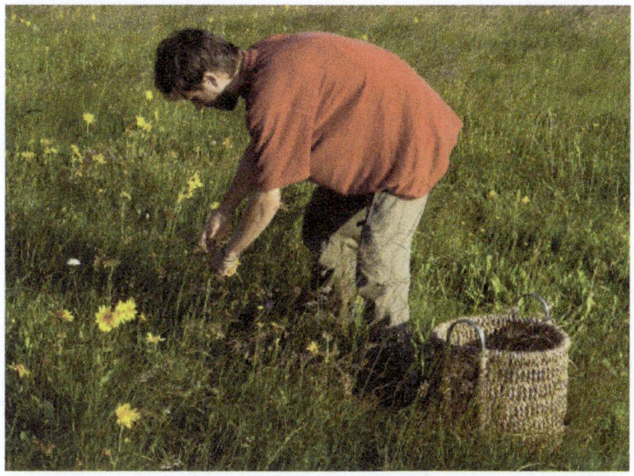

A herbalist gathers the flower heads of *Arnica montana*.

A herbalist is:

1. A person whose life is dedicated to the economic or medicinal uses of plants.
2. One skilled in the harvesting and collection of medicinal plants.
3. Traditional Chinese herbalist: one who is trained or skilled in the dispensing of herbal prescriptions; traditional Chinese herb doctor. Similarly, traditional Ayurvedic herbalist: one who is trained or skilled in the dispensing of herbal prescriptions in the Ayurvedic tradition.
4. One trained or skilled in the therapeutic use of medicinal plants.
5. One who is skilled in the preparation/manufacture of dried and/or liquid herbal products who possesses a pharmacognostic, formulary and/or clinical understanding of the products being prepared/manufactured.

Herbalists must learn many skills, including the wildcrafting or cultivation of herbs, diagnosis and treatment of conditions or dispensing herbal medication, and preparations of herbal medications. Education of herbalists varies considerably in different areas of the world. Lay herbalists and traditional indigenous medicine people generally rely upon apprenticeship and recognition from their communities in lieu of formal schooling.

In some countries formalized training and minimum education standards exist, although these are not necessarily uniform within or between countries. For example, in Australia the currently self-regulated status of the profession (as of April 2008) results in different associations setting different educational standards, and subsequently recognising an educational institution or course of training. The National Herbalists Association of Australia is generally recognised as having the most rigorous professional standard within Australia. In the United Kingdom, the training of medical herbalists is done by state funded Universities. For example, Bachelor of Science degrees in herbal medicine are offered at Universities such as University of East London, Middlesex University, University of Central Lancashire, University of Westminster, University of Lincoln and Napier University in Edinburgh at the present.

Government Regulations

The World Health Organization (WHO), the specialized agency of the United Nations (UN) that is concerned with international public health, published *Quality control methods for medicinal plant materials* in 1998 in order to support WHO Member States in establishing quality standards and specifications for herbal materials, within the overall context of quality assurance and control of herbal medicines.

In the European Union (EU), herbal medicines are now regulated under the European Directive on Traditional Herbal Medicinal Products.

In the United States, herbal remedies are regulated dietary supplements by the Food and Drug Administration under current good manufacturing practice (cGMP) policy for dietary supplements. Manufacturers of products falling into this category are not required to prove the safety or efficacy of their product so long as they don't make 'medical' claims or imply being other than for 'dietary supplement' use, though the FDA may withdraw a product from sale should it prove harmful.

The National Nutritional Foods Association, the industry's largest trade association, has run a program since 2002, examining the products and factory conditions of member companies, giving them the right to display the GMP (Good Manufacturing Practices) seal of approval on their products.

Some herbs, such as cannabis and coca, are outright banned in most countries though coca is legal in most of the South American countries where it is grown. The *Cannabis* plant is used as an herbal medicine, and as such is legal in some parts of the world. Since 2004, the sales of ephedra as a dietary supplement is prohibited in the United States by the Food and Drug Administration., and subject to Schedule III restrictions in the United Kingdom.

Traditional Herbal Medicine Systems

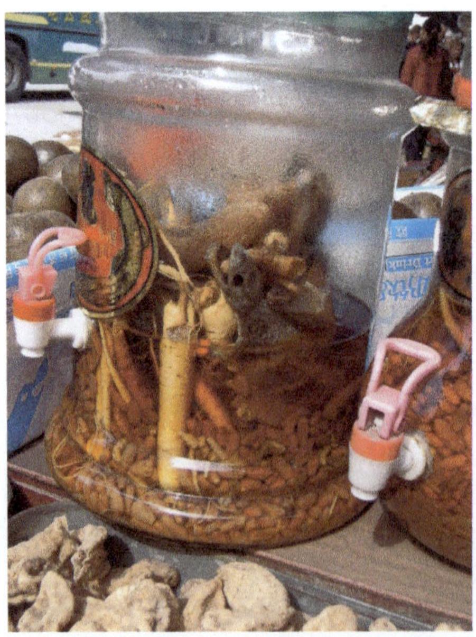

Ready to drink macerated medicinal liquor with goji berry, tokay gecko, and ginseng, for sale at a traditional medicine market in Xi'an, China.

Africa

Americas

Native Americans medicinally used about 2,500 of the approximately 20,000 plant species that are native to North America.

China

Some researchers trained in both western and traditional Chinese medicine have attempted to deconstruct ancient medical texts in the light of modern science. One idea is that the yin-yang balance, at least with regard to herbs, corresponds to the pro-oxidant and anti-oxidant balance. This interpretation is supported by several investigations of the ORAC ratings of various yin and yang herbs.

India

In India, Ayurvedic medicine has quite complex formulas with 30 or more ingredients, including a sizable number of ingredients that have undergone "alchemical processing", chosen to balance "Vata", "Pitta" or "Kapha".

In Ladakh, Lahul-Spiti and Tibet, the Tibetan Medical System is prevalent, also called the 'Amichi Medical System'. Over 337 species of medicinal plants have been documented by C.P. Kala. Those are used by Amchis, the practitioners of this medical system.

In Tamil Nadu, Tamils have their own medicinal system now popularly called Siddha medicine. The Siddha system is entirely in the Tamil language. It contains roughly 300,000 verses covering diverse aspects of medicine. This work includes herbal, mineral and metallic compositions used as medicine. Ayurveda is in Sanskrit, but Sanskrit was not generally used as a mother tongue and hence its medicines are mostly taken from Siddha and other local traditions.

Indonesia

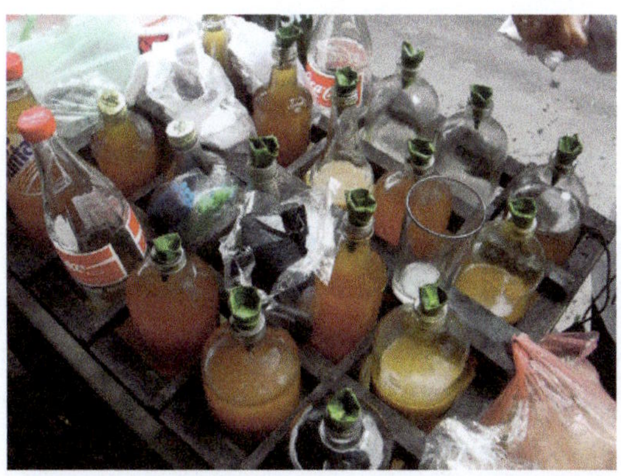

Different types of Indonesian jamu herbal medicines held in bottles.

In Indonesia, especially among the Javanese, the jamu traditional herbal medicine is an age old tradition preserved for centuries. Jamu is thought to have originated in the Mataram Kingdom era, some 1300 years ago. The bas-reliefs on Borobudur depicts the image of people ground herbs with stone mortar and pestle, drink seller, physician and masseuse treating their clients. All of these scenes might be interpreted as a traditional herbal medicine and health-related treatments in ancient Java. The Madhawapura inscription from Majapahit period mentioned a specific profession of herbs mixer and combiner (herbalist), called *Acaraki*. The medicine book from Mataram dated from circa 1700 contains 3,000 entries of jamu herbal recipes, while Javanese classical literature Serat Centhini (1814) describes some jamu herbal concoction recipes.

Though highly possible influenced by Indian Ayurveda system, Indonesia is a vast archipelago with numerous indigenous plants not to be found in India, which include plants similar to Australia beyond the Wallace Line. Indonesians might experimented and figure out the medicinal uses of these native herbal plants. Jamu may vary from region to region, and often not written down, especially in remote areas of the country. Although primarily herbal, materials acquired from animals, such as honey, royal jelly, milk and *ayam kampung* eggs are also often used in jamu.

Herbal Philosophy and Spiritual Practices

According to Eisenburg: "The Chinese and Western medical models are like two frames of reference in which identical phenomena are studied. Neither frame of reference provides an unobstructed view of health and illness. Each is incomplete and in need of refinement." Specifically, the traditional Chinese medical model could effect change on the recognized, and expected, phenomena of detachment to patients as people and estrangement unique to the clinical and impersonal relationships between patient and physician of the Western school of medicine.

Four approaches to the use of plants as medicine include:

1. The magical/shamanic—Almost all societies, with the exception of cultures influenced by Western-style industrialization, recognize this kind of use. The practitioner is regarded as endowed with gifts or powers that allow him/her to use herbs in a way that is hidden from the average person, and the herbs are said to affect the spirit or soul of the person.

2. The energetic—This approach includes the major systems of Traditional Chinese Medicine, Ayurveda, and Unani. Herbs are regarded as having actions in terms of their energies and affecting the energies of the body. The practitioner may have extensive training, and ideally be sensitive to energy, but need not have supernatural powers.

3. The functional dynamic—This approach was used by early physiomedical practitioners, whose doctrine forms the basis of contemporary practice in the UK. Herbs have a functional action, which is not necessarily linked to a physical compound, although often to a physiological function, but there is no explicit recourse to concepts involving energy.

4. The chemical—Modern practitioners - called Phytotherapists - attempt to explain herb actions in terms of their chemical constituents. It is generally assumed that the specific combination of secondary metabolites in the plant are responsible for the activity claimed or demonstrated, a concept called synergy.

Herbalists tend to use extracts from parts of plants, such as the roots or leaves but not isolate particular phytochemicals. Pharmaceutical medicine prefers single ingredients on the grounds that dosage can be more easily quantified. It is also possible to patent single compounds, and therefore generate income. Herbalists often reject the notion of a single active ingredient, arguing that the different phytochemicals present in many herbs will interact to enhance the therapeutic effects of the herb and dilute toxicity. Furthermore, they argue that a single ingredient may contribute to multiple effects. Herbalists deny that herbal synergism can be duplicated with synthetic chemicals They argue that phytochemical interactions and trace components may alter the drug response in ways that cannot currently be replicated with a combination of a few potentially active ingredients. Pharmaceutical researchers recognize the concept of drug synergism but note that clinical trials may be used to investigate the efficacy of a particular herbal preparation, provided the formulation of that herb is consistent.

In specific cases the claims of synergy and multifunctionality have been supported by science. The open question is how widely both can be generalized. Herbalists would argue that cases of synergy can be widely generalized, on the basis of their interpretation of evolutionary history, not necessarily shared by the pharmaceutical community. Plants are subject to similar selection pressures as humans and therefore they must develop resistance to threats such as radiation, reactive oxygen species and microbial attack in order to survive. Optimal chemical defenses have been selected for and have thus developed over millions of years. Human diseases are multifactorial and may be treated by consuming the chemical defences that they believe to be present in herbs. Bacteria, inflammation, nutrition and ROS (reactive oxygen species) may all play a role in arterial disease. Herbalists claim a single herb may simultaneously address several of these factors. Likewise a factor such as ROS may underlie more than one condition. In short herbalists view their field as the study of a web of relationships rather than a quest for single cause and a single cure for a single condition.

In selecting herbal treatments herbalists may use forms of information that are not applicable to pharmacists. Because herbs can moonlight as vegetables, teas or spices they have a huge consumer base and large-scale epidemiological studies become feasible. Ethnobotanical studies are another source of information. For example, when indigenous peoples from geographically dispersed areas use closely related herbs for the same purpose that is taken as supporting evidence for its efficacy. Herbalists contend that historical medical records and herbals are underutilized resources. They favor the use of convergent information in assessing the medical value of plants. An example would be when in-vitro activity is consistent with traditional use.

Uses of Herbal Medicines By Animals

Indigenous healers often claim to have learned by observing that sick animals change their food preferences to nibble at bitter herbs they would normally reject. Field biologists have provided corroborating evidence based on observation of diverse species, such as chickens, sheep, butterflies, and chimpanzee.The habit has been shown to be a physical means of purging intestinal parasites. Lowland gorillas take 90% of their diet from the fruits of *Aframomum melegueta*, a relative of the ginger plant, that is a potent antimicrobial and apparently keeps shigellosis and similar infections at bay. Current research focuses on the possibility that this plants also protects gorillas from fibrosing cardiomyopathy which has a devastating effect on captive animals.

Sick animals tend to forage plants rich in secondary metabolites, such as tannins and alkaloids. Since these phytochemicals often have antiviral, antibacterial, antifungal and antihelminthic properties, a plausible case can be made for self-medication by animals in the wild.

Herbal

A herbal is a book containing the names and descriptions of plants, usually with information on their medicinal, tonic, culinary, toxic, hallucinatory, aromatic, or magical powers, and the legends associated with them. A herbal may also classify the plants it describes, may give recipes for herbal extracts, tinctures, or potions, and sometimes include mineral and animal medicaments in addition to those obtained from plants. Herbals were often illustrated to assist plant identification.

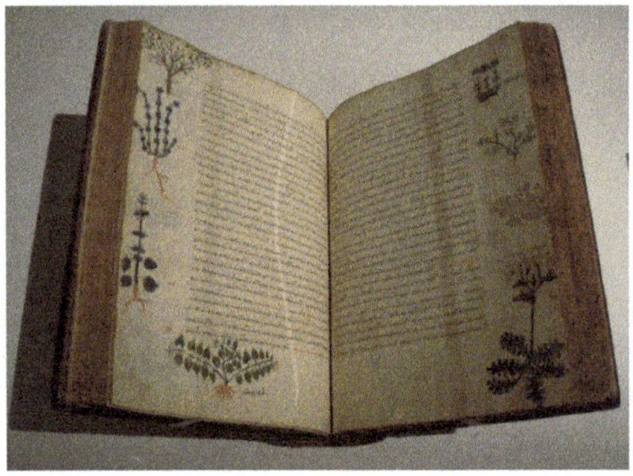

Dioscorides' *De Materia Medica*, Byzantium, 15th-century manuscript, by which time the text had been in circulation for about 1500 years

Herbals were among the first literature produced in Ancient Egypt, China, India, and Europe as the medical wisdom of the day accumulated by herbalists, apothecaries and physicians. Herbals were also among the first books to be printed in both China and Europe. In Western Europe herbals flourished for two centuries following the introduction of moveable type (c. 1470–1670).

In the late 17th century, the rise of modern chemistry, toxicology and pharmacology reduced the medicinal value of the classical herbal. As reference manuals for botanical study and plant identification herbals were supplanted by Floras – systematic accounts of the plants found growing in a particular region, with scientifically accurate botanical descriptions, classification, and illustrations. Herbals have seen a modest revival in the western world since the last decades of the 20th century, as herbalism and related disciplines (such as homeopathy and aromatherapy) became popular forms of alternative medicine.

History

The word *herbal* is derived from the mediaeval Latin *liber herbalis* ("book of herbs"): it is sometimes used in contrast to the word *florilegium*, which is a treatise on flowers with emphasis on their beauty and enjoyment rather than the herbal emphasis on their utility. Much of the information found in printed herbals arose out of traditional medicine and herbal knowledge that predated the invention of writing.

Before the advent of printing, herbals were produced as manuscripts, which could be kept as scrolls or loose sheets, or bound into codices. Early handwritten herbals were often illustrated with paintings and drawings. Like other manuscript books, herbals were "published" through repeated copying by hand, either by professional scribes or by the readers themselves. In the process of making a copy, the copyist would often translate, expand, adapt, or reorder the content. Most of the original herbals have been lost; many have survived only as later copies (of copies...), and others are known only through references from other texts.

As printing became available, it was promptly used to publish herbals, the first printed matter being known as incunabula. In Europe, the first printed herbal with woodcut (xylograph) illustrations, the *Puch der Natur* of Konrad of Megenberg, appeared in 1475. Metal-engraved plates were first used in about 1580. As woodcuts and metal engravings could be reproduced indefinitely they were traded among printers: there was therefore a large increase in the number of illustrations together with an improvement in quality and detail but a tendency for repetition.

As examples of some of the world's most important records and first printed matter, researchers will find herbals scattered through the world's most famous libraries including the Vatican Library in Rome, the Bodleian Library in Oxford, the Royal Library in Windsor, the British Library in London and the major continental libraries.

China, India, Mexico

Shen Nung Pen Ts'ao Ching of China

China is renowned for its traditional herbal medicines that date back thousands of years. Legend has it that mythical Emperor Shennong, the founder of Chinese herbal medicine, composed the *Shennong Bencao Jing* or *Great Herbal* in about 2700 BCE as the forerunner of all later Chinese herbals. It survives as a copy made c. 500 CE and describes about 365 herbs. High quality herbals and monographs on particular plants were produced in the period to 1250 CE including: the *Zhenlei bencao* written by Tang Shenwei in 1108, which passed through twelve editions until 1600; a monograph on the lychee by Cai Xiang in 1059 and one on the oranges of Wenzhhou by Han Yanzhi in 1178. In 1406 Ming dynasty prince Zhu Xiao (朱橚) published the *Jiuhuang Bencao* illustrated herbal for famine foods. It contained high quality woodcuts and descriptions of 414 species of plants of which 276 were described for the first time, the book pre-dating the first European printed book by 69 years. It was reprinted many times. Other herbals include *Bencao Fahui* in 1450 by Xu Yong and *Bencao Gangmu* of Li Shizhen in 1590.

Sushruta Samhita of India

Traditional herbal medicine of India, known as Ayurveda, possibly dates back to the second millennium BCE tracing its origins to the holy Hindu Vedas and, in particular, the Atharvaveda. One authentic compilation of teachings is by the surgeon Sushruta, available in a treatise called Sushruta Samhita. This contains 184 chapters and description of 1120 illnesses, 700 medicinal plants, 64 preparations from mineral sources and 57 preparations based on animal sources. Other early works of Ayurveda include the *Charaka Samhita*, attributed to Charaka. This tradition, however is mostly oral. The earliest surviving written material which contains the works of Sushruta is the *Bower Manuscript*—dated to the 4th century CE.

Hernandez – Rerum Medicarum and The Aztecs

An illustrated herbal published in Mexico in 1552, *Libellus de Medicinalibus Indorum Herbis* ("Book of Medicinal Herbs of the Indies"), is written in the Aztec Nauhuatl language by a native physician, Martín Cruz. This is probably an extremely early account of the medicine of the Aztecs although the formal illustrations, resembling European ones, suggest that the artists were following the traditions of their Spanish masters rather than an indigenous style of drawing. In 1570 Francisco Hernández (c.1514–1580) was sent from Spain to study the natural resources of New Spain (now Mexico). Here he drew on indigenous sources, including the extensive botanical gardens that had been established by the Aztecs, to record c. 1200 plants in his *Rerum Medicarum* of 1615. Nicolás Monardes' *Dos Libros* (1569) contains the first published illustration of tobacco.

Egypt, Mesopotamia, Greece and Rome

By about 2000 BCE, medical papyri in ancient Egypt included medical prescriptions based on plant matter and made reference to the herbalist's combination of medicines and magic for healing.

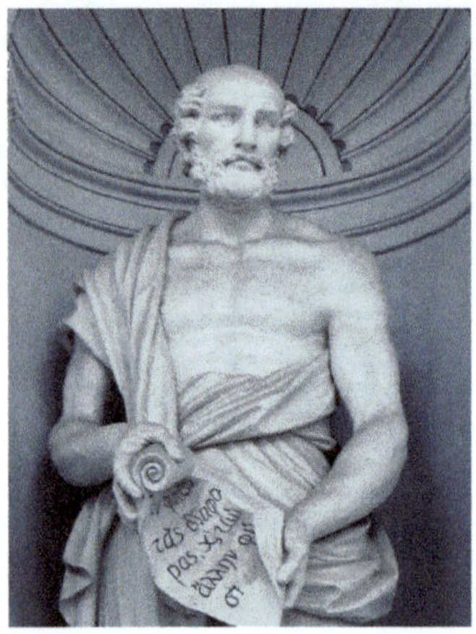

Statue of Theophrastus c. 371 – c. 287 BCE, Orto botanico di Palermo

Papyrus Ebers

The ancient Egyptian Papyrus Ebers is one of the earliest known herbals; it dates to 1550 BCE and is based on sources, now lost, dating back a further 500 to 2000 years. The earliest Sumerian herbal dates from about 2500 BCE as a copied manuscript of the 7th century BCE. Inscribed Assyrian tablets dated 668–626 BCE list about 250 vegetable drugs: the tablets include herbal plant names that are still in use today including: saffron, cumin, turmeric and sesame.

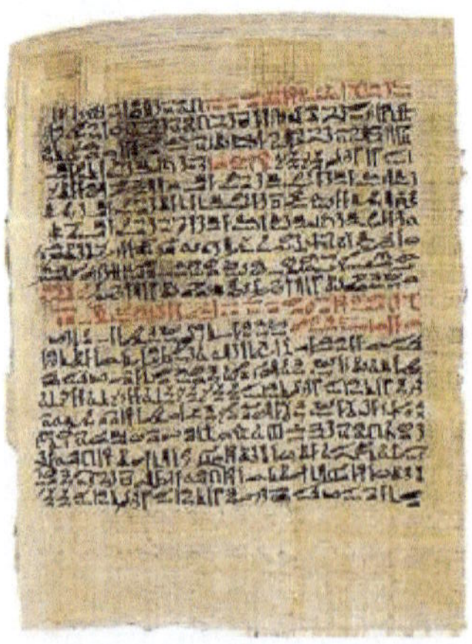

A page from the Ebers Papyrus, the most complete and extensive of surviving ancient herbals

The ancient Greeks gleaned much of their medicinal knowledge from Egypt and Mesopotamia. Hippocrates (460–377 BCE), the "father of medicine" (renowned for the eponymous Hippocratic oath), used about 400 drugs, most being of plant origin. However, the first Greek herbal of any note was written by Diocles of Carystus in the fourth century BC—although nothing remains of this except its mention in the written record. It was Aristotle's pupil Theophrastus (371–287 BCE) in his *Historia Plantarum*, (better known as the *Enquiry into Plants*) and *De Causis Plantarum* (*On the Causes of Plants*) that established the scientific method of careful and critical observation associated with modern botanical science. Based largely on Aristotle's notes, the Ninth Book of his *Enquiry* deals specifically with medicinal herbs and their uses including the recommendations of herbalists and druggists of the day, and his plant descriptions often included their natural habitat and geographic distribution. With the formation of the Alexandrian School c. 330 BCE medicine flourished and written herbals of this period included those of the physicians Herophilus, Mantias, Andreas of Karystos, Appolonius Mys, and Nicander. The work of rhizomatist (the rhizomati were the doctors of the day, berated by Theophrastus for their superstition) Krateuas (fl. 110 BCE) is of special note because he initiated the tradition of the illustrated herbal in the first century BCE.

Dioscorides – De Materia Medica

The *De Materia Medica* of Pedanios Dioscorides, a physician in the Roman army, was produced in about 65 CE. It was the single greatest classical authority on the subject and the most influential herbal ever written, serving as a model for herbals and pharmacopoeias, both oriental and occidental, for the next 1000 years up to the Renaissance. It drew together much of the accumulated herbal knowledge of the time, including some 500 medicinal plants. The original has been lost but a lavishly illustrated Byzantine copy known as the *Vienna Dioscurides* dating from about 512 CE remains.

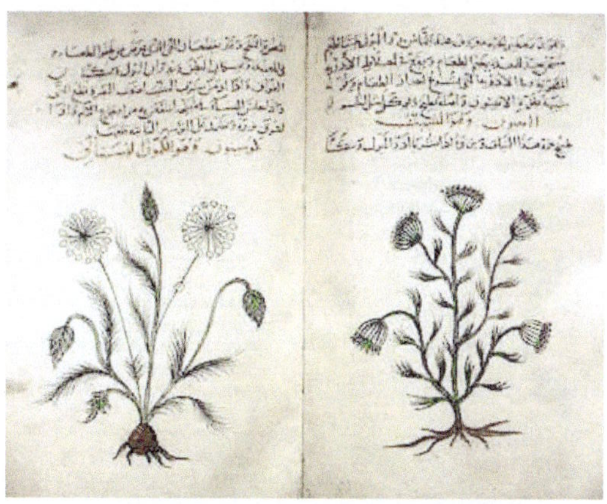

Arabic Book of Simple Drugs (c. 1334) from Dioscorides' *De Materia Medica*. British Museum

Pliny – Naturalis Historia

Pliny the Elder's (23–79 CE) encyclopaedic *Naturalis Historia* (c. 77–79 CE) is a synthesis of the information contained in about 2000 scrolls and it includes myths and folklore; there are about 200 extant copies of this work. It comprises 37 books of which sixteen (Books 12–27) are devoted to trees, plants and medicaments and, of these, seven describe medicinal plants. In medieval herbals, along with *De Materia Medica* it is Pliny's work that is the most frequently mentioned of the classical texts, even though the work *De Simplicibus* of Galen (131–201 CE) is more detailed and notable. Another Latin translation of Greek works that was widely copied in the Middle Ages, probably illustrated in the original, was that attributed to Apuleius and this also contained the alternative names for particular plants given in several languages. It dates to about 400 CE and a surviving copy dates to about 600 CE.

The Middle Ages and Arab World

During the 600 years of the European Middle Ages from 600 to 1200, the tradition of herbal lore fell to the monasteries. Many of the monks were skilled at producing books and manuscripts and tending both medicinal gardens and the sick, but written works of this period simply emulated those of the classical era.

Meanwhile, in the Arab world, by 900 the great Greek herbals had been translated and copies lodged in centres of learning in the Byzantine empire of the eastern Mediterranean including Byzantium, Damascus, Cairo and Baghdad where they were combined with the botanical and pharmacological lore of the Orient. In the medieval Islamic world, Muslim botanists and Muslim physicians made a major contribution to the knowledge of herbal medicines. Those associated with this period include Mesue Maior (Masawaiyh, 777–857) who, in his *Opera Medicinalia*, synthesised the knowledge of Greeks, Persians, Arabs, Indians and Babylonians, this work was complemented by the medical encyclopaedia of Avicenna (Ibn Sina, 980–1037). Avicenna's *Canon of Medicine* was used for centuries in both East and West. During this period Islamic science protected classical botanical knowledge that had been ignored in the West and Muslim pharmacy thrived.

Albertus Magnus – De Vegetabilibus

In the thirteenth century, scientific inquiry was returning and this was manifest through the production of encyclopaedias; those noted for their plant content included a seven volume treatise by Albertus Magnus (c. 1193–1280) a Suabian educated at the University of Padua and tutor to St Thomas Aquinas. It was called *De Vegetabilibus* (c. 1256 AD) and even though based on original observations and plant descriptions it bore a close resemblance to the earlier Greek, Roman and Arabic herbals. Other accounts of the period include *De Proprietatibus Rerum* (c. 1230–1240) of English Franciscan monk Bartholomaeus Anglicus and a group of herbals called *Tractatus de Herbis* written and pained between 1280 and 1300 by Matthaeus Platearius at the East-West cultural centre of Salerno Spain, the illustrations showing the fine detail of true botanical illustration.

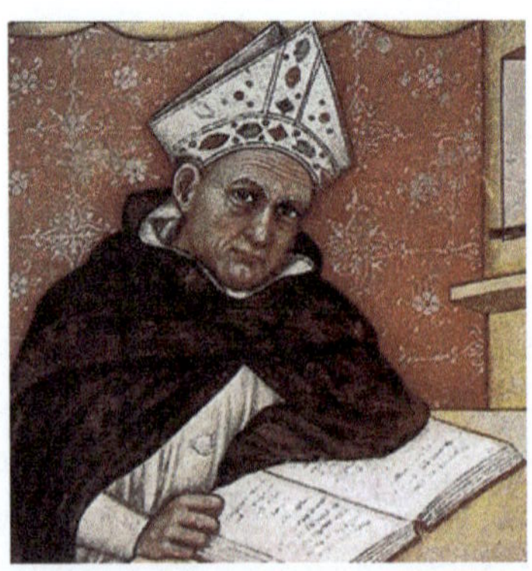

Albertus Magnus c. 1193–1280, author of *De Vegetabilibus*

Western Europe

Perhaps the best known herbals were produced in Europe between 1470 and 1670. The invention in Germany of printing from movable type in a printing press c. 1440 was a great stimulus to herbalism. The new herbals were more detailed with greater general appeal and often with Gothic script and the addition of woodcut illustrations that more closely resembled the plants being described.

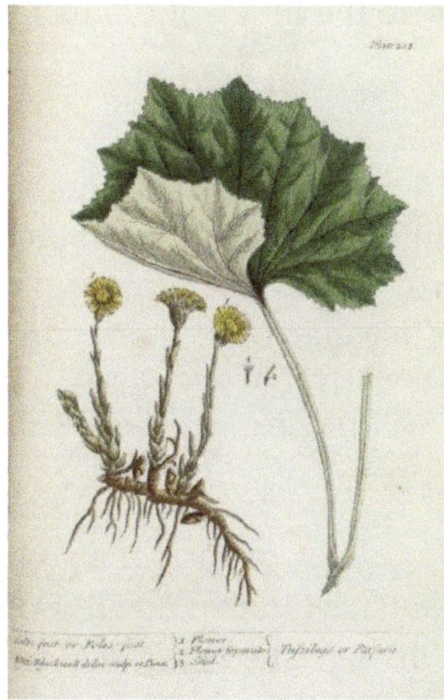

Illustration from Elizabeth Blackwell's *A Curious Herbal* (1737)

Three important herbals, all appearing before 1500, were printed in Mainz, Germany. Two of these were by Peter Schoeffer, his Latin *Herbarius* in 1484, followed by an updated and enlarged German version in 1485, these being followed in 1491 by the *Hortus Sanitatis* printed by Jacob Meyderbach. Other early printed herbals include the *Kreuterbuch* of Hieronymus Tragus from Germany in 1539 and, in England, the *New Herball* of William Turner in 1551 were arranged, like the classical herbals, either alphabetically, according to their medicinal properties, or as "herbs, shrubs, trees". Arrangement of plants in later herbals such as *Cruydboeck* of Dodoens and John Gerard's *Herball* of 1597 became more related to their physical similarities and this heralded the beginnings of scientific classification. By 1640 a herbal had been printed that included about 3800 plants – nearly all the plants of the day that were known.

In the Modern Age and Renaissance, European herbals diversified and innovated, and came to rely more on direct observation than being mere adaptations of traditional models. Typical examples from the period are the fully illustrated *De Historia Stirpium Commentarii Insignes* by Leonhart Fuchs (1542, with over 400 plants), the astrologically themed *Complete Herbal* by Nicholas Culpeper (1653), and the *Curious Herbal* by Elizabeth Blackwell (1737).

Anglo-saxon Herbals

Anglo-Saxon plant knowledge and gardening skills (the garden was called a *wyrtzerd*, literally, herb-yard) appears to have exceeded that on the continent. Our limited knowledge of Anglo-Saxon plant vernacular comes primarily from manuscripts that include: the Leechbook of Bald and the Lacnunga. The Leechbook of Bald (Bald was probably a friend of King Alfred of England) was painstakingly produced by the scribe Cild in about 900–950 CE. This was written in the vernacular (native) tongue and not derived from Greek texts. The oldest illustrated herbal from Saxon times is a translation of the Latin *Herbarius Apulei Platonici*, one of the most popular medical works of medieval times, the original dating from the fifth century; this Saxon translation was produced about 1000–1050 CE and is housed in the British Library. Another vernacular herbal was the *Buch der natur* or "Book of Nature" by Konrad von Megenberg (1309–1374) which contains the first two botanical woodcuts ever made; it is also the first work of its kind in the vernacular.

Anglo-norman Herbals

In the 12th and early 13th centuries, under the influence of the Norman conquest, the herbals produced in Britain fell less under the influence of France and Germany and more that of Sicily and the Near East. This showed itself through the Byzantine-influenced Romanesque framed illustrations. Anglo-Saxon herbals in the vernacular were replaced by herbals in Latin including Macers Herbal, *De Viribus Herbarum* (largely derived from Pliny), with the English translation completed in about 1373.

Fifteenth-century Incunabula

The earliest printed books and broadsheets are known as incunabula. The first printed herbal appeared in 1469, a version of Pliny's *Historia Naturalis*; it was published nine years before Dioscorides *De Materia Medica* was set in type. Important incunabula include the encyclopaedic *De Proprietatibus Rerum* of Franciscan monk Bartholomew Anglicus (c. 1203–1272) which, as a manuscript, had first appeared between 1248 and 1260 in at least six languages and after being first printed in 1470 ran to 25 editions. Assyrian physician Mesue (926–1016) wrote the popular *De Simplicibus*, *Grabadin* and *Liber Medicinarum Particularum* the first of his printings being in 1471. These were followed, in Italy, by the *Herbarium* of Apuleius Platonicus and three German works published in Mainz, the *Latin Herbarius* (1484), the first herbal published in Germany, *German Herbarius* (1485), the latter evolving into the *Ortus Sanitatis* (1491). To these can be added Macer's *De Virtutibus Herbarum*, based on Pliny's work; the 1477 edition is one of the first printed and illustrated herbals.

Fifteenth-century Manuscripts

In medieval times, medicinal herbs were generally referred to by the apothecaries (physicians or doctors) as "simples" or "officinals". Before 1542, the works principally used by apothecaries were the treatises on simples by Avicenna and Serapion's *Liber De Simplici Medicina*. The *De Synonymis* and other publications of Simon Januensis, the *Liber Servitoris* of Bulchasim Ben Aberazerim, which described the preparations made from plants, animals and minerals, provided a model for the chemical treatment of modern pharmacopoeias. There was also the *Antidotarium Nicolai* of Nicolaus de Salerno, which contained Galenical compounds arranged in alphabetical order.

Spain and Portugal – De Orta, Monardes, Hernandez

The Spaniards and Portuguese were explorers, the Portuguese to India (Vasco da Gama) and Goa where physician Garcia de Orta (1490–1570) based his work *Coloquios dos Simples* (1563). The first botanical knowledge of the New World came from Spaniard Nicolas Monardes (1493–1588) who published *Dos Libros* between 1569 and 1571. The work of Hernandez on the herbal medicine of the Aztecs has already been discussed.

Germany – Bock, Brunfels and Fuchs

Otto Brunfels (c. 1489–1534), Leonhart Fuchs (1501–1566) and Hieronymus Bock (1498–1554) were known as the "German fathers of botany" although this title belies the fact that they trod in the steps of the scientifically feted Hildegard of Bingen whose writings on herbalism were *Physica* and *Causae et Curae* (together known as *Liber subtilatum*) of 1150. The original manuscript is no longer in existence but a copy was printed in 1533. Another major herbalist was Valerius Cordus (1515–1544).

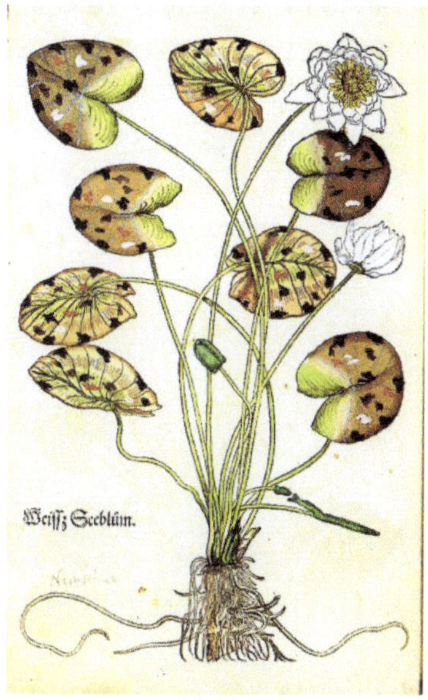

A Hans Weiditz hand-coloured woodcut from Otto Brunfels' *Herbarum Vivae Eicones*

The 1530, *Herbarum Vivae Eicones* of Brunfels contained the admired botanically accurate original woodcut colour illustrations of Hans Weiditz along with descriptions of 47 species new to science. Bock, in setting out to describe the plants of his native Germany, produced the *New Kreuterbuch* of 1539 describing the plants he had found in the woods and fields but without illustration; this was supplemented by a second edition in 1546 that contained 365 woodcuts. Bock was possibly the first to adopt a botanical classification in his herbal which also covered details of ecology and plant communities. In this, he was placing emphasis on botanical rather than medicinal characteristics, unlike the other German herbals and foreshadowing the modern Flora. *De Historia Stirpium* (1542 with a German version in 1843) of Fuchs was a later publication with 509 high quality woodcuts that again paid close attention to botanical detail: it included many plants introduced to Germany in the sixteenth century that were new to science. The work of Fuchs is regarded as being among the most accomplished of the Renaissance period.

Low Countries – Dodoens, Lobel, Clusius

The Flemish printer Christopher Plantin established a reputation publishing the works of Dutch herbalists Rembert Dodoens and Carolus Clusius and developing a vast library of illustrations.

Translations of early Greco-Roman texts published in German by Bock in 1546 as *Kreuterbuch* were subsequently translated into Dutch as *Pemptades* by Dodoens (1517–1585) who was a Belgian botanist of world renown. This was an elaboration of his first publication *Cruydeboeck* (1554). Matthias de Lobel (1538–1616) published his *Stirpium Adversaria Nova* (1570–1571) and a massive compilation of illustrations while Clusius's (1526–1609) magnum opus was *Rariorum Plantarum Historia* of 1601 which was a compilation of his Spanish and Hungarian floras and included over 600 plants that were new to science.

Italy – Mattioli, Calzolari, Alpino

In Italy, two herbals were beginning to include botanical descriptions. Notable herbalists included Pietro Andrea Mattioli (1501–1577), physician to the Italian aristocracy and his *Commentarii* (1544), which included many newly described species, and his more traditional herbal *Epistolarum Medicinalium Libri Quinque* (1561). Sometimes, the local flora was described as in the publication *Viaggio di Monte Baldo* (1566) of Francisco Calzolari. Prospero Alpino (1553–1617) published in 1592 the highly popular account of overseas plants *De Plantis Aegypti* and he also established a botanical garden in Padua in 1542, which together with those at Pisa and Florence, rank among the world's first.

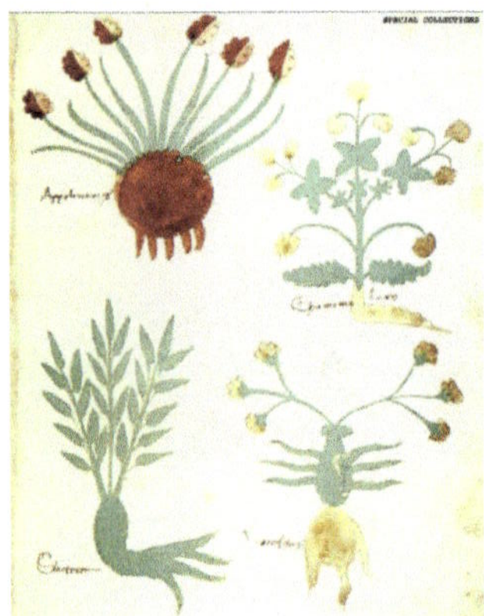

Early Italian manuscript herbal, c. 1500. Plants illustrated are *Appolinaris*, *Chamomeleon*, *Sliatriceo* and *Narcissus*

England – Turner, Gerard, Parkinson, Culpeper

The first true herbal printed in Britain was Richard Banckes' *Herball* of 1525 which, although popular in its day, was unillustrated and soon eclipsed by the most famous of the early printed herbals, Peter Treveris's *Grete Herball* of 1526 (derived in turn from the derivative French *Grand Herbier*).

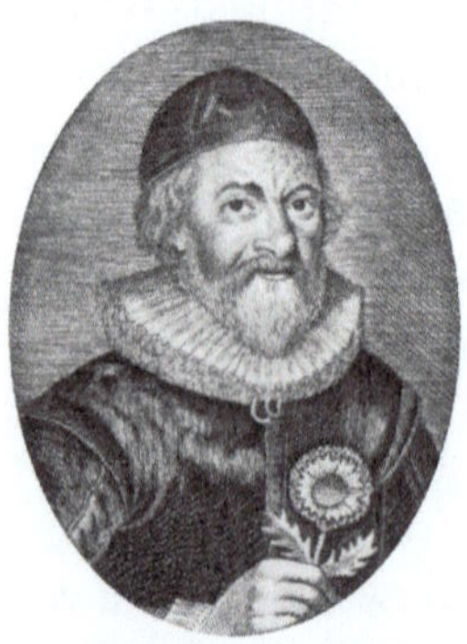

An engraving of Parkinson from his work *Theatrum Botanicum* (1640), reprinted in Agnes Arber's *Herbals*

William Turner (?1508–7 to 1568) was an English naturalist, botanist, and theologian who studied at Cambridge University and eventually became known as the "father of English botany." His 1538 publication *Libellus de re Herbaria Novus* was the first essay on scientific botany in English. His three-part *A New Herball* of 1551–1562–1568, with woodcut illustrations taken from Fuchs, was noted for its original contributions and extensive medicinal content; it was also more accessible to readers, being written in vernacular English. Turner described over 200 species native to England. and his work had a strong influence on later eminent botanists such as John Ray and Jean Bauhin.

John Gerard (1545–1612) is the most famous of all the English herbalists. His *Herball* of 1597 is, like most herbals, largely derivative. It appears to be a reformulation of Hieronymus Bock's *Kreuterbuch* subsequently translated into Dutch as *Pemptades* by Rembert Dodoens (1517–1585), and thence into English by Carolus Clusius, (1526–1609) then re-worked by Henry Lyte in 1578 as *A Nievve Herball*. This became the basis of Gerard's *Herball* or *General Historie of Plantes*. that appeared in 1597 with its 1800 woodcuts (only 16 original). Although largely derivative, Gerard's popularity can be attributed to his evocation of plants and places in Elizabethan England and to the clear influence of gardens and gardening on this work. He had published, in 1596, *Catalogus* which was a list of 1033 plants growing in his garden.

John Parkinson (1567–1650) was apothecary to James I and a founding member of the Worshipful Society of Apothecaries. He was an enthusiastic and skilful gardener, his garden in Long Acre being stocked with rarities. He maintained an active correspondence with important English and Continental botanists, herbalists and plantsmen importing new and unusual plants from overseas, in particular the Levant and Virginia. Parkinson is celebrated for his two monumental works, the first *Paradisi in Sole Paradisus Terrestris* in 1629: this was essentially a gardening book, a florilegium for which Charles I awarded him the title *Botanicus Regius Primarius* – Royal Botanist. The second was his *Theatrum Botanicum* of 1640, the largest herbal ever produced in the English language. It lacked the quality illustrations of Gerard's works, but was a massive and informative compendium including about 3800 plants (twice the number of Gerard's first edition *Herball*), over 1750 pages and over 2,700 woodcuts. This was effectively the last and culminating herbal of its kind and, although it included more plants of no discernible economic or medicinal use than ever before, they were nevertheless arranged according to their properties rather than their natural affinities.

Nicholas Culpeper (1616–1654) was an English botanist, herbalist, physician, apothecary and astrologer from London's East End. His published books were *A Physicall Directory* (1649), which was a pseudoscientific pharmacopoeia. *The English Physitian* (1652) and the *Complete Herbal* (1653), contain a rich store of pharmaceutical and herbal knowledge. His works lacked scientific credibility because of their use of astrology, though he combined diseases, plants and astrological prognosis into a simple integrated system that has proved popular to the present day.

Legacy

The legacy of the herbal extends beyond medicine to botany and horticulture. Herbal medicine is still practiced in many parts of the world but the traditional grand herbal, as described here, ended with the European Renaissance, the rise of modern medicine and the use of synthetic and industrialized drugs. The medicinal component of herbals has developed in several ways. Firstly, discussion of plant lore was reduced and with the increased medical content there emerged the official pharmacopoeia. The first British Pharmacopoeia was published in the English language in 1864, but gave such general dissatisfaction both to the medical profession and to chemists and druggists that the General Medical Council brought out a new and amended edition in 1867. Secondly, at a more popular level, there are the books on culinary herbs and herb gardens, medicinal and useful plants. Finally, the enduring desire for simple medicinal information on specific plants has resulted in contemporary herbals that echo the herbals of the past, an example being Maud Grieve's *A Modern Herbal*, first published in 1931 but with many subsequent editions.

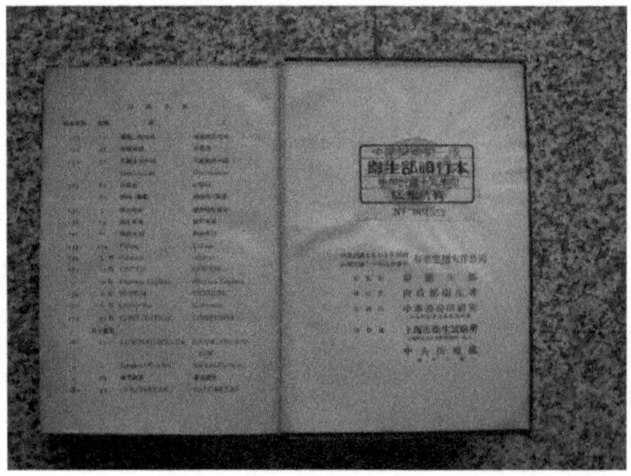

Back cover of the Chinese pharmacopoeia (1930)

The magical and mystical side of the herbal also lives on. Herbals often explained plant lore, displaying a superstitious or spiritual side. There was, for example, the fanciful doctrine of signatures, the belief that there were similarities in the appearance of the part of the body affected the appearance of the plant to be used as a remedy. The astrology of Culpeper can be seen in contemporary anthroposophy (biodynamic gardening) and alternative medical approaches like homeopathy, aromatherapy and other new age medicine show connections with herbals and traditional medicine.

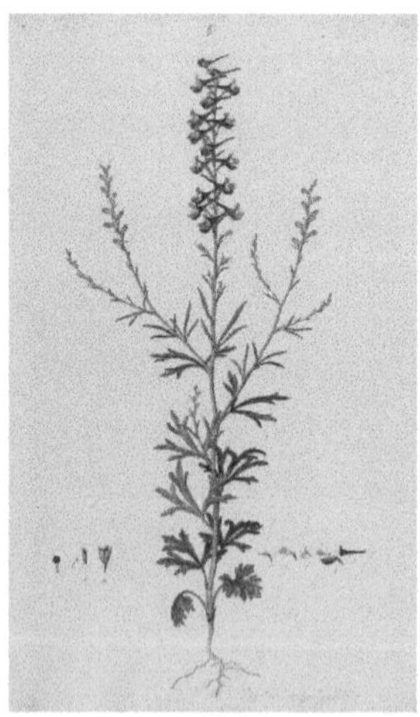

Illustration of *Delphinium peregrinum* in *Flora Graeca* by John Sibthorp and Ferdinand Bauer (1806–1840)

It is sometimes forgotten that the plants described in herbals were grown in special herb gardens (physic gardens). Such herb gardens were, for example, part of the medieval monastery garden that supplied the simples or officinals used to treat the sick being cared for within the monastery. Early physic gardens were also associated with institutes of learning, whether a monastery, university or herbarium. It was this medieval garden of the fourteenth to sixteenth centuries, attended by apothecaries and physicians, that established a tradition leading to the systems gardens of the eighteenth century (gardens that demonstrated the classification system of plants) and the modern botanical garden. The advent of printing, woodcuts and metal engraving improved the means of communication. Herbals prepared the ground for modern botanical science by pioneering plant description, classification and illustration. From the time of the ancients like Dioscorides through to Parkinson in 1629, the scope of the herbal remained essentially the same.

The greatest legacy of the herbal is to botany. Up to the seventeenth century, botany and medicine were one and the same but gradually greater emphasis was placed on the plants rather than their medicinal properties. During the seventeenth and eighteenth centuries, plant description and classification began to relate plants to one another and not to man. This was the first glimpse of non-anthropocentric botanical science since Theophrastus and, coupled with the new system of binomial nomenclature, resulted in "scientific herbals" called *Floras* that detailed and illustrated the plants growing in a particular region. These books were often backed by herbaria, collections of dried plants that verified the plant descriptions given in the Floras. In this way modern botany, especially plant taxonomy, was born out of medicine. As herbal historian Agnes Arber remarks – "Sibthorp's monumental *Flora Graeca* is, indeed, the direct descendant in modern science of the *De Materia Medica* of Dioscorides."

History of Herbalism

The history of herbalism is closely tied with the history of medicine from prehistoric times up until the development of the germ theory of disease in the 19th century. Modern medicine from the 19th century to today has been based on evidence gathered using the scientific method. Evidence-based use of pharmaceutical drugs has largely replaced herbal treatments in modern health care. However, many people continue to employ various forms of traditional or alternative medicine. These systems often have a significant herbal component. The history of herbalism also overlaps with food history, as many of the herbs and spices historically used by humans to season food yield useful medicinal compounds, and use of spices with antimicrobial activity in cooking is part of an ancient response to the threat of food-borne pathogens.

Prehistory

The use of plants as medicines predates written human history. Archaeological evidence indicates that humans were using medicinal plants during the Paleolithic, approximately 60,000 years ago. (Furthermore, other non-human primates are also known to ingest medicinal plants to treat illness) Plant samples gathered from prehistoric burial sites have been thought to support the claim that Paleolithic peoples had knowledge of herbal medicine. For instance, a 60,000-year-old Neanderthal burial site, "Shanidar IV", in northern Iraq has yielded large amounts of pollen from 8 plant species, 7 of which are used now as herbal remedies. More recently Paul B. Pettitt has written that "A recent examination of the microfauna from the strata into which the grave was cut suggests that the pollen was deposited by the burrowing rodent Meriones tersicus, which is common in the Shanidar microfauna and whose burrowing activity can be observed today". Medicinal herbs were found in the personal effects of *Ötzi the Iceman*, whose body was frozen in the Ötztal Alps for more than 5,000 years. These herbs appear to have been used to treat the parasites found in his intestines.

Ancient History

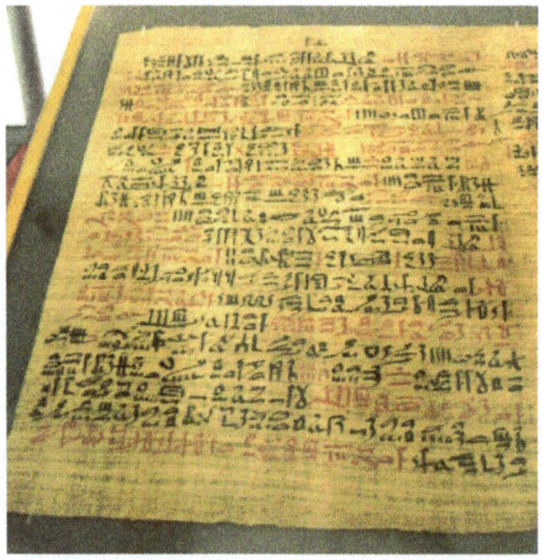

The Ebers Papyrus (c. 1550 BCE) from ancient Egypt has a prescription for *Cannabis sativa* (marijuana) applied topically for inflammation.

Mesopotamia

In Mesopotamia, the written study of herbs dates back over 5,000 years to the Sumerians, who created clay tablets with lists of hundreds of medicinal plants (such as myrrh and opium).

Ancient Egypt

Ancient Egyptian texts are of particular interest due to the language and translation controversies that accompany texts from this era and region. These differences in conclusions stem from the lack of complete knowledge of the Egyptian language: many translations are composed of mere approximations between Egyptian and modern ideas,and there can never be complete certainty of meaning or context. While physical documents are scarce, texts such as the Papyrus Ebers serve to illuminate and relieve some of the conjecture surrounding ancient herbal practices. The Papyrus consists of lists of ailments and their treatments, ranging from "disease of the limbs" to "diseases of the skin" and has information on over 850 plant medicines, including garlic, juniper, cannabis, castor bean, aloe, and mandrake. Treatments were mainly aimed at ridding the patient of the most prevalent symptoms because the symptoms were largely regarded as the disease itself. Knowledge of the collection and preparation of such remedies are mostly unknown, as many of the texts available for translation assume the physician already has some knowledge of how treatments are conducted and therefore such techniques would not need restating. Though modern understanding of Egyptian herbals stem form the translation of ancient texts, there is no doubt that trade and politics carried the Egyptian tradition to regions across the world, influencing and evolving many cultures medical practices and allowing for a glimpse into the world of ancient Egyptian medicine. Herbs used by Egyptian healers were mostly indigenous in origin, although some were imported from other regions like Lebanon. Other than papyri, evidence of herbal medicine has also been found in tomb illustrations or jars containing traces of herbs.

India

In India, Ayurveda medicine has used many herbs such as turmeric possibly as early as 4,000 BC. Earliest Sanskrit writings such as the Rig Veda, and Atharva Veda are some of the earliest available documents detailing the medical knowledge that formed the basis of the Ayurveda system. Many other herbs and minerals used in Ayurveda were later described by ancient Indian herbalists such as Charaka and Sushruta during the 1st millennium BC. The *Sushruta Samhita* attributed to Sushruta in the 6th century BC describes 700 medicinal plants, 64 preparations from mineral sources, and 57 preparations based on animal sources.

China

By 2,000 BC, Chinese started prescribing to herbal medicines. In China, seeds likely used for herbalism have also been found in the archaeological sites of Bronze Age China dating from the Shang Dynasty. The mythological Chinese emperor Shennong is said to have written the first Chinese pharmacopoeia, the "Shennong Ben Cao Jing". The "Shennong Ben Cao Jing" lists 365 medicinal plants and their uses - including Ephedra (the shrub that introduced the drug ephedrine to modern medicine), hemp, and chaulmoogra (one of the first effective treatments for leprosy). Succeeding generations augmented on the *Shennong Bencao Jing*, as in the *Yaoxing Lun* (*Treatise on the Nature of Medicinal Herbs*), a 7th-century Tang Dynasty treatise on herbal medicine.

Ancient Greece and Rome

Hippocrates

The *Hippocratic Corpus* serves as a collection of texts that are associated with the 'Father of Western Medicine', Hippocrates of Kos. Though the actual authorship of some of these texts is disputed, each reflects the general ideals put forth by Hippocrates and his followers. The recipes and remedies included in parts of the *Corpus* no doubt reveal popular and prevalent treatments of the early ancient Greek period.

Though any of the herbals included in the *Corpus* are similar to those practiced in the religious sectors of healing, they differ strikingly in the lack of rites, prayers, or chants used in the application of remedies. This distinction is truly indicative of the Hippocratic preference for logic and reason within the practices of medicine.

The ingredients mentioned in the *Corpus* consist of a myriad of herbs, both local to Greece and imported from exotic locales such as Arabia. While many imported goods would have been too expensive for common household use, some of the suggested ingredients include the more common and cheaper elderberries and St. John's Wort.

Galen

Galen of Pergamon, a Greek physician practicing in Rome, was certainly prolific in his attempt to write down his knowledge on all things medical – and in his pursuit, he wrote many texts regarding herbs and their properties, most notably his *Works of Therapeutics*. In this text, Galen outlines the merging of each discipline within medicine that combine to restore health and prevent disease. While the subject of therapeutics encompasses a wide array of topics, Galen's extensive work in the humors and four basic qualities helped pharmacists to better calibrate their remedies for the individual person and their unique symptoms.

Diocles of Carystus

The writings of Diocles of Carystus were also extensive and prolific in nature. With enough prestige to be referred to as "the second Hippocrates," his advice in herbalism and treatment was to be taken seriously. Though the original texts no longer exist, many medical scholars throughout the ages have quoted Diocles rather extensively, and it is in these fragments that we gain knowledge of his writings. It is purported that Diocles actually wrote the first comprehensive herbal- this work then cited numerous times by contemporaries such as Galen, Celsus, and Soranus.

Pliny

In what is one of the first encyclopedic texts, Pliny the Elder's *Natural History* serves as a comprehensive guide to nature and also presents an extensive catalog of herbs valuable in medicine. With over 900 drugs and plants listed, Pliny's writings provide a very large knowledge base upon which we may learn more about ancient herbalism and medical practices. Pliny himself referred to ailments as "the greatest of all the operations of nature," and the act of treatment via drugs as impacting the "state of peace or of war which exists between the various departments of nature".

Dioscordes

Much like Pliny, Pedanius Dioscorides constructed a pharmacopeia, *De Materia Medica*, consisting of over 1000 medicines produced form herbs, minerals, and animals. The remedies that comprise this work were widely utilized throughout the ancient period and Dioscorides remained the greatest expert on drugs for over 1,600 years.

Similarly important for herbalists and botanists of later centuries was Theophrastus' *Historia Plantarum*, written in the 4th century BC, which was the first systematization of the botanical world.

Middle Ages

While there are certainly texts from the medieval period that denote the uses of herbs, there has been a long-standing debate between scholars as to the actual motivations and understandings that underline the creation of herbal documents during the medieval period. The first point of view dictates that the information presented in these medieval texts were merely copied from their classical equivalents without much thought or understanding. The second viewpoint, which is gaining traction among modern scholars, states that herbals were copied for actual use and backed by genuine understanding.

Some evidence for the suggestion that herbals were utilized with knowledgeable intent, was the addition of several chapters of plants, lists of symptoms, habitat information, and plant synonyms added to texts such as the *Herbarium*. Notable texts utilized in this time period include Bald's Leechbook, the Lacnunga, the peri didaxeon, Herbarium Apulei, Da Taxone, and Madicina de Quadrupedidus, while the most popular during this time period were the Ex Herbis Femininis, the Herbarius, and works by Dioscorides.

Benedictine monasteries were the primary source of medical knowledge in Europe and England during the Early Middle Ages. However, most of these monastic scholars' efforts were focused on translating and copying ancient Greco-Roman and Arabic works, rather than creating substantial new information and practices. Many Greek and Roman writings on medicine, as on other subjects, were preserved by hand copying of manuscripts in monasteries. The monasteries thus tended to become local centers of medical knowledge, and their herb gardens provided the raw materials for simple treatment of common disorders. At the same time, folk medicine in the home and village continued uninterrupted, supporting numerous wandering and settled herbalists. Among these were the "wise-women" and "wise men", who prescribed herbal remedies often along with spells, enchantments, divination and advice. It was not until the late Middle Ages that women and men who were knowledgeable in herb lore became the targets of the witch hysteria. One of the most famous women in the herbal tradition was Hildegard of Bingen. A 12th-century Benedictine nun, she wrote a medical text called *Causae et Curae*.

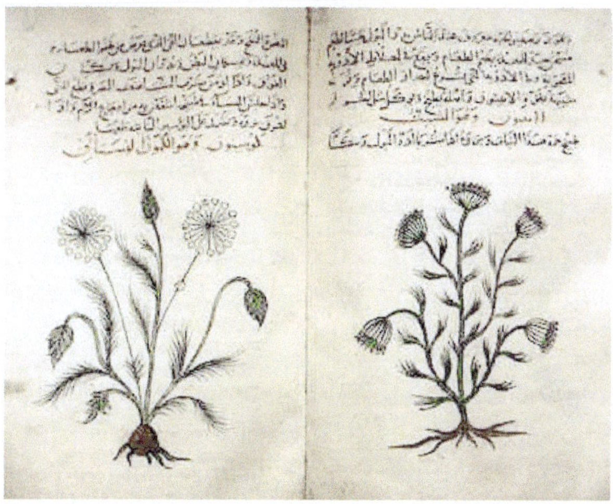

Dioscorides' *Materia Medica*, c. 1334 copy in Arabic, describes medicinal features of cumin and dill.

During this time, herbalism was mainly practiced by women, particularly among Germanic tribes. However, there were three major sources of information on healing at the time including the Arabian School, Anglo-Saxon Leechcraft, and Salerno. A great scholar of the Arabian School included Avicenna, who wrote *The Canon of Medicine* which became the standard medical reference work of the Arab world. "*The Canon of Medicine* is known for its introduction of systematic experimentation and the study of physiology, the discovery of contagious diseases and sexually transmitted diseases, the introduction of quarantine to limit the spread of infectious diseases, the introduction of experimental medicine, clinical trials, and the idea of a syndrome in the diagnosis of specific diseases. ...*The Canon* includes a description of some 760 medicinal plants and the medicine that could be derived from them." With Leechcraft, though bringing to mind part of their treatments, Leech was the English term for medical practitioner. Salerno was a famous school in Italy centered around health and medicine. A student of the school was Constantine the African, credited with bringing Arab medicine to Europe.

Translation of Herbals

During the Middle Ages, the study of plants began to be based on critical observations. "In the 16th and 17th century an interest in botany revived in Europe and spread to America by way of European conquest and colonization." Philosophers started to act as herbalists and academic professors studied plants with great depth. Herbalists began to explore the use of plants for both medicinal purposes and agricultural uses. Botanists in the Middle Ages were known as herbalists; they collected, grew, dried, stored, and sketched plants. Many became experts in identifying and describing plants according to their morphology and habitats, as well as their usefulness. These books, called herbals included beautiful drawings and paintings of plants as well as their uses.

At that time both botany and the art of gardening stressed the utility of plants for man; the popular herbal, described the medical uses of plants. During the Middle Ages, there was an expansion of book culture that spread through the medieval world. The phenomenon of translation is well-documented, from its beginnings as a scholarly endeavor in Baghdad as early as the eighth century to its expansion throughout European Mediterranean centers of scholarship by the eleventh and twelfth centuries. The process of translation is collaborative effort, requiring a variety of people to translate and add to them. However, how the Middle Ages viewed nature seems to be a mystery.

Translation of text and image has provided numerous versions and compilations of individual manuscripts from diverse sources, old and new. Translation is a dynamic process as well as a scholarly endeavor that contributed great to science in the Middle Ages; the process naturally entailed continuous revisions and additions. The Benedictine monasteries were known for their in-depth knowledge of herbals. These gardens grew the herbs which were considered to be useful for the treatment of the various human ills; the beginnings of modern medical education can be connected with monastic influence. Monastic academies were developed and monks were taught how to translate Greek manuscripts into Latin.

Knowledge of medieval botanicals was closely related to medicine because the plant's principal use was for remedies. Herbals were structured by the names of the plants, identifying features, medicinal parts of plant, therapeutic properties, and some included instructions on how to prepare and use them. For medical use of herbals to be effective, a manual was developed. Dioscorides' *De material medica* was a significant herbal designed for practical purposes.

Theophrastus wrote more than 200 papers describing the characteristics of over 500 plants. He developed a classification system for plants based on their morphology such as their form and structure. He described in detail pepper, cinnamon, bananas, asparagus, and cotton. Two of his best-known works, *Enquiry into Plants* and *The Causes of Plants*, have survived for many centuries and were translated into Latin. He has been referred to as the "grandfather of botany". Crateuas was the first to produce a pharmacological book for medicinal plants, and his book influenced medicine for many centuries. A Greek physician, Pedanius Dioscorides described over 600 different kinds of plants and describes their useful qualities for herbal medicine, and his illustrations were used for pharmacology and medicine as late as the Renaissance years.

Monasteries established themselves as centers for medical care. Information on these herbals and how to use them was passed on from monks to monks, as well as their patients. These illustrations were of no use to everyday individuals; they were intended to be complex and for people with prior knowledge and understanding of herbal. The usefulness of these herbals have been questioned because they appear to be unrealistic and several plants are depicted claiming to cure the same condition, as "the modern world does not like such impression." When used by experienced healers, these plants can provide their many uses. For these medieval healers, no direction was needed their background allowed them to choose proper plants to use for a variety of medical conditions. The monk's purpose was to collect and organize text to make them useful in their monasteries. Medieval monks took many remedies from classical works and adapted them to their own needs as well as local needs. This may be why none of the collections of remedies we have presently agrees fully with another.

Another form of translation was oral transmission; this was used to pass medical knowledge from generation to generation. A common misconception is that one can know early medieval medicine simply by identifying texts, but it is difficult to compose a clear understanding of herbals without prior knowledge. There are many factors that played in influenced in the translation of these herbals, the act of writing or illustrating was just a small piece of the puzzle, these remedies stems from many previous translations the incorporated knowledge from a variety of influences.

Early Modern Era

The 16th and 17th centuries were the great age of herbals, many of them available for the first time in English and other languages rather than Latin or Greek. The 18th and 19th centuries saw more incorporation of plants found in the Americas, but also the advance of modern medicine.

16th Century

The first herbal to be published in English was the anonymous *Grete Herball* of 1526. The two best-known herbals in English were *The Herball or General History of Plants* (1597) by John Gerard and *The English Physician Enlarged* (1653) by Nicholas Culpeper. Gerard's text was basically a pirated translation of a book by the Belgian herbalist Dodoens and his illustrations came from a German botanical work. The original edition contained many errors due to faulty matching of the two parts. Culpepper's blend of traditional medicine with astrology, magic, and folklore was ridiculed by the physicians of his day, yet his book - like Gerard's and other herbals - enjoyed phenomenal popularity. The Age of Exploration and the Columbian Exchange introduced new medicinal plants to Europe. The *Badianus Manuscript* was an illustrated Mexican herbal written in Nahuatl and Latin in the 16th century.

17th Century

The second millennium, however, also saw the beginning of a slow erosion of the pre-eminent position held by plants as sources of therapeutic effects. This began with the Black Death, which the then dominant Four Element medical system proved powerless to stop. A century later, Paracelsus introduced the use of active chemical drugs (like arsenic, copper sulfate, iron, mercury, and sulfur).

18th Century

In the Americas, herbals were relied upon for most medical knowledge with physicians being few and far between. These books included almanacs, Dodoens' *New Herbal, Edinburgh New Dispensatory,* Buchan's *Domestic Medicine,* and other works. Aside from European knowledge on American plants, Native Americans shared some of their knowledge with colonists, but most of these records were not written and compiled until the 19th century. John Bartram was a botanist that studied the remedies that Native Americans would share and often included bits of knowledge of these plants in printed almanacs.

19th Century

The formalization of pharmacology in the 19th century led to greater understanding of the specific actions drugs have on the body. At that time, Samuel Thompson was an uneducated but well respected herbalist who influenced professional opinions so much that Doctors and Herbalists would refer to themselves as Thompsonians. They distinguished themselves from "regular" doctors of the time who used calomel and bloodletting, and led to a brief renewal of the empirical method in herbal medicine.

Modern Era

Traditional herbalism has been officially regarded as a method of alternative medicine in the United States since the Flexner Report of 1910 led to the closing of the eclectic medical schools where botanical medicine was exclusively practiced. In China, Mao Zedong reintroduced Traditional Chinese Medicine, which relied heavily on herbalism, into the health care system in 1949. Since then, schools have been training thousands of practitioners – including Americans – in the basics of Chinese medicines to be used in hospitals. "The Chinese pharmacopeia is 5000 years old and contains substances that are transformed into effective but non-toxic medicines." While Britain in the 1930s was experiencing turbulence over the practice of herbalism, in the United States, government regulation began to prohibit the practice.

"The World Health Organization estimated that 80% of people worldwide rely on herbal medicines for some part of their primary health care. In Germany, about 600 to 700 plant based medicines are available and are prescribed by some 70% of German physicians." South African doctors use herbs to treat many patients, some patients finding the plants more useful than modern medicine previously prescribed to them.

The practice of prescribing treatments and cures to patients requires a legal medical license in the United States of America, and the licensing of these professions occurs on a state level. "There is currently no licensing or certification for herbalists in any state that precludes the rights of anyone to use, dispense, or recommend herbs."

"Traditional medicine is a complex network of interaction of both ideas and practices, the study of which requires a multidisciplinary approach." Many alternative physicians in the 21st century incorporate herbalism in traditional medicine due to the diverse abilities plants have and their low number of side effects.

List of Herbs with Known Adverse Effects

This is a partial list of herbs and herbal treatments with known or suspected adverse effects, either alone or in interaction with other herbs or drugs. Non-inclusion of an herb in this list does not imply that it is free of adverse effects. In general, the safety and effectiveness of alternative medicines have not been scientifically proven and remain largely unknown. Beyond adverse effects from the herb itself, “adulteration, inappropriate formulation, or lack of understanding of plant and drug interactions have led to adverse reactions that are sometimes life threatening or lethal.”

Most of the adverse effects stated in this list are associated with only a small percentage of cases; they should be understood as potential risks rather than as certainties.

Herbs, Treatments, and Constituents With Known or Suspected Adverse Effects

Name	Other common names	Scientific name	Adverse effects
Aconite	monkshood, wolfsbane, aconitum	Aconitum spp.	Heart palpitations and arrhythmias, hypotension, nausea, vomiting, abdominal pain, respiratory system paralysis, death
Aloe vera juice	medicinal aloe	Aloe vera	“abdominal pain, diarrhea, potentially carcinogenic, with others can potentiate cardiac glycosides and antiarrhythmic agents”
Anthranoid laxatives			“abdominal pain, diarrhea, potentially carcinogenic, with others can potentiate cardiac glycosides and antiarrhythmic agents”
Areca nut	Betel nut	Areca catechu	“deterioration of psychosis in patients with preexisting psychiatric disorders”; known carcinogen contributing to cancer of the mouth, pharynx, esophagus and stomach when chewed.
Aristolochic acid (contained in herbs in the genus *Aristolochia* e.g. *Aristolochia serpentaria* (Virginia snakeroot), *Aristolochia reticulata* (Texas snakeroot) and in Chinese herbs such as *Aristolochia fangchi* and *Aristolochia mandshurensis* (banned in China and withdrawn from Chinese Pharmacopoea 2005; *Stephania tetrandra* and *Magnolia officinalis* do not contain aristolochic acid).			Kidney toxicity associated with kidney failure; associated with development of cancer, particularly of the urinary tract, known carcinogen

Atractylate		Atractylis gummifera	Liver damage, nausea, vomiting, epigastric and abdominal pain, diarrhoea, anxiety, headache and convulsions, often followed by coma
Ayurvedic Herbo-mineral (Rasashastra) Medicines			Heavy metal contamination
Bitter orange			'Fainting, arrhythmia, heart attack, stroke, death'
Broom	Broom Flower, Dyers Broom, Dyer's Greenwood, Dyer's Weed, Dyer's Whin, Furze, Green Broom, Greenweed, Wood Waxen	Genista tinctoria	Uterotonic properties, nausea vomiting, and diarrhea, contraindicated for pregnancy and breast feeding
Buckthorn bark and berry		Rhamnus frangula	"abdominal pain, diarrhea, potentially carcinogenic, with others can potentiate cardiac glycosides and antiarrhythmic agents"
Cascara Sagrada bark		Rhamnus purshiana	"abdominal pain, diarrhea, potentially carcinogenic, with others can potentiate cardiac glycosides and antiarrhythmic agents"
Chaparral	creosote bush, gobernadora, larreastat	Larrea tridentata, Larrea divaricata	Liver damage, kidney problems, Hypotension in cancer patients
Chinese herbal mixtures			Heavy metal poisoning
Coltsfoot	coughwort, farfarae folium leaf, foalswort	Tussilago farfara	Liver damage, cancer
Comfrey	comphrey, blackwort, common comfrey, slippery root		Liver damage, cancer
Country mallow	heartleaf, silky white mallow	Sida cordifolia	"Heart attack, heart arrhythmia, stroke, death"
Dan Shen	Red sage, Chinese sage, tan shen	Salvia miltiorrhiza	Potentiates warfarin activity, leading to excessive anticoagulation and bleeding
Dong quai	female ginseng	Angelica sinensis	May induce uterine contractions; contraindicated when pregnant or nursing
European Mistletoe		Viscum album	Toxic to cardio and central nervous systems, gastrointestinal bleeding
Ephedra	ma huang	Ephedra sinica	Agitation and palpitations, "hypertension, irregular heart rate, insomnia, nervousness, tremors and seizures, paranoid psychoses, heart attacks, strokes, and death", kidney stones

Flavonoids (contained in many medicinal plants)	Vitamin P, citrin	Flavonoids, bioflavonoids	Hemolytic anemia, kidney damage
Germander		Teucrium	Liver damage
Ginger			May alter bleeding time
Ginkgo biloba			Bleeding
American Ginseng	American Ginseng, Canadian Ginseng, Ginseng, Ginseng Root, North American Ginseng, Occidental Ginseng, Ontario Ginseng, Panax quinquefolium, Panax quinquefolius, Red Berry, Ren Shen, Sang, Shang, Shi Yang Seng, Wisconsin Ginseng	Panax quinquefolius	"Hypertensive and chronotropic activities, may increase digoxin levels", diarrhea, itching, insomnia, headaches, nervousness, rapid heartbeat, hypertension or hypotension, breast tenderness, vaginal bleeding. Very rarely Stevens–Johnson syndrome, liver damage, severe allergy has been reported May lower blood sugar excessively in combination with diabetes medication. Contains a chemical linked to possible birth defects. May worsen hormone sensitive conditions such as breast cancer, uterine cancer, ovarian cancer, endometriosis, and uterine fibroids. Insomnia.
Goldenseal	Orange-root, Orangeroot,	Hydrastis canadensis	Uterotonic
Greater celandine	celandine	Chelidonium majus	Liver damage
Guarana		Paullinia cupana	Agitation and insomnia
Guar gum	guaran		Obstruction of gastrointestinal tract
Gugulipid	Guggal, Guggul, Mukul myrrh tree	Commiphora mukul	"Headache, nausea, hiccups, diminished efficacy of other cardiovascular drugs including diltiazem and propranolol"
Hawthorn	Common hawthorn, may, mayblossom, maythorn, quickthorn, whitethorn, motherdie, haw	Crataegus monogyna	"Potentiates digitalis activity, increases coronary dilation effects of theophylline, caffeine, papaverine, sodium nitrate, adenosine and epinephrine, increase barbiturate-induced sleeping times"
Horse chestnut	Conker	Aesculus hippocastanum	Liver toxicity, allergic reaction, anaphylaxis
Kava	awa, kava-kava	Piper methysticum	Potentates CNS sedatives, chronic use might cause a reversible dry skin condition.
Khat		Catha edulis	Chronic liver dysfunction
Liquorice root		Glycyrrhiza glabra	Hypokalemia, hypertension, arrhythmias, edema
Lobelia	asthma weed, pukeweed, vomit wort	Lobelia Inflata	Toxicity, rapid heartbeat, hypotension, coma, death
Milk thistle		Silybum marianum	Mild laxative, allergy

Pennyroyal		Mentha pulegium	Liver damage
Peony	Bai Shao, Chi Shao, Chinese Peony, Common Peony, Coral Peony, Cortex Moutan, European Peony, Jiu Chao Bai Shao, Moutan, Mu Dan PI, Peony Flower, Peony Root, Piney, Radix Peony, Red Peony, Shakuyaku, Shao Yao, Tree Peony, Ud Saleeb, Udsalam, Udsalap, White Peony	Radix Paeoniae, Radix Paeoniae Alba, Radix Paeoniae Rubra, Paeonia, Paeonia alba, Paeonia lactiflora, Paeonia mascula; Paeonia obovata; Paeonia officinalis; Paeonia suffruticosa, Paeonia veitchii, Paeoniae Flos, Paeoniae Radix	May slow clotting; contraindicated for people with bleeding disorders and before and after surgery. May induce uterine contractions; contraindicated when pregnant or nursing.
Pyrrolizidine alkaloids (contained in comfrey, borage, senecio, coltsfoot, and others)			Liver damage
Reserpine		Rauvolfia serpentina	"Sedation, inability to complete tasks, mental depression, nasal congestion, increased gastric secretion and mild diarrhea"
Safrole		Sassafras albidum	Liver damage
Saw palmetto		Serenoa repens	"rare and mild gastrointestinal upset, headaches, diarrhea, gynecomastia, paroxysmal atrial fibrillation, ventricular rupture and death in one patient"
Senna		Senna alexandrina (Cassia senna)	"abdominal pain, diarrhea, potentially carcinogenic, with others can potentiate cardiac glycosides and antiarrhythmic agents", liver damage
St John's wort	Tipton's weed, Klamath weed	Hypericum perforatum	Photosensitization, GI disturbances, "allergic reactions, fatigue, dizziness, confusion, dry mouth"
Valerian	garden valerian, garden heliotrope, all-heal	Valeriana officinalis	"drowsiness, GI upset, headache, palpitations, insomnia", oversedation, overstimulation
Vasambu	sweet flag	Acorus calamus	Vomiting and nausea
Yohimbe	yohimbine	Corynanthe yohimbe	rapid heart rate, hypertension, hypotension, heart problems, death

Herbs with Adverse Drug Interactions

Name	Other common names	Scientific name	Drug	Adverse effects
Cinchona bark		Cinchona pubescens	Warfarin	Possibly additive

Devil's Claw	grapple plant, wood spider	Harpagophytum	Warfarin	Additive effects
Ephedra			Caffeine, decongestants, stimulants	
Feverfew		Tanacetum parthenium	Aspirin	Additive effects
Garlic		Allium sativum	Warfarin	Additive effects
Ginger		Zingiber officinale	Warfarin	Additive effect, causes iris bleeding
Ginkgo biloba			Aspirin, warfarin, ticlopidine, clopidogrel, dipyridamole, garlic, vitamin E	With aspirin - retards aspirin absorption
Ginseng		Panax ginseng	Warfarin	
Papaya extract		Carica papaya	Warfarin	Damage to GI tract mucous membranes, Possibly additive, purpura
Kava			Sedatives, sleeping pills, antipsychotics, alcohol	
Pineapple enzyme		Ananas comosus	Bromelain	"Diarrhea, increased tendency for bleeding if used simultaneously with anticoagulants and inhibitors of thrombocytic aggregation due to modulation of the arachidonate cascade"
Psyllium seed		Plantago spp	Coumarin derivates	Retards absorption of drug
St John's wort	Tipton's weed, Klamath weed	Hypericum perforatum	Antidepressants, warfarin, protease inhibitors for HIV, birth control, some asthma drugs, and many other medications	

Herbal Plants Associated with Allergic Reactions

- Angelica
- Aniseed
- Apricot
- Arnica
- Artichoke
- Asafoetida
- Boneset
- Cassia
- Celery

- Cinnamon
- Cowslip
- Dandelion
- Elecampane
- Euphorbia
- Feverfew
- Fucus
- Gravel root
- Guaiacum
- Holy Thistle
- Hops
- Hydrangea
- Hydrocotyle
- Juniper
- Lady’s slipper
- Meadowsweet
- Milk thistle
- Motherwort
- Parsley
- Pilewort
- Plantain
- Pulsatilla
- Rosemary
- Tansy
- Vitex agnus-castus
- Wild carrot
- Yarrow

Zoopharmacognosy

Zoopharmacognosy is a behaviour in which non-human animals apparently self-medicate by selecting and ingesting or topically applying plants, soils, insects, and psychoactive drugs to prevent or reduce the harmful effects of pathogens and toxins. The term derives from Greek roots *zoo* ("animal"), *pharma* ("drug"), and *gnosy* ("knowing").

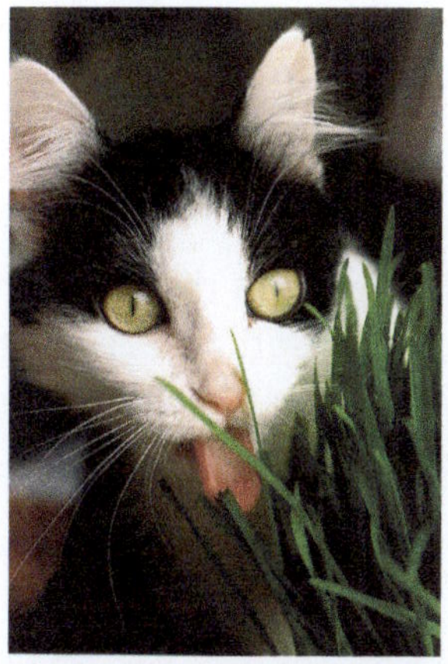

A cat eating grass - an example of zoopharmacognosy

A well-known example of zoopharmacognosy occurs when dogs eat grass to induce vomiting. However, the behaviour is more diverse than this. Animals ingest or apply non-foods such as clay, charcoal and even toxic plants and invertebrates, apparently to prevent parasitic infestation or poisoning.

Whether animals truly self-medicate remains a somewhat controversial subject because early evidence is mostly circumstantial or anecdotal, however, more recent examinations have adopted an experimental, hypothesis-driven approach.

The methods by which animals self-medicate vary, but can be classified according to function as prophylactic (preventative, before infection or poisoning) or therapeutic (after infection, to combat the pathogen or poisoning). The behaviour is believed to have widespread adaptive significance.

History and Etymology

In 1978, Janzen suggested that vertebrate herbivores might benefit medicinally from the secondary metabolites in their plant food.

In 1993, the term "zoopharmacognosy" was coined, derived from the Greek roots *zoo* ("animal"), *pharma* ("drug"), and *gnosy* ("knowing"). The term gained popularity from academic works and in a book by Cindy Engel entitled *Wild Health: How Animals Keep Themselves Well and What We Can Learn from Them.*

Mechanisms

The anti-parasitic effect of zoopharmacognosy could occur by at least two mechanisms. First, the ingested material may have pharmacological antiparasitic properties such that phytochemicals decrease the ability of worms to attach to the mucosal lining of the intestines, or chemotaxis attracts worms into the folds of leaves. Many ingested plants during purported zoopharmacognosy have a consistent physical property, e.g., the rough surface of the leaves sports many hooked and spiky hairs. So, parasites may became attached to the bristly surface or the coarse structure may function as a rasping plug, dislodging parasites from the intestines. The second possible mode of action is the material may initiate a purging response of the gastrointestinal tract by rapidly inducing diarrhea. This substantially decreases gut transit time, causes worm expulsion and interrupts the life cycle of parasites. This, or a similar, mechanism could explain undigested grass in the faeces of various animals such as birds, carnivores and primates.

Methods of Self-medication

Some animals ingest or apply the substance when they appear to be well, suggesting the behaviour is preventative or prophylactic. In other cases, animals ingest or apply the substance when unwell, suggesting the behaviour is therapeutic or curative. There are three methods of self-medication, namely, ingestion, absorption, or topical application.

Ingestion

Many examples of zoopharmacognosy involve an animal ingesting a substance with (potential) medicinal properties.

Ants

Ants infected with Beauveria bassiana, a fungus, selectively consume harmful substances (reactive oxygen species, ROS) upon exposure to a fungal pathogen, yet avoid these in the absence of infection.

Mammals

Great apes often consume plants that have no nutritional values but which have beneficial effects on gut acidity or combat intestinal parasitic infection.

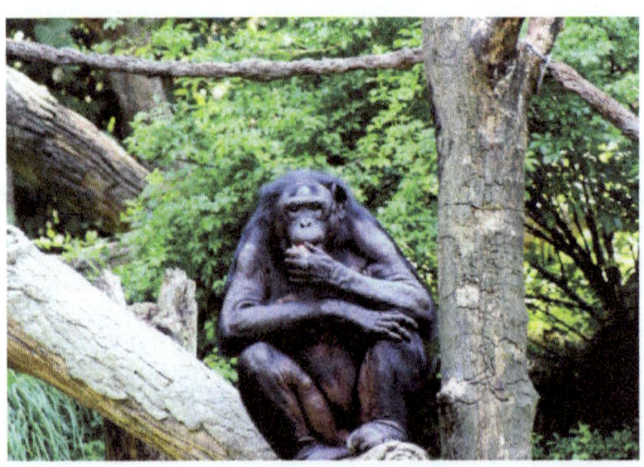

A variety of simian species have been observed to medicate themselves when ill using materials such as plants.

Chimpanzees sometimes select bitter leaves for chewing. Parasite infection drops noticeably after chimpanzees chew leaves of pith (*Vernonia amyddalina*), which have anti-parasitic activity against schistosoma, plasmodium and Leishmania. Chimpanzees don't consume this plant on a regular basis, but when they do eat it, it is often in small amounts by individuals that appear ill. Jane Goodall witnessed chimpanzees eating particular bushes, apparently to make themselves vomit. There are reports that chimpanzees swallow whole leaves of particular rough-leaved plants such as *Aneilema aequinoctiale*; these remove parasitic worms from their intestines.

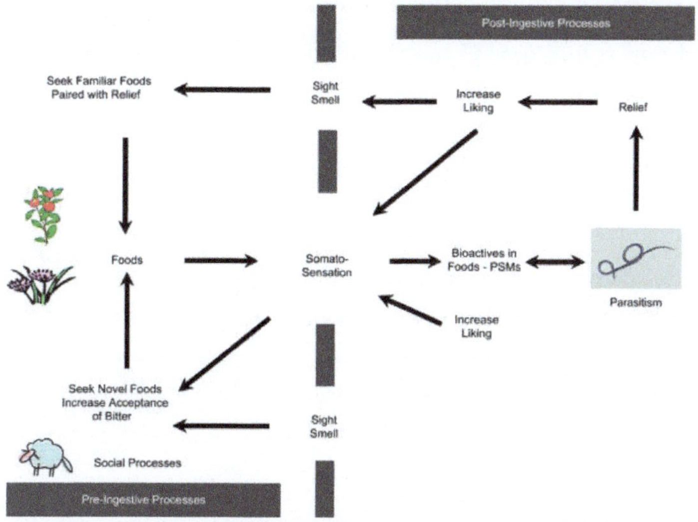

A conceptual representation of how pre- and post-ingestive events control the manifestation of self-medicative behavior in mammalian herbivores.

Chimpanzees sometimes eat the leaves of the herbaceous *Desmodium gangeticum*. Undigested, non-chewed leaves were recovered in 4% of faecal samples of wild chimpanzees and clumps of sharp-edged grass leaves in 2%. The leaves have a rough surface or sharp-edges and the fact they were not chewed and excreted whole indicates they were not ingested for nutritional purposes. Furthermore, this leaf-swallowing was restricted to the rainy season when parasite re-infections are more common, and parasitic worms (Oesophagostomum stephanostomum) were found together with the leaves.

Chimpanzees, bonobos, and gorillas eat the fruits of Aframomum angustifolium. Laboratory assays of homogenized fruit and seed extracts show significant anti-microbial activity. Illustrating the medicinal knowledge of some species, apes have been observed selecting a particular part of a medicinal plant by taking off leaves and breaking the stem to suck out the juice.

Anubis baboons (*Papio anubis*) and hamadryas baboons (*Papio hamadryas*) in Ethiopia use fruits and leaves of *Balanites aegyptiaca* to control schistosomiasis. Its fruits contain diosgenin, a hormone precursor that presumably hinders the development of schistosomes.

African elephants (*Loxodonta africana*) apparently self-medicate to induce birth by chewing on the leaves of a particular tree from the family Boraginaceae; Kenyan women brew a tea from this tree to induce childbirth.

White-nosed coatis (*Nasua narica*) in Panama take the menthol-scented resin from freshly scraped bark of *Trattinnickia aspera* (Burseraceae) and vigorously rub it into their own fur or that of other coatis, possibly to kill ectoparasites such as fleas, ticks, and lice, as well as biting insects such as mosquitoes; the resin contains triterpenes α - and β-amyrin, the eudesmane derivative β-selinene, and the sesquiterpene lactone 8β-hydroxyasterolide.

Domestic cats and dogs often select and ingest plant material, apparently to induce vomiting.

Indian wild boars selectively dig up and eat the roots of pigweed which humans use as an anthelmintic. Mexican folklore indicates that pigs eat pomegranate roots because they contain an alkaloid that is toxic to tapeworms.

A study on domestic sheep (*Ovis aries*) has provided clear experimental proof of self-medication via individual learning. Lambs in a treatment group were allowed to consume foods and toxins (grain, tannins, oxalic acid) that lead to malaise (negative internal states) and then allowed to eat a substance known to alleviate each malaise (sodium bentonite, polyethylene glycol and dicalcium phosphate, respectively). Control lambs ate the same foods and medicines, but this was disassociated temporally so they did not recuperate from the illness. After the conditioning, lambs were fed grain or food with tannins or oxalates and then allowed to choose the three medicines. The treatment animals preferred to eat the specific compound known to rectify the state of malaise induced by the food previously ingested. However, control animals did not change their pattern of use of the medicines, irrespective of the food consumed before the choice. Other ruminants learn to self-medicate against gastrointestinal parasites by increasing consumption of plant secondary compounds with antiparasitic actions.

Standard laboratory cages prevent mice from performing several natural behaviours for which they are highly motivated. As a consequence, laboratory mice sometimes develop abnormal behaviours indicative of emotional disorders such as depression and anxiety. To improve welfare, these cages are sometimes enriched with items such as nesting material, shelters and running wheels. Sherwin and Olsson tested whether such enrichment influenced the consumption of Midazolam, a drug widely used to treat anxiety in humans. Mice in standard cages, standard cages but with unpredictable husbandry, or enriched cages, were given a choice of drinking either non-drugged water or a solution of the Midazolam. Mice in the standard and unpredictable cages drank a greater proportion of the anxiolytic solution than mice from enriched cages, presumably because they had been experiencing greater anxiety. Early studies indicated that autoimmune (MRL/lpr) mice readily consume solutions with cyclophosphamide, an immunosuppressive drug that prevents inflammatory damage to internal organs. However, further studies provided contradictory evidence.

Geophagy

Many animals eat soil or clay, a behaviour known as *geophagy*. Clay is the primary ingredient of kaolin. It has been proposed that for primates, which can logically be extended to other animals, there are four hypotheses relating to geophagy in alleviating gastrointestinal disorders or upsets:

1. soils adsorb toxins such as phenolics and secondary metabolites
2. soil ingestion has an antacid action and adjusts the gut pH
3. soils act as an antidiarrhoeal agent
4. soils counteract the effects of endoparasites.

Furthermore, two hypotheses pertain to geophagy in supplementing minerals and/or elements:

5. soils supplement nutrient-poor diets

6. soils provide extra iron at high altitudes

Tapirs, forest elephants, colobus monkeys, mountain gorillas and chimpanzees seek out and eat clay, which absorbs intestinal bacteria and their toxins and alleviates stomach upset and diarrhoea. Cattle eat clay-rich termite mound soil, which deactivates ingested pathogens or fruit toxins.

Birds

Many parrot species in the Americas, Africa, and Papua New Guinea consume kaolin or clay, which both releases minerals and absorbs toxic compounds from the gut. Great bustards eat blister beetles of the genus *Meloe* to decrease parasite load in the digestive system; cantharidin, the toxic compound in blister beetles, can kill a great bustard if too many beetles are ingested.

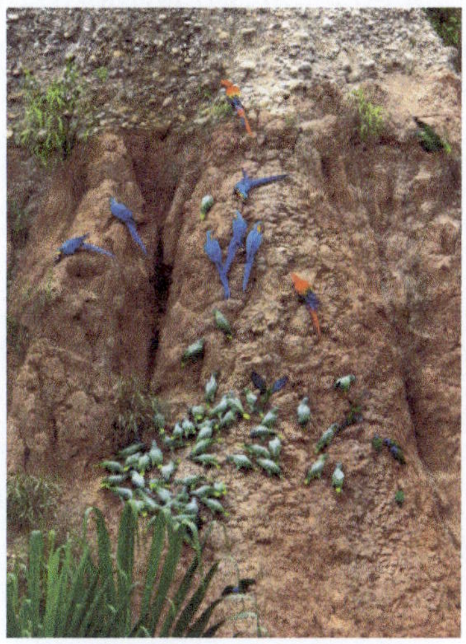

Parrots eating earth

Invertebrates

Woolly bear caterpillars (*Grammia incorrupta*) are sometimes lethally endoparasitised by tachinid flies. The caterpillars ingest plant toxins called pyrrolizidine alkaloids, which improve the survival of by conferring resistance against the flies. Crucially, parasitised caterpillars are more likely than non-parasitised caterpillars to specifically ingest large amounts of pyrrolizidine alkaloids, and excessive ingestion of these toxins reduces the survival of non-parasitised caterpillars. These three findings are all consistent with the adaptive plasticity theory.

The tobacco hornworm ingests nicotine which reduces colony growth and toxicity of *Bacillus thuringiensis*, leading to increased survival of the hornworm.

Absorption and Adsorption

The swallowing of whole leaves by apes without chewing has been observed for over 40 plant species.

Wild chimpanzees sometimes seek whole leaves of the *Aspilia* plant. These contain thiarubrine-A, a chemical active against intestinal nematode parasites, however, it is quickly broken-down by the stomach. The chimpanzees pick the *Aspilia* leaves and, rather than chewing them, they roll them around in their mouths, sometimes for as long as 25 seconds. They then swallow the capsule-like leaves whole. As many as 15 to 35 *Aspilia* leaves may be used in each bout of this behaviour, particularly in the rainy season when there are many parasitic larvae leading to an increased risk of infection.

Bonobos sometimes swallow non-chewed stem-strips of (*Manniophyton fulvum*). Despite the plant being abundantly available all year, *M. fulvum* is ingested only at specific times, in small amounts, and by a small proportion of bonobos in each group.

Topical Application

Some animals apply substances with medicinal properties to their skin. Again, this can be prophylactic or curative. In some cases, this is known as self-anointing.

Mammals

A female capuchin monkey in captivity was observed using tools covered in a sugar-based syrup to groom her wounds and those of her infant.

North American brown bears (*Ursos arctos*) make a paste of Osha roots (*Ligusticum porteri*) and saliva and rub it through their fur to repel insects or soothe bites. This plant, locally known as "bear root", contains 105 active compounds, such as coumarins that may repel insects when topically applied. Navajo Indians are said to have learned to use this root medicinally from the bear for treating stomach aches and infections.

A range of primates rub millipedes onto their fur and skin; millipedes contain benzoquinones, compounds known to be potently repellent to insects.

Tufted capuchins (*Cebus apella*) rub various parts of their body with carpenter ants (*Camponotus rufipes*) or allow the ants to crawl over them, in a behaviour called anting. The capuchins often combine anting with urinating into their hands and mixing the ants with the urine.

Birds

More than 200 species of song birds wipe ants perform anting. Birds either grasp ants in their bill and wipe them vigorously along the spine of each feather down to the base, or sometimes roll in ant hills twisting and turning so the ants crawl through their feathers. Birds most commonly use ants that spray formic acid. In laboratory tests, this acid is harmful to feather lice. Its vapour alone can kill them.

Some birds select nesting material rich in anti-microbial agents that may protect themselves and their young from harmful infestations or infections. European starlings (*Sturnus vulgaris*) preferentially select and line their nests with wild carrot (*Daucus carota*); chicks from nests lined with this have greater levels of haemoglobin compared to those from nests which are not, although there is no difference in the weight or feather development of the chicks. Laboratory studies show that wild carrot substantially reduces the emergence of the instars of mites. House sparrows (*Passer domesticus*) have been observed to line their nests with materials from the neem tree (*Azadirach-

ta indica) but change to quinine-rich leaves of the Krishnachua tree (*Caesalpinia pulcherrima*) during an outbreak of malaria; quinine controls the symptoms of malaria.

Social Zoopharmacognosy

Zoopharmacognosy is not always exhibited in a way that benefits the individual. Sometimes the target of the medication is the group or the colony.

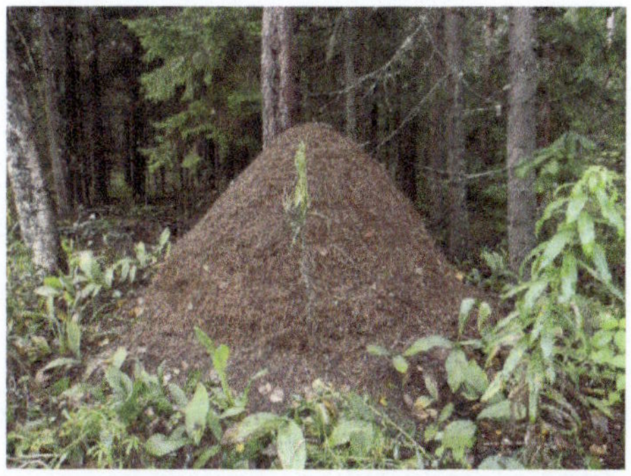

Wood ants incorporate resin into their nest to inhibit the growth of microorganisms

Wood ants (Formica paralugubris) often incorporate large quantities of solidified conifer resin into their nests. Laboratory studies have shown this resin inhibits the growth of bacteria and fungi in a context mimicking natural conditions. The ants show a strong preference for resin over twigs and stones, which are building materials commonly available in their environment. There is seasonal variation in the foraging of ants: the preference for resin over twigs is more pronounced in spring than in summer, whereas in autumn the ants collect twigs and resin at equal rates. The relative collection rate of resin versus stones does not depend on infection with the entomopathogenic fungus *Metarhizium anisopliae* in laboratory conditions, indicating the resin collection is prophylactic rather than therapeutic.

Honey bees also incorporate plant-produced resins into their nest architecture, which can reduce chronic elevation of an individual bee's immune response. When colonies of honey bees are challenged with the fungal parasite (Ascophaera apis), the bees increase their resin foraging. Additionally, colonies experimentally enriched with resin have decreased infection intensities of the fungus.

Transgenerational Zoopharmacognosy

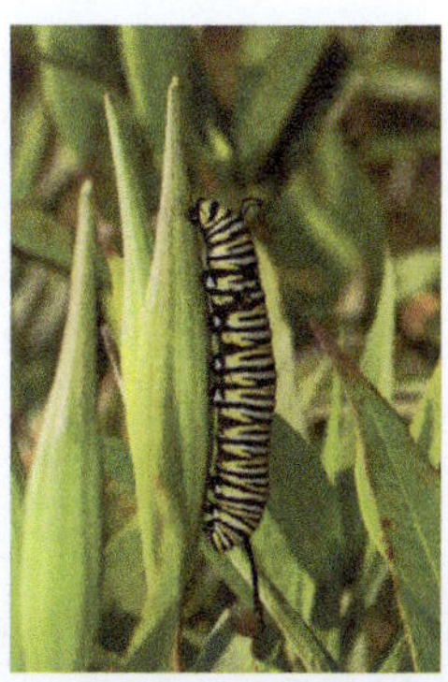

Adult monarch butterflies lay their eggs on toxic plants to reduce parasite growth and disease in their offspring

Zoopharmacognosy can be classified depending on the target of the medication. Some animals lay their eggs in such a way that their offspring are the target of the medication.

Adult monarch butterflies preferentially lay their eggs on toxic plants such as milkweed which reduce parasite growth and disease in their offspring caterpillars. This has been termed *transgenerational therapeutic medication.*

When fruit flies detect the presence of parasitoid wasps, they preferentially lay their eggs in high-ethanol food; this reduces infection risk in their offspring. This has been termed *transgenerational prophylaxis.*

Value to Humans

In an interview with Neil Campbell, Rodriguez describes the importance of biodiversity to medicine:

> "Some of the compounds we've identified by zoopharmacognosy kill parasitic worms, and some of these chemicals may be useful against tumors. There is no question that the templates for most drugs are in the natural world."

Media

- 2002 British documentary television series *Weird Nature* episode 6 *Peculiar Potions* documents variety of animals engaging in intoxication or zoopharmacognosy.

References

- Unschuld, Pual (2003). Huang Di Nei Jing: Nature, Knowledge, Imagery in an Ancient Chinese Medical Text. University of California Press. p. 286. ISBN 978-0-520-92849-7.
- Robson, Barry & Baek, O.K. (2009). The Engines of Hippocrates: From the Dawn of Medicine to Medical and Pharmaceutical Informatics. John Wiley & Sons. p. 50. ISBN 9780470289532.
- Saad, Bashar & Said, Omar (2011). Greco-Arab and Islamic Herbal Medicine: Traditional System, Ethics, Safety, Efficacy, and Regulatory Issues. John Wiley & Sons. p. 80. ISBN 9780470474211.
- Green, James (2000). The Herbal Medicine Maker's Handbook: A Home Manual. Chelsea Green Publishing. p. 168. ISBN 9780895949905.
- Moerman, Daniel E. (1997). "Ethnobotany in North America". In Selin, Helaine. Encyclopaedia of the History of Science, Technology, and Medicine in Non-Western Cultures. Springer. p. 321. ISBN 9780792340669.
- Engel, Cindy (2002). Wild Health: How Animals Keep Themselves Well and What We Can Learn From Them. Houghton Mifflin. ISBN 0-618-07178-4.
- Susan G. Wynn; Barbara Fougère (2007). Veterinary Herbal Medicine. Elsevier Health Sciences. p. 60. ISBN 0323029981.
- hood, Lucy (2013-11-26). Leddy & Pepper's Conceptual Bases of Professional Nursing. Lippincott Williams & Wilkins. p. 35. ISBN 9781469831916.
- Totelin, Laurence M.V (2009). Hippocratic Recipes: Oral and Written Transmission of Pharmacological Knowledge in Fifth and Fourth Century Greece. Leiden and Boston: Brill. p. 125. ISBN 978-90-474-2486-4.
- Hankinson, R.J (2008). "Therapeutics- Van Der Eijk". The Cambridge Companion to Galen. Cambridge: Cambridge University Press. ISBN 978-1-139-82691-4.

- Hankinson, R.J (2008). “Drugs and Pharmacology- Vogt”. The Cambridge Companion to Galen. Cambridge: Cambridge University Press. ISBN 9781139826914.
- Eijk, Philip J (2000). Diocles of Carystus: A Collection of the Fragments with Translation and Commentary. Brill. pp. vii. ISBN 978-90-04-10265-1.
- Grene, Marjorie (2004). The philosophy of biology: an episodic history. Cambridge University Press. p. 11. ISBN 978-0-521-64380-1.
- Arsdall, Anne V. (2002). Medieval Herbal Remedies: The Old English Herbarium and Anglo-Saxon Medicine. Psychology Press. pp. 70–71. ISBN 9780415938495.
- Mills, Frank A. (2000). “Botany”. In Johnston, William M. Encyclopedia of Monasticism: M-Z. Taylor & Francis. p. 179. ISBN 9781579580902.
- Lozano, G.A. (1998). “Parasitic stress and self-medication in wild animals”. Advances in the Study of Behavior. 27: 291–317. doi:10.1016/s0065-3454(08)60367-8. ISBN 9780120045273.
- Reynolds, Vernon (2005). The chimpanzees of the Budongo Forest: ecology, behaviour, and conservation. Oxford University Press. pp. 41–43. ISBN 978-0-19-851545-6.
- Campbell, N.A. (1996). An interview with Eloy Rodriguez. Biology (4th edition). Benjamin Cummings, NY. p. 23. ISBN 0-8053-1957-3.
- Linden, Eugene (2002). The Octopus and the Orangutan: More Tales of Animal Intrigue, Intelligence and Ingenuity. New York City: Plume. pp. 16–17, 104–105, 191. ISBN 0-452-28411-2. OCLC 49627740.

7

Osteopathy: An Alternative Medicine

Osteopathy focuses on massages and other physical manipulation of muscle tissues. Craniosacral therapy is a form of alternative therapy that is used in gently manipulating the joints of the cranium. Muscle energy technique, joint manipulation, osteopathic manipulative medicine and osteopathic medicine in the United States have been explained in the following chapter.

Osteopathy

Osteopathy is a type of alternative medicine that emphasizes massage and other physical manipulation of muscle tissue and bones.

In the United States, osteopathic physicians are trained and are certified to practice medicine. They represent a branch of medicine called Osteopathic Medicine. Osteopaths trained elsewhere are trained only in manual osteopathic treatment, generally to relieve muscular and skeletal conditions, and are referred to as osteopathic practitioners. They are not allowed to call themselves Osteopaths in the United States to avoid confusion with certified physicians. In the United Kingdom, France, Germany, Australia and New Zealand osteopaths are registered and regulated by law as therapists but may not practice medicine (although Germany, like Canada, allows US-trained osteopathic physicians to practice).

Thus Britain's National Health Service advises that, while there is "good" evidence for osteopathy as a treatment for low back pain and "limited evidence to suggest it may be effective for some types of neck, shoulder or lower limb pain and recovery after hip or knee operations", there is no, or insufficient, evidence that osteopathy is effective as a treatment for health conditions "unrelated" to the bones and muscles, "such as headaches, migraines, painful periods, digestive disorders, depression and excessive crying in babies (colic)"; an explicit reference to the claims of osteopathic manipulative medicine. Osteopaths are not certified for medical practice in Britain, while European osteopaths are not allowed to practice in the USA lest they be mistaken for physicians who are still commonly called osteopaths there. Hence studies prepared in different countries must be applied with care in reference to one another.

Furthermore, although there have been several studies and data meta-analyses according to different criteria, research on osteopathic treatment is unable to employ double-blind, placebo-controlled trials since researchers are unable to blind both the practitioner and the patient.

History

The practice of osteopathy began in the United States in 1874. The term "osteopathy" was coined by Andrew Taylor Still, MD, DO. Still was a physician and surgeon, Kansas state and territorial legislator, a free state leader, and one of the founders of Baker University, who lived near Baldwin City, Kansas at the time of the American Civil War. In Baldwin, he developed the practice of osteopathy.

Still named his new school of medicine "osteopathy," reasoning that "the bone, osteon, was the starting point from which [he] was to ascertain the cause of pathological conditions." Still founded the American School of Osteopathy (now A.T. Still University of the Health Sciences) in Kirksville, Missouri, for the teaching of osteopathy on 10 May 1892. While the state of Missouri granted the right to award the MD degree, he remained dissatisfied with the limitations of conventional medicine and instead chose to retain the distinction of the DO degree. In 1898 the American Institute of Osteopathy started the *Journal of Osteopathy* and by that time four states recognized osteopathy as a profession.

Osteopathy Worldwide

The osteopathic profession has evolved into two branches, non-physician manual medicine osteopaths and full scope of medical practice osteopathic physicians. These groups are so distinct that in practice they function as separate professions. The regulation of non-physician manual medicine osteopaths varies greatly between jurisdictions. In Australia, the UK, and New Zealand the non-physician manual medicine osteopaths are regulated by statute and practice requires registration with the relevant regulatory authority. The Osteopathic International Alliance has a country guide with details of registration and practice rights and the International Osteopathic Association has a list of all accredited osteopathic colleges.

Several international and national organizations exist relating to osteopathic education and political advocacy. Similarly, there is also an international organization of organizations for national osteopathic and osteopathic medical associations, statutory regulators, and universities/medical schools offering osteopathic and osteopathic medical education, known as the Osteopathic International Alliance (OIA).

The following sections describe the legal status of *osteopathy* and *osteopathic medicine* in each country listed.

Australia

Osteopaths work in private practice, and the majority of private health insurance providers cover treatment performed by osteopaths. In addition, treatment performed by osteopaths is covered by the public health care system in Australia (Medicare) under the Chronic Disease Management plan.

Osteopaths in Australia undertake a minimum of five years' university training in anatomy, physiology, pathology, general medical diagnosis and osteopathic techniques to be eligible to practice.

Osteopathy Australia (formerly the Australian Osteopathic Association) is a national organization representing the interests of Australian osteopaths, osteopathy as a profession in Australia, and consumers' right to access osteopathic services. Originally founded in 1955 in Victoria, the Australian Osteopathic Association became a national body in 1991 and became Osteopathy Australia in 2014. and is a member of the Osteopathic International Alliance.

The Osteopathy Board of Australia is part of the Australian Health Practitioner Regulation Agency which is the regulatory body for all recognized health care professions in Australia. The Osteopathic Board of Australia is separate from the Medical Board of Australia which is the governing body that regulates medical practitioners. Osteopaths trained internationally may be eligible for registration in Australia, dependent on their level of training and following relevant competency assessment.

Canada

In Canada, the titles "osteopath" and "osteopathic physician" are protected in some provinces by the medical regulatory college for physicians and surgeons. As of 2011, there were approximately 20 U.S.-trained osteopathic physicians, all of which held a Doctor of Osteopathic Medicine degree, practicing in all of Canada. As of 2014, no training programs have been established for osteopathic physicians in Canada.

The non-physician manual practice of osteopathy is practiced in most Canadian provinces. As of 2014, manual osteopathic practice is not a government-regulated health profession in any province, and those interested in pursuing osteopathic studies must register in private osteopathy schools. It is estimated that there are over 1,300 osteopathic manual practitioners in Canada, most of whom practice in Quebec and Ontario. Some sources indicate that there are between 1,000 and 1,200 osteopaths practicing in the province of Quebec, and although this number might seem quite elevated, many osteopathy clinics are adding patients on waiting lists due to a shortage of osteopaths in the province.

Attempt to Create A Professional Osteopathy Program in Quebec, Canada

Beginning in 2009, Université laval in Quebec City was working with the *Collège d'études ostéopathiques* in Montreal on a project to implement a professional osteopathy program consisting of a bachelor's degree followed by a professional master's degree in osteopathy as manual therapy. However, due to the many doubts concerning the scientific credibility of osteopathy from the university's faculty of medicine, the program developers decided to abandon the project in 2011, after 2 ½ years of discussion, planning, and preparation for the program implementation. There was some controversy with the final decision of the university's committee regarding the continuous undergraduate and professional graduate program in osteopathy because the Commission of studies, which is in charge of evaluating new training programs offered by the university, had judged that the program had its place at Université Laval before receiving the unfavourable support decision from the faculty of medicine. Had the program been implemented, Université Laval would have been the first university institution in Quebec to offer a professional program in osteopathy as a manual therapy.

European Union

There is no universal regulatory authority for the practice of *osteopathy* or *osteopathic medicine* within the European Union; it is on a country-by-country basis. The UK's General Osteopathic Council, a regulatory body set up under the country's Osteopaths Act 1993, has issued a position paper on European regulation of osteopathy.

France

Osteopathy is a governmentally recognized profession and has title protection, *autorisation d'utiliser le titre d'ostéopathe*. The most recent decree regarding osteopathy was enacted in 2007.

Germany

Germany has both *osteopathy* and *osteopathic medicine*. There is a difference in the osteopathic education between non-physician osteopaths, physiotherapists, and medical physicians.

Physiotherapists are a recognized health profession and can achieve a degree of "Diploma in Osteopathic Therapy (D.O.T.)." Non-physician *osteopaths* are not medically licensed. They have an average total of 1200 hours of training, roughly half being in manual therapy and osteopathy, with no medical specialization before they attain their degree. Non-physician osteopaths in Germany officially work under the "Heilpraktiker" law. Heilpraktiker is a separate profession within the health care system. There are many schools of osteopathy in Germany; most are moving toward national recognition although such recognition does not currently exist. In Germany there are rules (at the country level) under which persons (non-physicians) may call themselves osteopaths.

New Zealand

The practice of *osteopathy* is regulated by law, under the terms of the Health Practitioners Competence Assurance Act 2003 which came into effect on 18 September 2004. Under the Act, it is a legal requirement to be registered with the Osteopathic Council of New Zealand (OCNZ), and to hold an annual practicing certificate issued by them, in order to practice as an osteopath. Each of the fifteen health professions regulated by the HPCA Act work within the "Scope of Practice" determined and published by its professional Board or Council. Osteopaths in New Zealand are not fully licensed physicians. In New Zealand, in addition to the general scope of practice, osteopaths may also hold the Scope of Practice for Osteopaths using Western Medical Acupuncture and Related Needling Techniques.

In New Zealand a course is offered at Unitec. Australasian courses consist of a bachelor's degree in clinical science (osteopathy) followed by a master's degree. The Unitec New Zealand double degree programme is the OCNZ prescribed qualification for registration in the scope of practice: Osteopath, Australian qualifications accredited by the Australian and New Zealand Osteopathic Council are also prescribed qualifications.

Osteopaths registered and in good standing with the Australian Health Practitioner Regulation Agency – Osteopathy Board of Australian are eligible to register in New Zealand under the mutual recognition system operating between the two countries. Graduates from programs in every other country are required to complete an assessment procedure.

The scope of practice for US-trained *osteopathic physicians* is unlimited on an *exceptions* basis. Full licensure to practice medicine is awarded on an exceptions basis following a hearing before the licensing authorities in New Zealand. Both the Medical Council of New Zealand and the Osteopathic Council of New Zealand [OCNZ] regulate osteopathic physicians in New Zealand. Currently, the country has no recognized osteopathic medical schools.

United Kingdom

The practice of *osteopathy* has a long history in the United Kingdom. The first school of osteopathy was established in London in 1917 by John Martin Littlejohn a pupil of A. T. Still, who had been Dean of The Chicago College of Osteopathic Medicine. After many years of existing outside the mainstream of health care provision, the osteopathic profession in the UK was accorded formal recognition by Parliament in 1993 by the Osteopaths Act. This legislation now provides the profession of osteopathy the same legal framework of statutory self-regulation as other healthcare professions such as medicine and dentistry.

The General Osteopathic Council (GOsC) regulates the practice of osteopathy under the terms of the Osteopaths Act 1993. Under British law, an osteopath must be registered with the GOsC to practice in the United Kingdom. The General Osteopathic Council has a statutory duty to promote, develop and regulate the profession of osteopathy in the UK. It fulfills its duty to protect the interests of the public by ensuring that all osteopaths maintain high standards of safety, competence and professional conduct throughout their professional lives. In order to be registered with the General Osteopathic Council an osteopath must hold a recognized qualification that meets the standards as set out by law in the GOsC's Standard of Practice. This Act provides for "protection of title" A person who, whether expressly or implication describes himself as an osteopath, osteopathic practitioner, osteopathic physician, osteopathist, osteotherapist, or any kind of osteopath is guilty of an offence unless he is registered as an osteopath. There are currently more than five thousand osteopaths registered in the UK.

Osteopathic medicine is regulated by the General Osteopathic Council (GOsC) under the terms of the Osteopaths Act 1993 and statement from the GMC. Practising osteopaths will usually have a B.S. or M.Sc. in osteopathy. Accelerated courses leading to accreditation are available for those with an M.D. and physiotherapists. The London College of Osteopathic Medicine, teaches osteopathy only to those who are already physicians.

United States

Licensure or registration of non-physician *osteopaths* is not permitted anywhere in the United States. European-style osteopaths are prohibited from calling themselves osteopaths. To avoid confusion, the American Osteopathic Association and the American Association of Colleges of Osteopathic Medicine recommend using the terms *osteopathic physician* (U.S.-trained only) and *osteopathic medicine* in reference to osteopathic medicine as practised in the United States. In contrast, osteopathic physicians earn the degree of Doctor of Osteopathic Medicine (D.O.), a degree equivalent, though different in certain aspects, to that of Doctor of Medicine (M.D.).

Osteopathic medicine in the United States has always meant a physician trained in and entitled to the full scope of medical practice. *Osteopathy* or *osteopath* as written in some U.S. state and federal laws refers only to *osteopathic medicine* or *osteopathic physicians,* respectively. With the increased internationalization of the profession, these older terms have fallen out of favor as generally accepted use due to the confusion they may cause.

Egypt and The Middle East

Hesham Khalil introduced osteopathy in the Middle East at a local physical therapy conference in Cairo, Egypt in 2005 with a lecture titled "The global Osteopathic Concept / Holistic approach in

Somatic Dysfunction". Since then he has toured the Middle East to introduce osteopathy in other Middle Eastern and North African countries, including Sudan, Jordan, Saudi Arabia, Qatar, UAE, Kuwait and Oman. In December 2007 the first Workshop on Global osteopathic approach was held at the Nasser Institute Hospital for Research and Treatment, sponsored by the Faculty of Physical Therapy, University of Cairo, Egypt. On August 6, 2010, the Egyptian Osteopathic Society (OsteoEgypt) was founded. OsteoEgypt promotes a two-tier model of osteopathy in Egypt and the Middle East. The event was timed to coincide with the birthday of A. T. Still.

Craniosacral Therapy

Craniosacral therapy (CST) is a form of bodywork or alternative therapy using gentle touch to manipulate the synarthrodial joints of the cranium. A practitioner of cranial-sacral therapy may also apply light touches to a patient's spine and pelvis. Practitioners believe that this manipulation regulates the flow of cerebrospinal fluid and aids in "primary respiration". Craniosacral therapy was developed by John Upledger, D.O. in the 1970s, as an offshoot osteopathy in the cranial field, or cranial osteopathy, which was developed in the 1930s by William Garner Sutherland.

According to the American Cancer Society, although CST may relieve the symptoms of stress or tension, "available scientific evidence does not support claims that craniosacral therapy helps in treating cancer or any other disease". CST has been characterized as pseudoscience and its practice has been called quackery. Cranial osteopathy has received a similar assessment, with one 1990 paper finding there was no scientific basis for any of the practitioners' claims the paper examined.

Etymology

The term craniosacral or cranial-sacral are based on the terms cranium and sacrum, a bone of the pelvis which connects the lowest lumbar vertebra to the two hip bones and the tailbone.

History and Conceptual Basis

Cranial osteopathy, a forerunner of CST, was originated by osteopath William Sutherland (1873–1954) in 1898–1900. While looking at a disarticulated skull, Sutherland was struck by the idea that the cranial sutures of the temporal bones where they meet the parietal bones were "beveled, like the gills of a fish, indicating articular mobility for a respiratory mechanism."

John Upledger devised CST. Comparing it to cranial osteopathy he wrote: "Dr. Sutherland's discovery regarding the flexibility of skull sutures led to the early research behind CranioSacral Therapy – and both approaches affect the cranium, sacrum and coccyx – the similarities end there." However, modern day cranial osteopaths largely consider the two practices to be the same, but that cranial osteopathy has "been taught to non-osteopaths under the name CranialSacro therapy."

From 1975 to 1983, Upledger and neurophysiologist and histologist Ernest W. Retzlaff worked at Michigan State University as clinical researchers and professors. They assembled a research team to investigate the purported pulse and further study Sutherland's theory of cranial bone movement. Upledger and Retzlaff went on to publish their results, which they interpreted as support for both the concept of cranial bone movement, and the concept of a cranial rhythm. Later reviews of these studies have concluded that their research did not meet enduring standards to offer conclusive proof for the effectiveness of craniosacral therapy and the existence of cranial bone movement.

Practitioners of both cranial osteopathy and craniosacral therapy assert that there are small, rhythmic motions of the cranial bones attributed to cerebrospinal fluid pressure or arterial pressure. The premise of CST is that palpation of the cranium can be used to detect this rhythmic movement of the cranial bones and selective pressures may be used to manipulate the cranial bones to achieve a therapeutic result. However, the degree of mobility and compliance of the cranial bones is considered controversial and is a critically important concept in craniosacral therapy.

Primary Respiratory Mechanism

The *Primary Respiratory Mechanism* (PRM), the mechanism originally proposed by Sutherland, has been summarized in five ideas:

1. Inherent motility of the central nervous system
2. Fluctuation of the cerebrospinal fluid
3. Mobility of the intracranial and intraspinal dural membranes
4. Mobility of the cranial bones
5. Involuntary motion of the sacrum between the ilia

Inherent Motility of The Central Nervous System

The postulated intracranial fluid fluctuation is described by practitioners as an interaction between four main components: arterial blood, capillary blood (brain volume), venous blood and cerebrospinal fluid (CSF).

Fluctuation of The Cerebrospinal Fluid

There is research which demonstrates examiners are unable to measure craniosacral motion reliably, as indicated by a lack of inter-rater agreement among examiners. The authors of this research conclude this "measurement error may be sufficiently large to render many clinical decisions potentially erroneous". Alternative medicine practitioners have interpreted this result as a product of entrainment between patient and practitioner, a principle which lacks scientific support. Whether craniosacral motion can be reliably palpated remains a subject of debate with studies producing mixed results.

Mobility of The Intracranial and Intraspinal Dural Membranes

In 1970, Upledger observed during a surgical procedure on the neck what he described as a slow pulsating movement within the spinal meninges. He attempted to hold the membrane still and found that he could not due to the strength of the action behind the movement.

Mobility of The Cranial Bones

The extent to which cranial bones are able to move is considered controversial and studies of the existence and degree of cranial motion have yielded mixed findings. Cranial sutures are the areas in which the eight cranial bones are joined. During infancy, the cranial bones are not rigidly fused to each other, but are instead bound together by a membrane known as a fontanelle where two sutures join. Between the first and second year of life, the cranial bones begin to move together and fuse as a normal part of development. Studies examining the age of the closure of the cranial sutures have reported mixed findings. Closure has been reported to occur during adolescence while other studies indicate greater individual variability in the timing of this closure with fusion of the lambdoid suture, sagittal suture, and coronal sutures taking place in the fourth decade of life, but complete fusion of all sutures not occurring until advanced age (the eighth decade of life has been reported); some studies have found that the sutures never rigidly fuse. According to Gray's Anatomy, "[w]hen such sutures are tied by sutural ligament and periosteum, almost complete immobility results".

Treatment

The therapist lightly palpates the patient's body, and focuses intently on the communicated movements. A practitioner's feeling of being in tune with a patient is described as *entrainment*. Patients often report feelings of deep relaxation during and after the treatment session, and may feel light-headed. While sometimes thought to be caused by an increase in endorphins, research shows the effects may actually be brought about by the endocannabinoid system.

There are few reports of adverse events from CST treatment. In one study of craniosacral manipulation in patients with traumatic brain syndrome, the incidence of adverse effects from treatment was 5%.

Reception

According to the American Cancer Society, although CST may relieve the symptoms of stress or tension, "available scientific evidence does not support claims that craniosacral therapy helps in treating cancer or any other disease". Cranial osteopathy has received a similar assessment, with one 1990 paper finding there was no scientific basis for any of the practitioners' claims the paper examined.

In October 2012 Edzard Ernst conducted a systematic review of randomized clinical trials of craniosacral therapy. He concluded that "the notion that CST is associated with more than non-specific effects is not based on evidence from rigorous randomised clinical trials." Commenting specifically on this conclusion Ernst commented on his blog that he had chosen the wording as "a polite and scientific way of saying that CST is bogus." Ernst also commented that the quality of five of the six trials he had reviewed was "deplorably poor," a sentiment which echoed an August 2012 review that noted the "moderate methodological quality of the included studies."

Ernst criticized a 2011 systematic review performed by Jakel and von Hauenschild for inclusion of observational studies and including studies with healthy volunteers. This review concluded that the evidence base surrounding craniosacral therapy and its efficacy was sparse and composed of studies with heterogeneous design. The authors of this review stated that currently available evidence was insufficient to draw conclusions.

The evidence base for CST is sparse and lacks a demonstrated biologically plausible mechanism. In the absence of rigorous, well-designed randomized controlled trials, it has been characterized as pseudoscience, and its practice called quackery.

Muscle Energy Technique

Muscle Energy Techniques (METs) describes a broad class of manual therapy techniques directed at improving musculoskeletal function or joint function, and improving pain. METs are commonly used by Manual Therapists, Osteopaths, Physical Therapists, Chiropractors, Athletic Trainers, osteopathic physicians, and Massage Therapists.

Historically, the concept emerged as a form of osteopathic manipulative diagnosis and treatment in which the patient's muscles are actively used on request, from a precisely controlled position, in a specific direction, and against a distinctly executed physician counterforce. It was first described in 1948 by Fred Mitchell, Sr, D.O. Muscle energy techniques are used to treat somatic dysfunction, especially decreased range of motion, muscular hypertonicity, and pain.

Pathophysiology

Injury can occur as a result of trauma, accidents, overuse, strain/sprain, etc., not all of which should be treated with muscle energy. These techniques are most appropriate for the following injury patterns:

- Decreased range of motion secondary to muscular spasticity, rigidity, hypertonicity or hypotonicity. Hypertonicity often follows overuse and can result in altered joint position, increased irritability and decreased elasticity. This injury pattern is often accompanied by a non-specific muscle ache in the area of injury.
- Interneuronal injury—when dysfunction occurs at one joint or segment, the related agonist muscles are also affected. If uncorrected, the antagonistic muscles eventually become involved as well, leading to dysfunction of both muscle groups. This presents as decreased range of motion with pain and/or tenderness in the area.

Mechanism of Action for Muscle Energy Techniques

Muscle energy is a direct and active technique; meaning it engages a restrictive barrier and requires the patient's participation for maximal effect. As the patient performs an isometric contraction, the following physiologic changes occur:

- Golgi tendon organ activation results in direct inhibition of agonist muscles
- A reflexive reciprocal inhibition occurs at the antagonistic muscles
- As the patient relaxes, agonist and antagonist muscles remain inhibited allowing the joint to be moved further into the restricted range of motion.

Despite the many claims made regarding the efficacy of these techniques, there are only two peer-reviewed studies that have shown that muscle energy techniques can significantly decrease disability and improve functionality in patients with disorders such as low back pain.

Indications and Contraindications

Muscle energy techniques can be employed to reposition a dysfunctional joint and treat the affected musculature. Indications include, but are not limited to: muscular shortening, low back pain, pelvic imbalance, edema, limited range of motion, somatic dysfunction, respiratory dysfunction, cervicogenic headaches, and many others.

These techniques are inappropriate when a patient has injuries such as fractures, avulsion injuries, severe osteoporosis, open wounds, or has metastatic disease. Additionally, because these techniques require active patient participation, they are inappropriate for any patient that is unable to cooperate.

Techniques

Muscle energy techniques can be applied to most areas of the body.According to one textbook, each technique requires 8 essential steps:

1. Perform and obtain an accurate structural diagnosis.
2. Engage the restrictive barrier in as many planes as possible.
3. Physician and patient engage in an unyielding counterforce where the patient's force matches the physician's force.
4. The patient's isometric contraction has the correct amount of force, the correct direction of effort (away from the restrictive barrier), and the correct duration (3–5 seconds).
5. Complete relaxation occurs after the muscular effort.
6. The patient is repositioned into the new restrictive barrier in as many planes as possible.
7. Steps 3-6 are repeated approximately 3-5 times or until no further improvement in range of motion is observed.
8. The structural diagnosis is repeated to evaluate if the dysfunction has resolved or improved.

Joint Manipulation

Joint manipulation is a type of passive movement of a skeletal joint. It is usually aimed at one or more 'target' synovial joints with the aim of achieving a therapeutic effect.

Practice of Manipulation

A modern re-emphasis on manipulative therapy occurred in the late 19th century in North America with the emergence of osteopathic medicine and chiropractic medicine. In the context of healthcare, joint manipulation is performed by several professional groups. In North America and Europe, joint manipulation is most commonly performed by chiropractors (estimated to perform over 90% of all manipulative treatments), American-trained osteopathic physicians, occupational therapists, physiotherapists, and European osteopaths. When applied to joints in the spine, it is referred to as spinal manipulation.

Terminology

Manipulation is known by several other names. Historically, general practitioners and orthopaedic surgeons have used the term "manipulation". Chiropractors refer to manipulation of a spinal joint as an 'adjustment'. Following the labelling system developed by Geoffery Maitland, manipulation is synonymous with Grade V mobilization, a term commonly used by physical therapists. Because of its distinct biomechanics, the term high velocity low amplitude (HVLA) thrust is often used interchangeably with manipulation.

Biomechanics of Joint Manipulation

Manipulation can be distinguished from other manual therapy interventions such as joint mobilization by its biomechanics, both kinetics and kinematics.

Kinetics

Until recently, force-time histories measured during spinal manipulation were described as consisting of three distinct phases: the preload (or prethrust) phase, the thrust phase, and the resolution phase. Evans and Breen added a fourth 'orientation' phase to describe the period during which the patient is oriented into the appropriate position in preparation for the prethrust phase.

When individual peripheral synovial joints are manipulated, the distinct force-time phases that occur during spinal manipulation are not as evident. In particular, the rapid rate of change of force that occurs during the thrust phase when spinal joints are manipulated is not always necessary. Most studies to have measured forces used to manipulate peripheral joints, such as the metacarpophalangeal (MCP) joints, show no more than gradually increasing load. This is probably because there are many more tissues restraining a spinal motion segment than an independent MCP joint.

Kinematics

The kinematics of a complete spinal motion segment when one of its constituent spinal joints are manipulated are much more complex than the kinematics that occur during manipulation of an independent peripheral synovial joint. Even so, the motion that occurs between the articular surfaces of any individual synovial joint during manipulation should be very similar and is described below.

Early models describing the kinematics of an individual target joint during the various phases of manipulation (notably Sandoz 1976) were based on studies that investigated joint cracking in MCP joints. The cracking was elicited by pulling the proximal phalanx away from the metacarpal bone (to separate, or 'gap' the articular surfaces of the MCP joint) with gradually increasing force until a sharp resistance, caused by the cohesive properties of synovial fluid, was met and then broken.

These studies were therefore never designed to form models of therapeutic manipulation, and the models formed were erroneous in that they described the target joint as being configured at the end range of a rotation movement, during the orientation phase. The model then predicted that this end range position was maintained during the prethrust phase until the thrust phase where it was moved beyond the 'physiologic barrier' created by synovial fluid resistance; conveniently within the limits of anatomical integrity provided by restraining tissues such as the joint capsule and ligaments. This model still dominates the literature. However, after re-examining the original studies on which the kinematic models of joint manipulation were based, Evans and Breen argued that the optimal prethrust position is actually the equivalent of the neutral zone of the individual joint, which is the motion region of the joint where the passive osteoligamentous stability mechanisms exert little or no influence. This new model predicted that the physiologic barrier is only confronted when the articular surfaces of the joint are separated (gapped, rather than the rolling or sliding that usually occurs during physiological motion), and that it is more mechanically efficient to do this when the joint is near to its neutral configuration.

Cracking Joints

Joint manipulation is characteristically associated with the production of an audible 'clicking' or 'popping' sound. This sound is believed to be the result of a phenomenon known as cavitation occurring within the synovial fluid of the joint. When a manipulation is performed, the applied force separates the articular surfaces of a fully encapsulated synovial joint. This deforms the joint capsule and intra-articular tissues, which in turn creates a reduction in pressure within the joint cavity. In this low pressure environment, some of the gases that are dissolved in the synovial fluid (which are naturally found in all bodily fluids) leave solution creating a bubble or cavity, which rapidly collapses upon itself, resulting in a 'clicking' sound. The contents of this gas bubble are thought to be mainly carbon dioxide. The effects of this process will remain for a period of time termed the 'refractory period', which can range from a few minutes to more than an hour, while it is slowly reabsorbed back into the synovial fluid. There is some evidence that ligament laxity around the target joint is associated with an increased probability of cavitation.

Clinical Effects and Mechanisms of Action

The clinical effects of joint manipulation have been shown to include:

- Temporary relief of musculoskeletal pain.
- Shortened time to recover from acute back sprains (Rand).
- Temporary increase in passive range of motion (ROM).
- Physiological effects upon the central nervous system.
- No alteration of the position of the sacroiliac joint.

Common side effects of spinal manipulative therapy (SMT) are characterized as mild to moderate and may include: local discomfort, headache, tiredness, or radiating discomfort.

Shekelle (1994) summarised the published theories for mechanism(s) of action for how joint manipulation may exert its clinical effects as the following:

- Release of entrapped synovial folds or plica
- Relaxation of hypertonic muscle
- Disruption of articular or periarticular adhesions
- Unbuckling of motion segments that have undergone disproportionate displacement

Safety Issues

As with all interventions, there are risks associated with joint manipulation, especially manipulation of spinal joints. Infrequent, but potentially serious side effects, include: vertebrobasilar accidents (VBA), strokes, spinal disc herniation, vertebral and rib fractures, and cauda equina syndrome.

In a 1993 study, J.D. Cassidy, DC, and co-workers concluded that the treatment of lumbar intervertebral disk herniation by side posture manipulation is "both safe and effective."

Risks of Upper Cervical Manipulation

The degree of serious risks associated with manipulation of the cervical spine is uncertain, with widely differing results being published.

A 2008 study in the journal "Spine", JD Cassidy, E Boyle, P Cote', Y He, et al. investigated 818 VBA strokes that were hospitalized in a population of more than 100 million person-years. In those aged <45 years, cases were about three times more likely to see a chiropractor or a PCP before their stroke than controls. Results were similar in the case control and case cross over analyses. There was no increased association between chiropractic visits and VBA stroke in those older than 45 years. Positive associations were found between PCP visits and VBA stroke in all age groups. The study concluded that VBA stroke is a very rare event in the population. The increased risks of VBA stroke associated with chiropractic and PCP visits is likely due to patients with headache and neck pain from VBA dissection seeking care before their stroke. The study found no evidence of excess risk of VBA stroke associated chiropractic care compared to primary care.

A 1996 Danish chiropractic study confirmed the risk of stroke to be low, and determined that the greatest risk is with manipulation of the first two vertebra of the cervical spine, particularly passive rotation of the neck, known as the "master cervical" or "rotary break."

Serious complications after manipulation of the cervical spine are estimated to be 1 in 4 million manipulations or fewer. A RAND Corporation extensive review estimated "one in a million." Dvorak, in a survey of 203 practitioners of manual medicine in Switzerland, found a rate of one serious complication per 400,000 cervical manipulations, without any reported deaths, among an estimated 1.5 million cervical manipulations. Jaskoviak reported approximately 5 million cervical manipulations from 1965 to 1980 at The National College of Chiropractic Clinic in Chicago, without a single case of vertebral artery stroke or serious injury. Henderson and Cassidy performed a survey at the Canadian Memorial Chiropractic College outpatient clinic where more than a half-million treatments were given over a nine-year period, again without serious incident. Eder offered a report of 168,000 cervical manipulations over a 28-year period, again without a single significant complication. After an extensive literature review performed to formulate practice guidelines, the authors concurred that "the risk of serious neurological complications (from cervical manipulation) is extremely low, and is approximately one or two per million cervical manipulations."

In comparison, there is a 3-4% rate of complications for cervical spinal surgery, and 4,000-10,000 deaths per million neck surgeries.

Understandably, vascular accidents are responsible for the major criticism of spinal manipulative therapy. However, it has been pointed out that "critics of manipulative therapy emphasize the possibility of serious injury, especially at the brain stem, due to arterial trauma after cervical manipulation. It has required only the very rare reporting of these accidents to malign a therapeutic procedure that, in experienced hands, gives beneficial results with few adverse side effects". In very rare instances, the manipulative adjustment to the cervical spine of a vulnerable patient becomes the final intrusive act which results in a very serious consequence.

Potential for Incident Underreporting

Statistics on the reliability of incident reporting for injuries related to manipulation of the cervical spine vary. The RAND study assumed that only 1 in 10 cases would have been reported. However, Prof Ernst surveyed neurologists in Britain for cases of serious neurological complications occurring within 24 hours of cervical spinal manipulation by various types of practitioners; 35 cases had been seen by the 24 neurologists who responded, but none of the cases had been reported. He concluded that underreporting was close to 100%, rendering estimates "nonsensical." He therefore suggested that *"clinicians might tell their patients to adopt a cautious approach and avoid the type of spinal manipulation for which the risk seems greatest: forceful manipulation of the upper spine with a rotational element."* The NHS Centre for Reviews and Dissemination stated that the survey had methodological problems with data collection. Both NHS and Ernst noted that bias is a problem with the survey method of data collection.

A 2001 study in the journal *Stroke* found that vertebrobasilar accidents (VBAs) were five times more likely in those aged less than 45 years who had visited a chiropractor in the preceding week, compared to controls who had not visited a chiropractor. No significant associations were found for those over 45 years. The authors concluded: *"While our analysis is consistent with a positive association in young adults... The rarity of VBAs makes this association difficult to study despite high volumes of chiropractic treatment."* The NHS notes that this study collected data objectively by using administrative data, involving less recall bias than survey studies, but the data were collected retrospectively and probably contained inaccuracies.

In 1996, Coulter *et al.* had a multidisciplinary group of 4 MDs, 4 DCs and 1 MD/DC look at 736 conditions where it was used. Their job was to evaluate the appropriateness of manipulation or mobilization of the cervical spine in those cases (including a few cases not performed by chiropractors).

"According to the report ... 57.6% of reported indications for cervical manipulation was considered inappropriate, with 31.3% uncertain. Only 11.1% could be labeled appropriate. A panel of chiropractors and medical practitioners concluded that '. . . much additional scientific data about the efficacy of cervical spine manipulation are needed.'"

Misattribution Problems

Studies of stroke and manipulation do not always clearly identify what professional has performed the manipulation. In some cases this has led to confusion and improper placement of blame. In a 1995 study, chiropractic researcher Allan Terrett, DC, pointed to this problem:

> "The words chiropractic and chiropractor have been incorrectly used in numerous publications dealing with SMT injury by medical authors, respected medical journals and medical organizations. In many cases, this is not accidental; the authors had access to original reports that identified the practitioner involved as a nonchiropractor. The true incidence of such reporting cannot be determined. Such reporting adversely affects the reader's opinion of chiropractic and chiropractors."

This error was taken into account in a 1999 review of the scientific literature on the risks and benefits of manipulation of the cervical spine (MCS). Special care was taken, whenever possible, to correctly identify all the professions involved, as well as the type of manipulation responsible for any injuries and/or deaths. It analyzed 177 cases that were reported in 116 articles published between 1925 and 1997, and summarized:

> "The most frequently reported injuries involved arterial dissection or spasm, and lesions of the brain stem. Death occurred in 32 (18%) of the cases. Physical therapists were involved in less than 2% of the cases, and no deaths have been attributed to MCS provided by physical therapists. Although the risk of injury associated with MCS appears to be small, this type of therapy has the potential to expose patients to vertebral artery damage that can be avoided with the use of mobilization (nonthrust passive movements)."

In Figure 1 in the review, the types of injuries attributed to manipulation of the cervical spine are shown, and Figure 2 shows the type of practitioner involved in the resulting injury. For the purpose of comparison, the type of practitioner was adjusted according to the findings by Terrett.

The review concluded:

> "The literature does not demonstrate that the benefits of MCS outweigh the risks. Several recommendations for future studies and for the practice of MCS are discussed."

Edzard Ernst has written:

> "...there is little evidence to demonstrate that spinal manipulation has any specific therapeutic effects. On the other hand, there is convincing evidence to show that it is associated with frequent, mild adverse effects as well as with serious complications of unknown incidence. Therefore, it seems debatable whether the benefits of spinal manipulation outweigh its risks. Specific risk factors for vascular accidents related to spinal manipulation have not been identified, which means that any patient may be at risk, particularly those below 45 years of age. Definitive, prospective studies that can overcome the limitations of previous investigations are now a matter of urgency. Until they are available, clinicians might tell their patients to adopt a cautious approach and avoid the type of spinal manipulation for which the risk seems greatest: forceful manipulation of the upper spine with a rotational element."

Emergency Medicine

In emergency medicine joint manipulation can also refer to the process of bringing fragments of fractured bone or dislocated joints into normal anatomical alignment (otherwise known as 'reducing' the fracture or dislocation). These procedures have no relation to the HVLA thrust procedure.

Osteopathic Manipulative Medicine

Osteopathic manipulative medicine is a core set of techniques of osteopathy and osteopathic medicine distinguishing these fields from the rest of medicine. Parts of osteopathy, such as cranial therapy have been labeled pseudoscience and are said to have no therapeutic value. The techniques are based on an ideology created by Andrew Taylor Still (1828–1917) which posits the existence of a myofascial continuity – a tissue layer that connects all parts of the body. Non-physician osteopaths and osteopathic physicians attempt to diagnose and treat somatic dysfunction by manipulating a person's bones and muscles and therefore address a variety of ailments. OMT techniques are most commonly used to treat back pain and other musculoskeletal issues, and are less commonly used to treat systemic conditions such as asthma and Parkinson's disease.

Osteopathic Medicine in The United States
Andrew Taylor Still (founder)
Doctor of Osteopathic Medicine (DO)
Medicine · US Medical education

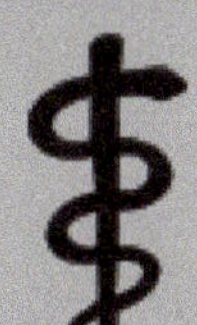

Schools · Physicians
Osteopathic Manipulative Medicine
AOA · AACOM · AAO · COMLEX
MD & DO Comparison
Specialty Colleges · AOA BOS

OMT is based on the idea that a myofascial continuity "links every part of the body with every other part"; a practitioner, through a "skillful and dexterous use of the hands" treats what was originally called "the osteopathic lesion", but which is now named "somatic dysfunction". The most commonly treated ailment is back pain, although some practitioners claim OMT can be used to treat a wide range of conditions.

History

Andrew Taylor Still, M.D., D.O. was a 19th-century American physician and Civil War surgeon who founded osteopathic medicine. Following the loss of three of his children to spinal meningitis,

Still became dissatisfied with contemporary medical practices and sought to further medical understanding and treatment. Still claimed that human illness was rooted in problems with the musculoskeletal system, and that hands-on manipulations could solve these problems and so effect a cure by harnessing the body's own self-repairing potential. Still's proposed treatment regime also included as strong dose of healthy living: he advocated abstinence from alcohol, and patients were forbidden from taking medicine.

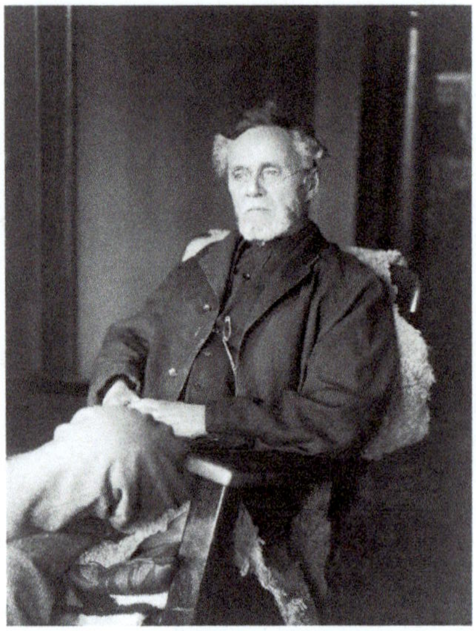

Andrew Taylor Still in 1914

Clinical Practice

According to the American Osteopathic Association (AOA), osteopathic manipulative treatment is considered to be only one component of osteopathic medicine and may be used alone or in combination with pharmacotherapy, rehabilitation, surgery, patient education, diet, and exercise. OMT techniques are not necessarily unique to osteopathic medicine; other disciplines, such as physical therapy or chiropractic, use similar techniques.

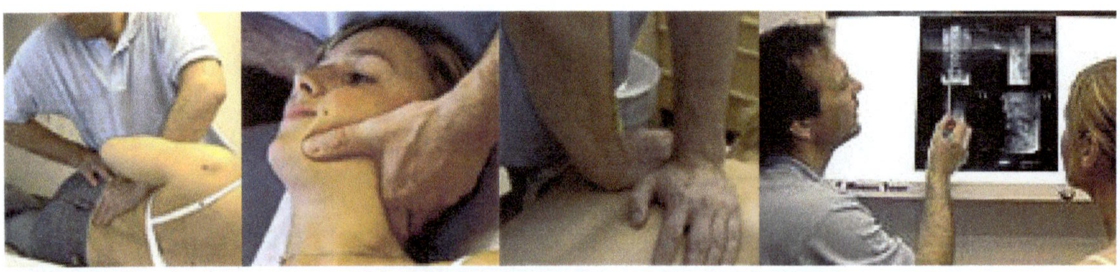

Osteopathic manipulative treatment (OMT) involves palpation and manipulation of bones, muscles, joints, and fasciae.

One key concept osteopathic medical students learn is that structure influences function. Thus, if there is a problem in one part of the body's structure, function in that area, and possibly in other areas, may be affected. Another integral tenet of osteopathic medicine is the body's innate ability to heal itself. Many of osteopathic medicine's manipulative techniques are aimed at reducing or eliminating the impediments to proper structure and function so the self-healing mechanism can assume its role in restoring a person to health.

Osteopathic medicine defines a concept of health care that embraces the concept of the unity of the living organism's structure (anatomy) and function (physiology). The American Osteopathic Association (AOA) state that the four major principles of osteopathic medicine are the following:

1. The body is an integrated unit of mind, body, and spirit.
2. The body possesses self-regulatory mechanisms, having the inherent capacity to defend, repair, and remodel itself.
3. Structure and function are reciprocally interrelated.
4. Rational therapy is based on consideration of the first three principles.

These principles are not held by Doctors of Osteopathic Medicine to be empirical laws; they serve, rather, as the underpinnings of the osteopathic approach to health and disease.

Muscle Energy

Muscle energy techniques address somatic dysfunction through stretching and muscle contraction. For example, if a person is unable to fully abduct her arm, the treating physician raises the patient's arm near the end of the patient's range of motion, also called the edge of the restrictive barrier. The patient then tries to lower her arm, while the physician provides resistance. This resistance against the patient's motion allows for isometric contraction of the patient's muscle. Once the patient relaxes, her range of motion increases slightly. The repetition of alternating cycles of contraction and subsequent relaxation help the treated muscle improve its range of motion. Muscle energy techniques are contraindicated in patients with fractures, crush injuries, dislocations, joint instability, severe muscle spasms or strains, severe osteoporosis, severe whiplash injury, vertebrobasilar insufficiency, severe illness, and recent surgery.

Counterstrain

Counterstrain is a system of diagnosis and treatment that considers the physical dysfunction to be a continuing, inappropriate strain reflex, which is inhibited during treatment by applying a position of mild strain in the direction exactly opposite to that of the reflex. After a counterstrain point tender to palpation has been diagnosed, the identified tender point is treated by the osteopathic physician who, while monitoring the tender point, positions the patient such that the point is no longer tender to palpation. This position is held for ninety seconds and the patient is subsequently returned to her normal posture. Most often this position of ease is usually achieved by shortening the muscle of interest. Improvement or resolution of the tenderness at the identified counterstrain point is the desired outcome. The use of counterstrain technique is contraindicated in patients with severe osteoporosis, pathology of the vertebral arteries, and in patients who are very ill or cannot voluntarily relax during the procedure.

High-velocity, Low-amplitude

High velocity, low amplitude (HVLA) is a technique which employs a rapid, targeted, therapeutic force of brief duration that travels a short distance within the anatomic range of motion of a joint and engages the restrictive barrier in one or more places of motion to elicit release of restriction. The use of HVLA is contraindicated in patients with Down syndrome due to instability of the atlantoaxial joint which may stem from ligamentous laxity, and in pathologic bone conditions such as fracture, history of a pathologic fracture, osteomyelitis, osteoporosis, and severe cases of rheumatoid arthritis. HVLA is also contraindicated in patients with vascular disease such as aneurysms, or disease of the carotid arteries or vertebral arteries. People taking ciprofloxacin or anticoagulants, or who have local metastases should not receive HVLA.

Myofascial Release

Myofascial release is a form of soft tissue therapy used to treat somatic dysfunction and the resultant pain and restriction of motion. Treatment requires continual palpatory feedback to achieve release of myofascial tissues. This is accomplished by relaxing contracted muscles, increasing circulation and lymphatic drainage, and stimulating the stretch reflex of muscles and overlying fascia.

Fascia is the soft tissue component of the connective tissue that provides support and protection for most structures within the human body, including muscle. This soft tissue can become restricted due to psychogenic disease, overuse, trauma, infectious agents, or inactivity, often resulting in pain, muscle tension, and corresponding diminished blood flow. Although fascia and its corresponding muscle are the main targets of myofascial release, other tissue may be affected as well, including other connective tissue.

Lymphatic Pump Treatment

Lymphatic pump treatment (LPT) is a manual technique intended to encourage lymph flow in a person's lymphatic system. The first modern lymphatic pump technique was developed in 1920, although osteopathic physicians used various forms of lymphatic techniques as early as the late 19th century.

Relative contraindications for the use of lymphatic pump treatments include fractures, abscesses or localized infections, and severe bacterial infections with body temperature elevated higher than 102 °F (39 °C).

Effectiveness

In 2014, a systematic review and meta-analysis of 15 randomized controlled trials found moderate-quality evidence that OMT reduces pain and improves functional status in acute and chronic nonspecific low back pain. The same analysis also found moderate-quality evidence for pain reduction for nonspecific low back pain in postpartum women and low-quality evidence for pain reduction in nonspecific low back pain in pregnant women. A 2013 systematic review found insufficient evidence to rate osteopathic manipulation for chronic nonspecific low back pain. In 2011, a systematic review found no compelling evidence that osteopathic manipulation was effective for the treatment of musculoskeletal pain.

In 2013, a Cochrane Review reviewed six randomized controlled trials which investigated the effect of four types of chest physiotherapy (including OMT) as adjunctive treatments for pneumonia in adults and concluded that "based on current limited evidence, chest physiotherapy might not be recommended as routine additional treatment for pneumonia in adults." A 2013 systematic review of the use of OMT for treating pediatric conditions concluded that its effectiveness was unproven.

With respect to irritable bowel syndrome, a 2014 review found that there had been a limited number of studies done and that all these studies had small sample sizes; with that caveat, it found preliminary evidence that osteopathic manipulation may be beneficial in this condition.

Earlier Research

A 2005 systematic review of OMT's use in treating asthma concluded: "There is insufficient evidence to support the use of manual therapies for patients with asthma."

Criticism

Initially, D.O.s were regarded by M.D.s as "cultists" whose treatments were rooted in "pseudoscientific dogma", and tensions between the two continued for many years.

In 1988, Petr Skrabanek classified osteopathy as one of the "paranormal" forms of alternative medicine, commenting that it has a view of disease which had no meaning outside its own closed system.

In a 1995 conference address, the president of the Association of American Medical Colleges, Jordan J. Cohen, pinpointed OMT as a defining difference between M.D.s and D.O.s; while he saw there was no quarrel in the appropriateness of manipulation for musculoskeletal treatment, the difficulty centered on "applying manipulative therapy to treat other systemic diseases" – at that point, Cohen maintained, "we enter the realm of skepticism on the part of the allopathic world."

In 1998 Stephen Barrett of Quackwatch posted a highly critical article online entitled "Dubious Osteopathic Practices", in which he said that the worth of manipulative therapy had been exaggerated and that the American Osteopathic Association (AOA) was acting unethically by failing to condemn craniosacral therapy. The article attracted a letter from the law firm representing the AOA accusing Barrett of libel and demanding an apology to avert legal action. In response Barrett made some slight modifications to his text, while maintaining its overall stance; he queried the AOA's reference to "the body's natural tendency toward good health" and challenged them to "provide [him] with adequate scientific evidence showing how this belief has been tested and demonstrated to be true." Barrett has been quoted as saying "the pseudoscience within osteopathy can't compete with the science".

In 1999, Joel D. Howell noted that osteopathy and medicine as practiced by M.D.s were becoming increasingly convergent. He suggested that this raised a paradox:

if osteopathy has become the functional equivalent of allopathy, what is the justification for its continued existence? And if there is value in therapy that is uniquely osteopathic – that is, based on osteopathic manipulation or other techniques – why should its use be limited to osteopaths?

In 2004, the osteopathic physician Bryan E. Bledsoe, a professor of emergency medicine, wrote disparagingly of the "pseudoscience" at the foundation of OMT. In his view, "OMT will and should follow homeopathy, magnetic healing, chiropractic, and other outdated practices into the pages of medical history".

In 2010, Steven Salzberg wrote that OMT was promoted as a special distinguishing element of DO training, but that it amounted to no more than "'extra' training in pseudoscientific practices".

Osteopathic Medicine in The United States

Osteopathic Medicine is a branch of the medical profession in the United States. Osteopathic physicians (D.O.s) are equivalent to Doctors of Medicine (M.D.s) and are considered fully licensed physicians (medical doctors) to practice medicine and surgery in all 50 states and are recognized in 65 other countries, including all Canadian provinces.

Andrew Taylor Still (founder)
Doctor of Osteopathic Medicine (DO)
Medicine · US Medical education

Schools · Physicians
Osteopathic Manipulative Medicine
AOA · AACOM · AAO · COMLEX
MD & DO Comparison
Specialty Colleges · AOA BOS

Frontier physician Andrew Taylor Still founded the profession as a rejection of the prevailing system of medical thought of the 19th century. Still's techniques relied on manipulation of joints and bones, to diagnose and treat illness, and he called his practices "osteopathy". By the middle of the 20th century, the profession had moved closer to mainstream medicine, adopting modern public health and biomedical principles. American "osteopaths" became "osteopathic medical doctors", ultimately achieving full practice rights as medical doctors in all 50 states, including serving in the U.S. armed forces as physicians.

In the 21st century, the training of osteopathic medical physicians in the United States is equivalent to the training of Doctors of Medicine (M.D.s). Osteopathic medical physicians attend four years of medical school followed by an internship and a minimum two years of residency. They use all conventional methods of diagnosis and treatment. Though still trained in osteopathic manipulative treatment (OMT), the modern derivative of Still's techniques, they work in all specialties of medicine. OMT is a skill they use often in family practice, sports medicine, emergency medicine, but OMT is not commonly used in specialties such as dermatology, surgery, or other fields that do not lend themselves to correcting the body with their hands.

In modern medicine, any distinction between the M.D. and the D.O. professions has eroded steadily; diminishing numbers of D.O. graduates enter primary care fields, fewer use OMT, and increasing numbers of osteopathic graduates choose to train in non-osteopathic residency programs. An osteopathic physician (DO) is a fully licensed, patient-centered medical doctor. DO has full medical practice rights throughout the United States and in 44 countries abroad.

Discussions about the future of modern medicine frequently debate the utility of maintaining separate, distinct pathways for educating physicians in the United States.

Nomenclature

Physicians and surgeons who graduate from osteopathic medical schools are known as physicians or osteopathic medical doctors. Upon graduation, they are conferred a professional doctorate, the Doctor of Osteopathic Medicine (D.O.).

Osteopathic curricula in other countries differ from those in the United States. European-trained practitioners of osteopathic manipulative techniques are referred to as "osteopaths": their scope of practice excludes most medical therapies and relies more on osteopathic manipulative medicine and alternative medical modalities. While it was once common for D.O. graduates in the United States to refer to themselves as 'osteopaths,' this term is now considered archaic and those holding the Doctor of Osteopathic Medicine degree are commonly referred to as 'osteopathic medical physicians'.

Demographics

Currently, there are 30 accredited osteopathic medical schools offering education in 42 locations across the United States and 141 accredited U.S. M.D. medical schools.

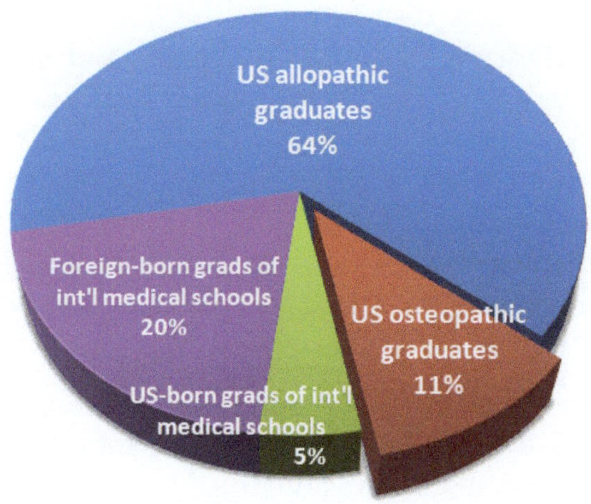

Physicians entering U.S. workforce by education, 2005

- In 1960, there were 13,708 physicians who were graduates of the 5 osteopathic medical schools.
- In 2002, there were 49,210 physicians from 19 osteopathic medical schools.
- Between 1980 and 2005, the number of osteopathic graduates per year increased over 250 percent from about 1,000 to 2,800. This number is expected to approach 5,000 by 2015.
- In 2015, there were 31 colleges of osteopathic medicine in 45 locations. One in four medical students in the United States is enrolled in an osteopathic medical school.
- As of 2015, there are more than 96,000 osteopathic medical physicians in the United States.
- By 2020, the number of osteopathic medical physicians will be over 100,000, say expert predictions, according to the American Medical Association.

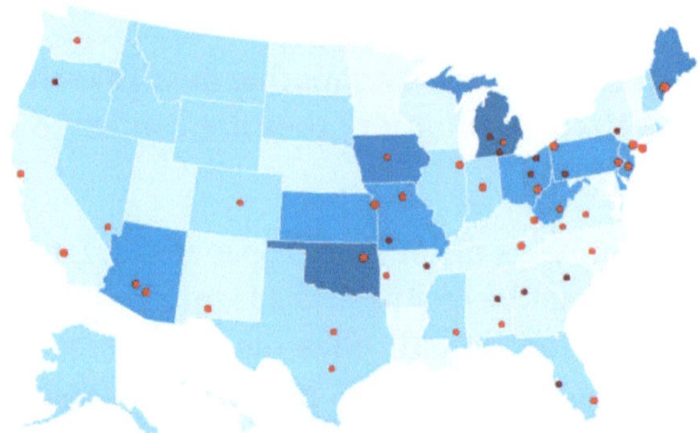

Geographic distribution of osteopathic physicians as a percentage of all physicians, by the state. Locations of osteopathic medical schools are in red.

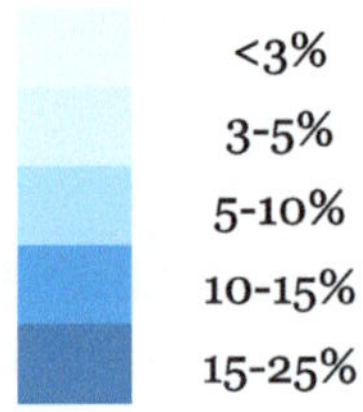

Osteopathic physicians are not evenly distributed in the United States. States with the highest concentration of osteopathic medical physicians are Oklahoma, Iowa, and Michigan where osteopathic medical physicians comprise 17-20% of the total physician workforce. The state with the greatest number of osteopathic medical physicians is Pennsylvania, with 7,260 DOs in active practice in 2011. The states with the lowest concentrations of DOs are Louisiana, Massachusetts and Vermont where only 1–3% of physicians have an osteopathic medical degree. Public awareness of osteopathic medicine likewise varies widely in different regions. People living in the midwest states are the most likely to be familiar with osteopathic medicine. In the Northeastern United States, osteopathic medical physicians provide more than one third of general and family medicine patient visits.

Between 2010 and 2015 twelve states experienced greater than 50% growth in the number of DOs—Virginia, South Carolina, Utah, Tennessee, North Dakota, Kentucky, South Dakota, Wyoming, Oregon, North Carolina, Minnesota, Washington.

Osteopathic Principles

Osteopathic medical students take the Osteopathic Oath, similar to the Hippocratic oath, to maintain and uphold the "core principles" of osteopathic medical philosophy. Revised in 1953, and again in 2002, the core principles are:

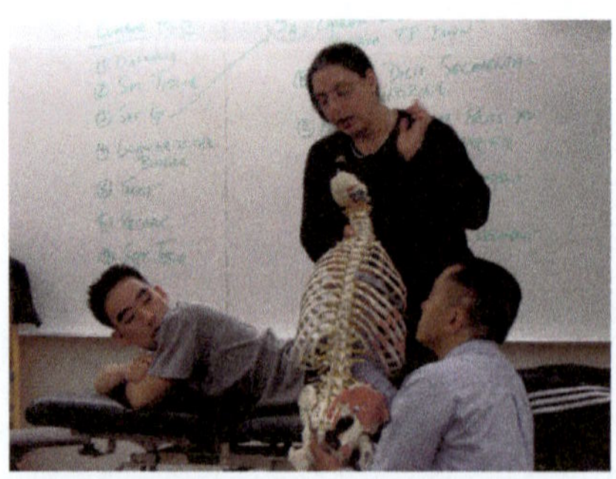

A physician demonstrates an OMT technique to medical students at an osteopathic medical school.

1. The body is a unit; a person is a unit of body, mind, and spirit.
2. The body is capable of self-regulation, self-healing, and health maintenance.
3. Structure and function are reciprocally interrelated.
4. Rational treatment is based on an understanding of these principles: body unity, self-regulation, and the interrelationship of structure and function.

Contemporary osteopathic physicians practice evidence-based medicine, indistinguishable from their MD colleagues.

Significance

There are different opinions on the significance of these principles. Some note that the osteopathic medical philosophy is akin to the tenets of holistic medicine, suggestive of a kind of social movement within the field of medicine, one that promotes a more patient-centered, holistic approach to medicine, and emphasizes the role of the primary care physician within the health care system. Others point out that there is nothing in the principles that would distinguish D.O. from M.D. training in any fundamental way. One study, published in *The Journal of the American Osteopathic Association* found a majority of M.D. medical school administrators and faculty saw nothing objectionable in the core principles listed above, and some endorse them generally as broad medical principles.

History

19th Century, A New Movement Within Medicine

Frontier physician Andrew Taylor Still, M.D., DO, founded the American School of Osteopathy (now the A.T. Still University-Kirksville (Mo.) College of Osteopathic Medicine) in Kirksville, MO, in 1892 as a radical protest against the turn-of-the-century medical system. A. T. Still believed that the conventional medical system lacked credible efficacy, was morally corrupt, and treated effects rather than causes of disease. He founded osteopathic medicine in rural Missouri at a time when medications, surgery, and other traditional therapeutic regimens often caused more harm than good. Some of the medicines commonly given to patients during this time were arsenic, castor oil, whiskey, and opium. In addition, unsanitary surgical practices often resulted in more deaths than cures.

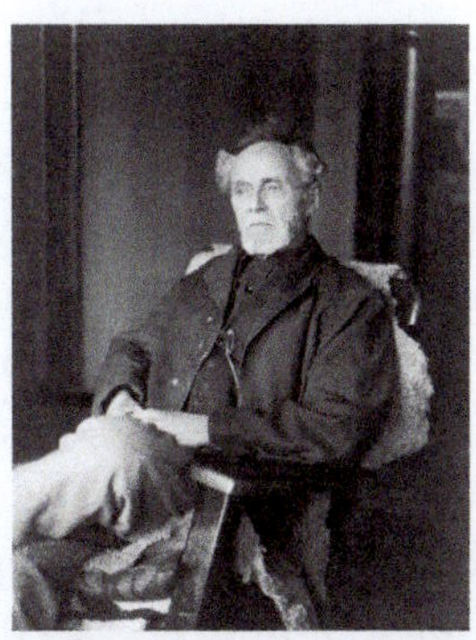

Andrew Taylor Still, founder of osteopathic medicine

"To find health should be the object of the doctor. Anyone can find disease."

Andrew Taylor Still, 1874

Dr. Still intended his new system of medicine to be a reformation of the existing 19th-century medical practices. He imagined that someday "rational medical therapy" would consist of manipulation of the musculoskeletal system, surgery, and very sparingly used drugs. He invented the name "osteopathy" by blending two Greek roots *osteon-* for bone and *-pathos* for suffering in order to communicate his theory that disease and physiologic dysfunction were etiologically grounded in a disordered musculoskeletal system. Thus, by diagnosing and treating the musculoskeletal system, he believed that physicians could treat a variety of diseases and spare patients the negative side-effects of drugs.

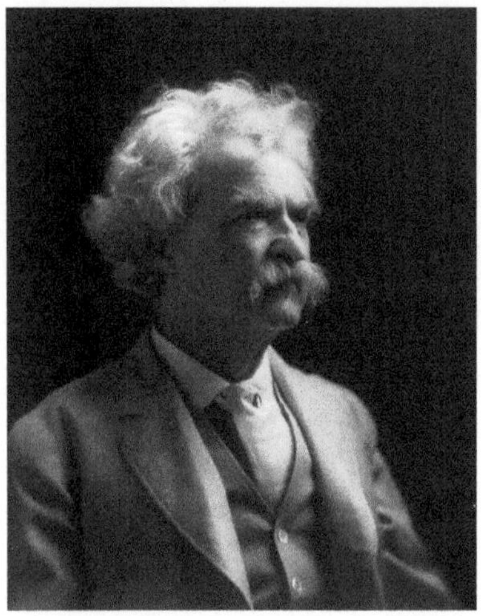

Mark Twain was a vocal supporter of the early osteopathic movement.

The new profession faced stiff opposition from the medical establishment at the time. The relationship of the osteopathic and medical professions was often "bitterly contentious" and involved "strong efforts" by medical organizations to discredit osteopathic medicine. Throughout the first half of the twentieth century, the policy of the American Medical Association labeled osteopathic medicine as a cult and osteopaths were seen as "cultist." The AMA code of ethics declared it unethical for a medical physician to voluntarily associate with an osteopath.

"To ask a doctor's opinion of osteopathy is equivalent to going to Satan for information about Christianity."

Mark Twain, 1901

One notable advocate for the fledgling movement was Mark Twain. Manipulative treatments had purportedly alleviated the symptoms of his daughter Jean's epilepsy as well as Twain's own chronic bronchitis. In 1909, he spoke before the New York State Assembly at a hearing regarding the practice of osteopathy in the state. "I don't know as I cared much about these osteopaths until I heard you were going to drive them out of the state, but since I heard that I haven't been able to sleep." Philosophically opposed to the American Medical Association's stance that its own type of medical practice was the only legitimate one, he spoke in favor of licensing for osteopaths. Physicians from the New York County Medical Society responded with a vigorous attack on Twain, who retorted with "[t]he physicians think they are moved by regard for the best interests of the public. Isn't there a little touch of self-interest back of it all?" "... The objection is, people are curing people without a license and you are afraid it will bust up business."

Evolution of osteopathic medicine's mission and identity	
Years	**Identity & Mission**
1892 to 1950	Manual medicine
1951 to 1970	Family practice / manual therapy
1971 to present	Full service care / multispeciality orientation

1916–1966, Federal Recognition

Recognition by the U.S. federal government was a key goal of the osteopathic medical profession in its effort to establish equivalency with its M.D. counterparts. Between 1916 and 1966, the profession engaged in a "long and tortuous struggle" for the right to serve as physicians and surgeons in the U.S. Military Medical Corps. On May 3, 1966 Secretary of Defense Robert McNamara authorized the acceptance of osteopathic physicians into all the medical military services on the same basis as MDs. The first osteopathic physician to take the oath of office to serve as a military physician was Harry J. Walter. The acceptance of osteopathic physicians was further solidified in 1996 when Ronald Blanck, DO was appointed to serve as Surgeon General of the Army, the only osteopathic physician to hold the post.

1962, California

In the 1960s in California, the American Medical Association (AMA) spent nearly $8 million to end the practice of osteopathic medicine in the state. In 1962, Proposition 22, a statewide ballot initiative in California, eliminated the practice of osteopathic medicine in the state. The California Medical Association (CMA) issued M.D. degrees to all DOs in the state of California for a nominal fee. "By attending a short seminar and paying $65, a doctor of osteopathy (D.O.) could obtain an M.D. degree; 86 percent of the DOs in the state (out of a total of about 2000) chose to do so." Immediately following, the AMA re-accredited the University of California at Irvine College of Osteopathic Medicine as the University of California, Irvine School of Medicine, an M.D. medical school. It also placed a ban on issuing physician licenses to DOs moving to California from other states. However, the decision proved to be controversial. In 1974, after protests and lobbying by influential and prominent DOs, the California Supreme Court ruled in Osteopathic Physicians and Surgeons of California v. California Medical Association, that licensing of DOs in that state must be resumed. Four years later, in 1978, the College of Osteopathic Medicine of the Pacific opened in Pomona, and in 1997 Touro University California opened in Vallejo. As of 2012, there were 6,368 D.O.s practicing in California.

1969, AMA House of Delegates Approval

In 1969, the American Medical Association (AMA) approved a measure allowing qualified osteopathic physicians as full and active members of the Association. The measure also allowed osteopathic physicians to participate in AMA-approved intern and residency programs. However, the American Osteopathic Association rejected this measure, claiming it was an attempt to eliminate the distinctiveness of osteopathic medicine. In 1970, AMA President Dwight L. Wilbur, M.D. sponsored a measure in the AMA's House of Delegates permitting the AMA Board of Trustees' plan for the merger of D.O. and M.D. professions. Today, a majority of osteopathic physicians are trained alongside MDs, in residency programs governed by the ACGME, an independent board of the AMA.

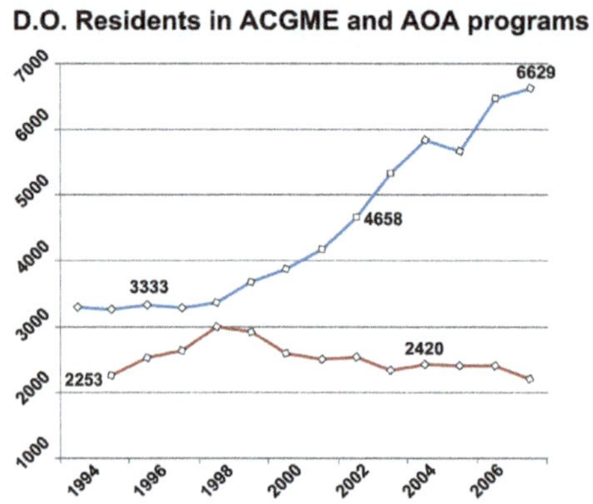

Total number of DOs in residency programs, by year.

DO residents in ACGME (M.D.) programs
DO residents in AOA (D.O.) programs.

1993, First African-american Woman to Serve as Dean of A U.S. Medical School

In 1993, Barbara Ross-Lee, DO was appointed to the position of dean of the Ohio University College of Osteopathic Medicine; she was the first African-American woman to serve as the dean of a U.S. medical school. Ross-Lee now is the dean of the NYIT College of Osteopathic Medicine at Arkansas State University in Jonesboro, Arkansas.

Non-discrimination Policies

Recent years have seen a professional rapprochement between the two groups. DOs have been admitted to full active membership in the American Medical Association since 1969. The AMA has invited a representative of the American Osteopathic Association to sit as a voting member in the AMA legislative body, the house of delegates.

2006, American Medical Student Association

In 2006, during the presidency of an osteopathic medical student, the American Medical Student Association (AMSA) adopted a policy regarding the membership rights of osteopathic medical students in their main policy document, the "Preamble, Purposes and Principles."

AMSA RECOGNIZES the equality of osteopathic and allopathic medical degrees within the organization and the healthcare community as a whole. As such, DO students shall be entitled to the same opportunities and membership rights as allopathic students.

—PPP, AMSA

2007, AMA

In recent years, the largest M.D. organization in the U.S., the American Medical Association, adopted a fee non-discrimination policy discouraging differential pricing based on attendance of an M.D. or D.O. medical school.

In 2006, calls for an investigation into the existence of differential fees charged for visiting D.O. and M.D. medical students at American medical schools were brought to the American Medical Association. After an internal investigation into the fee structure for visiting D.O. and M.D. medical students at M.D. medical schools, it was found that one institution of the 102 surveyed charged different fees for D.O. and M.D. students. The house of delegates of the American Medical Association adopted resolution 809, I-05 in 2007.

Our AMA, in collaboration with the American Osteopathic Association, discourages discrimination against medical students by institutions and programs based on osteopathic or allopathic training.

—*AMA policy H-295.876*

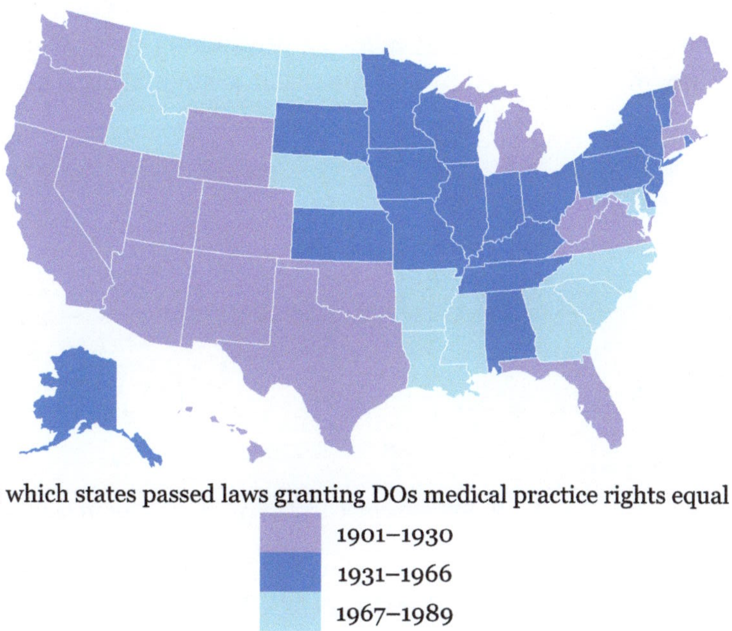

Years in which states passed laws granting DOs medical practice rights equal to MDs

State Licensing of Practice Rights

In the United States, laws regulating physician licenses are governed by the states. Between 1901 and 1989, osteopathic physicians lobbied state legislatures to pass laws giving those with a D.O. degree the same legal privilege to practice medicine as those with an M.D. degree. In many states, the debate was long and protracted. Both the AOA and the AMA were heavily involved in influencing the legislative process. The first state to pass such a law was California in 1901, the last was Nebraska in 1989.

Current Status

Education and Training

According to Harrison's Principles of Internal Medicine, "the training, practice, credentialing, licensure, and reimbursement of osteopathic physicians is virtually indistinguishable from those of (MD) physicians, with 4 years of osteopathic medical school followed by specialty and subspecialty training and [board] certification."

D.O.-granting U.S. medical schools have curricula identical for the most part to those of M.D.-granting schools. Generally, the first two years are classroom-based, while the third and fourth years consist of clinical rotations through the major specialties of medicine. Some schools of Osteopathic Medicine have been criticized by the osteopathic community for relying too heavily on clinical rotations with private practitioners, who may not be able to provide sufficient instruction to the rotating student. Other D.O.-granting and M.D.-granting schools place their students in hospital-based clinical rotations where the attending physicians are faculty of the school, and who have a clear duty to teach medical students while treating patients.

Graduate Medical Education

Upon graduation, most osteopathic medical physicians pursue residency training programs. Depending on state licensing laws, osteopathic medical physicians may also complete a one-year rotating internship at a hospital approved by the American Osteopathic Association (AOA).

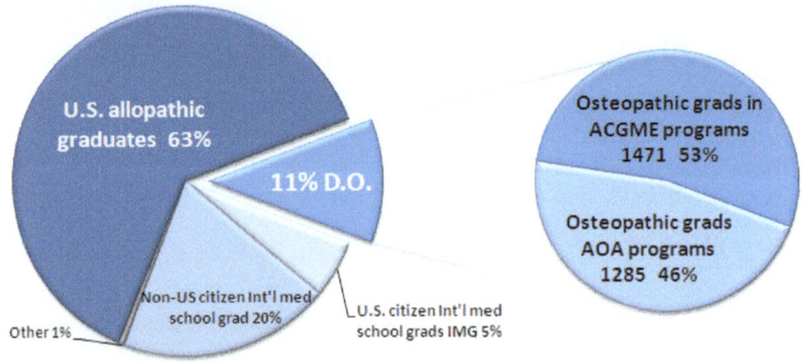

Sources of the 24,012 medical school graduates entering U.S. physician training programs in 2004.

Osteopathic physicians may apply to residency programs accredited by either the AOA or the Accreditation Council for Graduate Medical Education (ACGME). Currently, osteopathic physicians participate in more ACGME programs than in programs approved by the American Osteopathic Association (AOA). By June 30, 2020, all AOA residencies will also be required to have ACGME accreditation, and the AOA will cease accreditation activities.

Osteopathic Manipulative Treatment (OMT)

Within the osteopathic medical curriculum, manipulative treatment is taught as an adjunctive measure to other biomedical interventions for a number of disorders and diseases. However, a 2001 survey of osteopathic physicians found that more than 50% of the respondents used OMT on less than 5% of their patients. The survey follows many indicators that osteopathic physicians have become more like M.D. physicians in every respect —few perform OMT, and most prescribe medications or suggest surgery as the first line of treatment. The American Osteopathic Association has made an effort in recent years to support scientific inquiry into the effectiveness of osteopathic manipulation as well as to encourage osteopathic physicians to consistently offer manipulative treatments to their patients. However, the number of osteopathic physicians who report consistently prescribing and performing manipulative treatment has been falling steadily. Medical historian and sociologist Norman Gevitz cites poor educational quarters and few full-time OMT instructors as major factors for the decreasing interest of medical students in OMT. He describes problems with "the quality, breadth, nature, and orientation of OMM instruction," and he claims that the teaching of osteopathic medicine has not changed sufficiently over the years to meet the intellectual and practical needs of students.

In their assigned readings, students learn what certain prominent DOs have to say about various somatic dysfunctions. There is often a theory or model presented that provides conjectures and putative explanations about why somatic dysfunction exists and what its significance is. Instructors spend the bulk of their time demonstrating osteopathic manipulative (OM) techniques without providing evidence that the techniques are significant and efficacious. Even worse, faculty members rarely provide instrument-based objective evidence that somatic dysfunction is present in the first place.

At the same time, recent studies show an increasingly positive attitude of patients and physicians (M.D. and D.O.) towards the use of manual therapy as a valid, safe and effective treatment modality. One survey, published in the *Journal of Continuing Medical Education*, found that a majority of physicians (81%) and patients (76%) felt that manual manipulation (MM) was safe, and over half (56% of physicians and 59% of patients) felt that manipulation should be available in the primary care setting. Although less than half (40%) of the physicians reported any educational exposure to MM and less than one-quarter (20%) have administered MM in their practice, most (71%) respondents endorsed desiring more instruction in MM. Another small study examined the interest and ability of M.D. residents in learning osteopathic principles and skills, including OMT. It showed that after a 1-month elective rotation, the M.D. residents responded favorably to the experience.

Professional Attitudes

In 1998, a New York Times article described the increasing numbers, public awareness, and mainstreaming of osteopathic medical physicians, illustrating an increasingly cooperative climate between the D.O. and M.D. professions.

In 2005, during his tenure as president of the American Association of Medical Colleges, Jordan Cohen described a climate of cooperation between D.O. and M.D. practitioners:

"We now find ourselves living at a time when osteopathic and allopathic graduates are both sought after by many of the same residency programs; are in most instances both licensed by the same licensing boards; are both privileged by many of the same hospitals; and are found in appreciable numbers on the faculties of each other's medical schools".

Elsewhere, he has remarked that osteopathic manipulative medicine (OMT) "can be an aid to the physician in fostering a relationship with the patient."

International Practice Rights

Each country has different requirements and procedures for licensing or registering osteopathic physicians and osteopaths. The only osteopathic practitioners that the U.S. Department of Education recognizes as physicians are graduates of osteopathic medical colleges in the United States. Therefore, osteopaths who have trained outside the United States are not eligible for medical licensure in the United States. On the other hand, U.S.-trained DOs are currently able to practice in 45 countries with full medical rights and in several others with restricted rights.

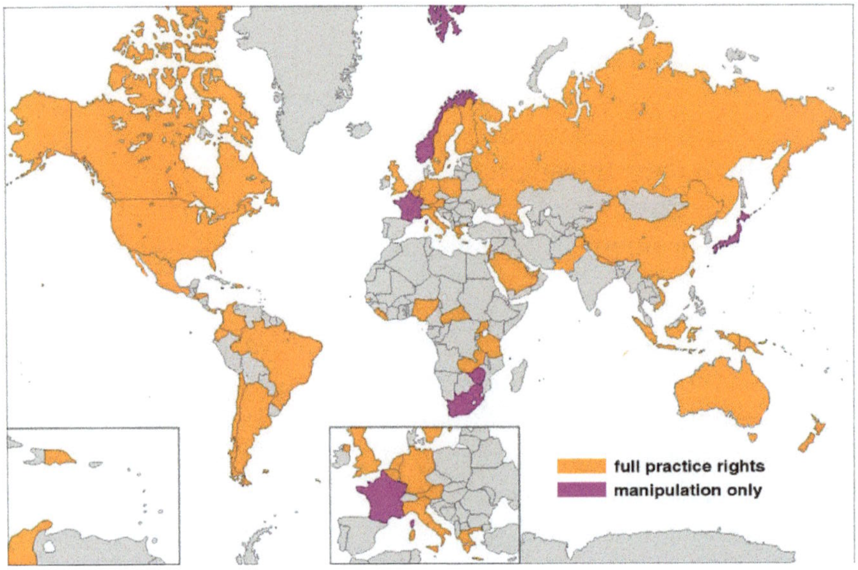

International practice rights of U.S. trained DOs

The *Bureau on International Osteopathic Medical Education and Affairs* (BIOMEA) is an independent board of the American Osteopathic Association. The BIOMEA monitors the licensing and registration practices of physicians in countries outside of the United States and advances the recognition of American-trained DOs. Towards this end, the BIOMEA works with international health organizations like the World Health Organization (WHO), the Pan American Health Organization (PAHO) as well as other groups.

The procedure by which countries consider granting physician licensure to foreigners varies widely. For U.S. trained physicians, the ability to qualify for "unlimited practice rights" also varies according to one's degree, M.D. or D.O. Many countries recognize U.S.-trained MDs as applicants for licensure, granting successful applicants "unlimited" practice rights. The American Osteopathic Association has lobbied the governments of other countries to recognize U.S.-trained DOs similarly to their M.D. counterparts, with some success.

Osteopathic Medicine & Osteopathy
Osteopathy in Australia & New Zealand
Osteopathic medicine in Canada
Osteopathy in Europe • Osteopathy in the UK
Osteopathic medicine in the United States

In over 65 countries, U.S.-trained DOs have unlimited practice rights. In 2005, after one year of deliberations, the General Medical Council announced that U.S.-trained DOs will be accepted for full medical practice rights in the United Kingdom. According to Josh Kerr of the AOA, "some countries don't understand the differences in training between an osteopathic physician and an osteopath." The American Medical Student Association strongly advocates for U.S.-trained D.O. international practice rights "equal to that" of M.D. qualified physicians.

Osteopathic Medicine and Primary Care

Osteopathic physicians have historically entered primary care fields at a higher rate than their M.D. counterparts. Some osteopathic organizations make claims to a greater emphasis on the importance of primary care within osteopathic medicine. However, the proportion of osteopathic students choosing primary care fields, like that of their M.D. peers, is declining. Currently, only one in five osteopathic medical students enters a family medicine residency (the largest primary care field). In 2004, only 32% of osteopathic seniors planned careers in any primary care field; this percentage was down from a peak in 1996 of more than 50%.

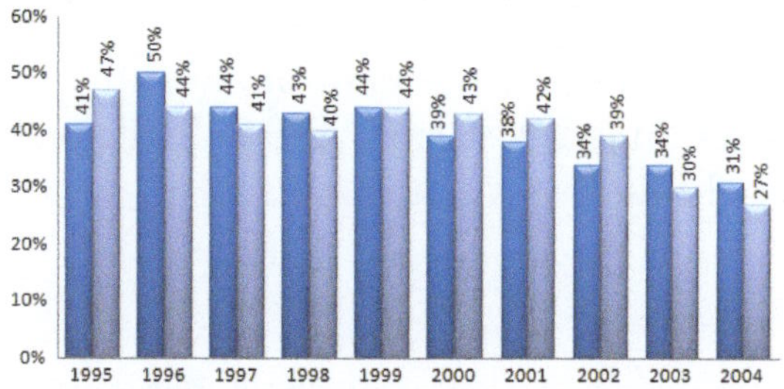

Trends in primary care as a career choice of osteopathic medical students
4th year students 1st year students

Criticism and Internal Debate

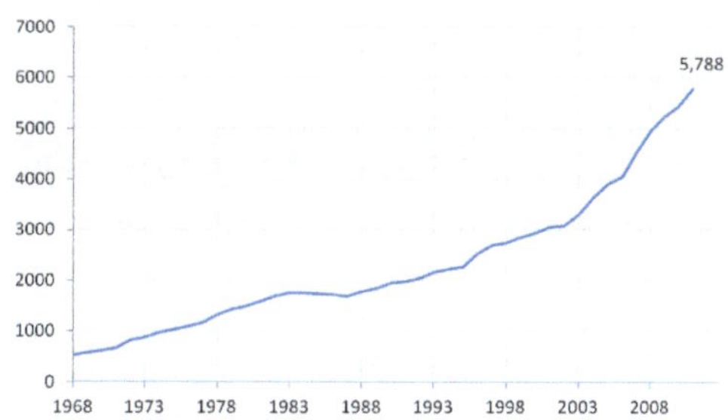

First-year enrollment at osteopathic medical schools, 1968–2011

OMT

Traditional osteopathic medicine, specifically OMT, has been criticized for many techniques such as cranial and cranio-sacral manipulation. A study performed in the early 2000s questioned the therapeutic utility of osteopathic manipulative treatment modalities. Also, New York University health information website claims that "it is difficult to properly ascertain the effectiveness of a hands-on therapy like OMT."

Research Emphasis

Another area of criticism has been the relative lack of research and lesser emphasis on scientific inquiry at D.O. schools in comparison with M.D. schools.

The inability to institutionalize research, particularly clinical research, at osteopathic institutions has, over the years, weakened the acculturation, socialization, and distinctive beliefs and practices of osteopathic students and graduates.

Identity Crisis

There is currently a debate within the osteopathic community over the feasibility of maintaining osteopathic medicine as a distinct entity within U.S. health care. JD Howell, author of *The Paradox of Osteopathy,* notes claims of a "fundamental yet ineffable difference" between MD and DO qualified physicians are based on practices such as "preventive medicine and seeing patients in a sociological context" that are "widely encountered not only in osteopathic medicine but also in allopathic medicine." Studies have confirmed the lack of any "philosophic concept or resultant practice behavior" that would distinguish a D.O. from an M.D. Howell summarizes the questions framing the debate over the future of osteopathic distinctiveness thus:

If osteopathy has become the functional equivalent of allopathy [meaning the MD profession], what is the justification for its continued existence? And if there is value in therapy that is uniquely osteopathic, why should its use be limited to osteopaths?

Rapid Expansion

As the number of osteopathic schools has increased, the debate over distinctiveness has often seen the leadership of the American Osteopathic Association at odds with the community of osteopathic physicians.

within the osteopathic community, the growth is drawing attention to the identity crisis faced by [the profession]. While osteopathic leaders emphasize osteopaths' unique identity, many osteopaths would rather not draw attention to their uniqueness.

The rapid expansion has raised concerns about the number of available faculty at osteopathic schools and the role that those faculty play in maintaining the integrity of the academic program of the schools. Norman Gevitz, author of the leading text on the history of osteopathic medicine, recently published,

DO schools are currently expanding their class sizes much more quickly than are their MD counterparts. Unlike MD colleges, where it is widely known that academic faculty members—fearing dilution of quality as well as the prospect of an increased teaching workload—constitute a powerful inhibiting force to expand the class size, osteopathic faculty at private osteopathic schools have traditionally had little or no input on such matters. Instead, these decisions are almost exclusively the responsibility of college administrators and their boards of trustees, who look at such expansion from an entrepreneurial as well as an educational perspective. Osteopathic medical schools can keep the cost of student body expansion relatively low compared with that of MD institutions. Although the standards of the Commission on Osteopathic College Accreditation ensure that there will be enough desks and lab spaces to accommodate all new students, they do not mandate that an osteopathic college must bear the expense of maintaining a high full-time-faculty:student ratio.

The president of the American Association of Colleges of Osteopathic Medicine commented on the current climate of crisis within the profession.

The simultaneous movement away from osteopathic medicine's traditionally separate training and practice systems, when coupled with its rapid growth, has created a sense of crisis as to its future. The rapid rate of growth has raised questions as to the availability of clinical and basic science faculty and clinical resources to accommodate the increasing load of students.

References

- Russell J, Rovere A, eds. (2009). "Craniosacral Therapy". American Cancer Society Complete Guide to Complementary and Alternative Cancer Therapies (2nd ed.). American Cancer Society. pp. 187–189. ISBN 9780944235713.
- Aronoff, George R., ed. (1999). Evaluation and Treatment of Chronic Pain (3rd ed.). Lippincott Williams and Wilkins. p. 571. ISBN 978-0-683-30149-6.
- Williams, P L; Warwick, R; Dyson, M; Bannister, L H. (1989). Gray's Anatomy (37th ed.). Edinburgh: Churchill Livingstone. p. 468. ISBN 0-443-02588-6.
- Vincent C, Furnham A (1997). Manipulative Therapies: Osteopathy and Chiropractic. Complementary Medicine: A Research Perspective. John Wiley & Sons. p. 15. ISBN 978-0-471-96645-6.
- DiGiovanna, Eileen L.; Schiowitz, Stanley; Dowling, Dennis J. (2004). An Osteopathic Approach to Diagnosis and Treatment (3 ed.). Lippincott Williams & Wilkins. ISBN 978-0-7817-4293-1.
- Oths, Kathryn S.; Servando Z. Hinojosa. (2004). "Divergences in the evolution of Osteopathy". Healing by Hand: Manual Medicine and Bonesetting in Global Perspective. Rowman Altamira. pp. 67–68. ISBN 0-7591-0393-3.
- Gevitz, Norman (2004). The DO's: osteopathic medicine in America. Baltimore, Maryland: Johns Hopkins University Press. ISBN 0-8018-7833-0.
- Robert, Ward (2002). Foundations for Osteopathic Medicine: The research status of somatic dysfunction (2nd ed.). Philadelphia: Lippincott Williams & Wilkins. pp. 1188–1193. ISBN 978-0781734974.
- "The Difference Between U.S.-Trained Osteopathic Physicians and Osteopaths Trained Abroad". AACOM. Retrieved August 21, 2016.

- Russell J, Rovere A, eds. (2009). "Craniosacral Therapy". American Cancer Society Complete Guide to Complementary and Alternative Cancer Therapies (2nd ed.). American Cancer Society. pp. 187–189. ISBN 9780944235713.
- Aronoff, George R., ed. (1999). Evaluation and Treatment of Chronic Pain (3rd ed.). Lippincott Williams and Wilkins. p. 571. ISBN 978-0-683-30149-6.
- Williams, P L; Warwick, R; Dyson, M; Bannister, L H. (1989). Gray's Anatomy (37th ed.). Edinburgh: Churchill Livingstone. p. 468. ISBN 0-443-02588-6.
- Vincent C, Furnham A (1997). Manipulative Therapies: Osteopathy and Chiropractic. Complementary Medicine: A Research Perspective. John Wiley & Sons. p. 15. ISBN 978-0-471-96645-6.
- DiGiovanna, Eileen L.; Schiowitz, Stanley; Dowling, Dennis J. (2004). An Osteopathic Approach to Diagnosis and Treatment (3 ed.). Lippincott Williams & Wilkins. ISBN 978-0-7817-4293-1.
- Oths, Kathryn S.; Servando Z. Hinojosa. (2004). "Divergences in the evolution of Osteopathy". Healing by Hand: Manual Medicine and Bonesetting in Global Perspective. Rowman Altamira. pp. 67–68. ISBN 0-7591-0393-3.
- Gevitz, Norman (2004). The DO's: osteopathic medicine in America. Baltimore, Maryland: Johns Hopkins University Press. ISBN 0-8018-7833-0.
- Robert, Ward (2002). Foundations for Osteopathic Medicine: The research status of somatic dysfunction (2nd ed.). Philadelphia: Lippincott Williams & Wilkins. pp. 1188–1193. ISBN 978-0781734974.
- "The Difference Between U.S.-Trained Osteopathic Physicians and Osteopaths Trained Abroad". AACOM. Retrieved August 21, 2016.

8

An Integrated Study of Chiropractic Treatment

Chiropractic is one of the many forms of alternative medicine. It helps in the curing of the disorders of the musculoskeletal system. This treatment majorly uses manipulation of the spine. The safety of this treatment has been debated as it certainly has adverse effects, and can also cause death in rare cases. The section focuses on the use of the chiropractic treatment and helps the readers in understanding the effects of this treatment.

Chiropractic

Chiropractic is a form of alternative medicine concerned with the diagnosis and treatment of unproven mechanical disorders of the musculoskeletal system, especially the spine, under the belief that such a disorder affects general health via the nervous system. The main chiropractic treatment technique involves manual therapy, especially spinal manipulation therapy (SMT), manipulations of other joints and soft tissues. The "specific focus of chiropractic practice" is chiropractic subluxation, an unproven concept that has no scientific basis. Chiropractors often also offer conventional therapies such as physical therapy and lifestyle counseling, and it may for the lay person be difficult to distinguish the unscientific from the scientific. The underlying philosophy as well as certain practices employed by chiropractors are pseudoscience and anti-scientific.

Numerous controlled clinical studies of treatments used by chiropractors have been conducted, with conflicting results. Systematic reviews of this research have not found evidence that chiropractic manipulation is effective, with the possible exception of treatment for back pain. A critical evaluation found that collectively, spinal manipulation was ineffective at treating any condition. A Cochrane review found very low to moderate evidence that spinal manipulation therapy was any more effective than inert interventions, sham SMT or as an adjunct therapy for acute low back pain. Spinal manipulation may be cost-effective for sub-acute or chronic low back pain but the results for acute low back pain were insufficient. The efficacy and cost-effectiveness of maintenance chiropractic care are unknown. There is not sufficient data to establish the safety of chiropractic manipulations. The rate of adverse events is unknown as they are under–reported. It is frequently associated with mild to moderate adverse effects. The incidence of serious complications which can lead to permanent disability or death is probably rare. There is controversy regarding the degree of risk of vertebral artery dissection, which can lead to stroke and death, from cervical manipulation. Several deaths have been associated with this technique and it is suggested that the relationship is causative. This is disputed by many chiropractors who believe it is unproven.

Many chiropractors describe themselves as primary care providers, but the chiropractic clinical training does not support the requirements to be considered primary care providers, so their role on primary care is limited and disputed. Chiropractic is well established in the United States, Canada, and Australia. It overlaps with other manual-therapy professions, including massage therapy, osteopathy, and physical therapy. Most who seek chiropractic care do so for low back pain, and back and neck pain are considered the specialties of chiropractic, but many chiropractors treat ailments other than musculoskeletal issues. A considerable number of chiropractors fear that if they do not separate themselves from the traditional vitalistic concept of "innate intelligence", chiropractic will continue to be seen as a fringe profession. Chiropractic has two main groups: "straights", now the minority, emphasize vitalism, "innate intelligence" and spinal adjustments, and consider vertebral subluxations to be the cause of all disease; "mixers", the majority, are more open to mainstream views and conventional medical techniques, such as exercise, massage, and ice therapy.

D. D. Palmer founded chiropractic in the 1890s, and his son B. J. Palmer helped to expand it in the early 20th century. Throughout its history, chiropractic has been controversial. Its foundation is at odds with mainstream medicine, and has been sustained by pseudoscientific ideas such as subluxation and innate intelligence that are not based on sound science because they do not exist. Neither the concept of subluxation nor spinal manipulation has any scientific basis. It is classified as a field of pseudomedicine. Despite the overwhelming evidence that vaccination is an effective public health intervention, among chiropractors there are significant disagreements over the subject, which has led to negative impacts on both public vaccination and mainstream acceptance of chiropractic. The American Medical Association called chiropractic an "unscientific cult" in 1966 and boycotted it until losing an antitrust case in 1987. Chiropractic has had a strong political base and sustained demand for services; in recent decades, it has gained more legitimacy and greater acceptance among conventional physicians and health plans in the U.S., and evidence-based medicine has been used to review research studies and generate practice guidelines.

Conceptual Basis

Philosophy

Chiropractic is a form of alternative medicine which focuses on manipulation of the musculoskeletal system, especially the spine. Its founder, D.D. Palmer, called it "a science of healing without drugs".

Two chiropractic belief system constructs	
The testable principle	**The untestable metaphor**
Chiropractic adjustment ↓ Restoration of structural integrity ↓ Improvement of health status	Universal intelligence ↓ Innate intelligence ↓ Body physiology
Materialistic:	*Vitalistic:*
• Operational definitions possible • Lends itself to scientific inquiry	• Origin of holism in chiropractic • Cannot be proven or disproven
Taken from Mootz & Phillips 1997	

Chiropractic's origins lie in the folk medicine of bonesetting, and as it evolved it incorporated vitalism, spiritual inspiration and rationalism. Its early philosophy was based on deduction from irrefutable doctrine helped distinguish chiropractic from medicine, provided it with legal and political defenses against claims of practicing medicine without a license, and allowed chiropractors to establish themselves as an autonomous profession. This "straight" philosophy, taught to generations of chiropractors, rejects the inferential reasoning of the scientific method, and relies on deductions from vitalistic first principles rather than on the materialism of science. However, most practitioners tend to incorporate scientific research into chiropractic, and most practitioners are "mixers" who attempt to combine the materialistic reductionism of science with the metaphysics of their predecessors and with the holistic paradigm of wellness. A 2008 commentary proposed that chiropractic actively divorce itself from the straight philosophy as part of a campaign to eliminate untestable dogma and engage in critical thinking and evidence-based research.

Although a wide diversity of ideas exist among chiropractors, they share the belief that the spine and health are related in a fundamental way, and that this relationship is mediated through the nervous system. Some chiropractors claim spinal manipulation can have an effect of a variety of ailments such as irritable bowel syndrome and asthma.

Chiropractic Philosophy Includes The Following Perspectives:

Holism assumes that health is affected by everything in an individual's environment; some sources also include a spiritual or existential dimension. In contrast, reductionism in chiropractic reduces causes and cures of health problems to a single factor, vertebral subluxation. Homeostasis emphasizes the body's inherent self-healing abilities. Chiropractic's early notion of innate intelligence can be thought of as a metaphor for homeostasis.

A variant of chiropractic called naprapathy originated in Chicago in the early twentieth century. It holds that manual manipulation of soft tissue can reduce "interference" in the body and thus improve health.

Straights and Mixers

Range of belief perspectives in chiropractic

Perspective attribute	**Potential belief endpoints**	
Scope of practice:	narrow ("straight") ←	→ broad ("mixer")
Diagnostic approach:	intuitive ←	→ analytical
Philosophic orientation:	vitalistic ←	→ materialistic
Scientific orientation:	descriptive ←	→ experimental
Process orientation:	implicit ←	→ explicit
Practice attitude:	doctor/model-centered ←	→ patient/situation-centered
Professional integration:	separate and distinct ←	→ integrated into mainstream

Taken from Mootz & Phillips 1997

Straight chiropractors adhere to the philosophical principles set forth by D.D. and B.J. Palmer, and retain metaphysical definitions and vitalistic qualities. Straight chiropractors believe that vertebral subluxation leads to interference with an "innate intelligence" exerted via the human nervous system and is a primary underlying risk factor for many diseases. Straights view the medical diagnosis of patient complaints (which they consider to be the "secondary effects" of subluxations) to be unnecessary for chiropractic treatment. Thus, straight chiropractors are concerned primarily with the detection and correction of vertebral subluxation via adjustment and do not "mix" other types of therapies into their practice style. Their philosophy and explanations are metaphysical in nature and they prefer to use traditional chiropractic lexicon terminology (e.g., perform spinal analysis, detect subluxation, correct with adjustment). They prefer to remain separate and distinct from mainstream health care. Although considered the minority group, "they have been able to transform their status as purists and heirs of the lineage into influence dramatically out of proportion to their numbers."

Mixer chiropractors "mix" diagnostic and treatment approaches from chiropractic, medical and/or osteopathic viewpoints and make up the majority of chiropractors. Unlike straight chiropractors, mixers believe subluxation is one of many causes of disease, and hence they tend to be open to mainstream medicine. Many of them incorporate mainstream medical diagnostics and employ conventional treatments including techniques of physical therapy such as exercise, stretching, massage, ice packs, electrical muscle stimulation, therapeutic ultrasound, and moist heat. Some mixers also use techniques from alternative medicine, including nutritional supplements, acupuncture, homeopathy, herbal remedies, and biofeedback.

Although mixers are the majority group, many of them retain belief in vertebral subluxation as shown in a 2003 survey of 1100 North American chiropractors, which found that 88% wanted to retain the term "vertebral subluxation complex", and that when asked to estimate the percent of disorders of internal organs (such as the heart, the lungs, or the stomach) that subluxation significantly contributes to, the mean response was 62%. A 2008 survey of 6,000 American chiropractors demonstrated that most chiropractors seem to believe that a subluxation-based clinical approach may be of limited utility for addressing visceral disorders, and greatly favored non-subluxation-based clinical approaches for such conditions. The same survey showed that most chiropractors generally believed that the majority of their clinical approach for addressing musculoskeletal/biomechanical disorders such as back pain was based on subluxation.

Vertebral Subluxation

Palmer hypothesized that vertebral joint misalignments, which he termed *vertebral subluxations*, interfered with the body's function and its inborn ability to heal itself. D. D. Palmer repudiated his earlier theory that vertebral subluxations caused pinched nerves in the intervertebral spaces in favor of subluxations causing altered nerve vibration, either too tense or too slack, affecting the tone (health) of the end organ. D. D. Palmer, using a vitalistic approach, imbued the term *subluxation* with a metaphysical and philosophical meaning. He qualified this by noting that knowledge of innate intelligence was not essential to the competent practice of chiropractic. This concept was later expanded upon by his son, B. J. Palmer, and was instrumental in providing the legal basis of differentiating chiropractic from conventional medicine. In 1910, D. D. Palmer theorized that the nervous system controlled health:

> "Physiologists divide nerve-fibers, which form the nerves, into two classes, afferent and efferent. Impressions are made on the peripheral afferent fiber-endings; these create sensations that are transmitted to the center of the nervous system. Efferent nerve-fibers carry

impulses out from the center to their endings. Most of these go to muscles and are therefore called motor impulses; some are secretory and enter glands; a portion are inhibitory, their function being to restrain secretion. Thus, nerves carry impulses outward and sensations inward. The activity of these nerves, or rather their fibers, may become excited or allayed by impingement, the result being a modification of functionality—too much or not enough action—which is disease."

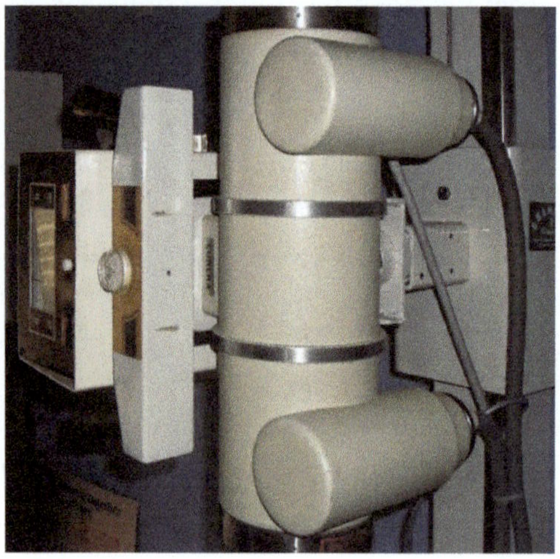

Chiropractors use x-ray radiography to examine the bone structure of a patient.

Vertebral subluxation, a core concept of traditional chiropractic, remains unsubstantiated and largely untested, and a debate about whether to keep it in the chiropractic paradigm has been ongoing for decades. In general, critics of traditional subluxation-based chiropractic (including chiropractors) are skeptical of its clinical value, dogmatic beliefs and metaphysical approach. While straight chiropractic still retains the traditional vitalistic construct espoused by the founders, evidence-based chiropractic suggests that a mechanistic view will allow chiropractic care to become integrated into the wider health care community. This is still a continuing source of debate within the chiropractic profession as well, with some schools of chiropractic still teaching the traditional/ straight subluxation-based chiropractic, while others have moved towards an evidence-based chiropractic that rejects metaphysical foundings and limits itself to primarily neuromusculoskeletal conditions.

In 2005, the chiropractic subluxation was defined by the World Health Organization as "a lesion or dysfunction in a joint or motion segment in which alignment, movement integrity and/or physiological function are altered, although contact between joint surfaces remains intact. It is essentially a functional entity, which may influence biomechanical and neural integrity." This differs from the medical definition of subluxation as a significant structural displacement, which can be seen with static imaging techniques such as X-rays. The 2008 book *Trick or Treatment* states "X-rays can reveal neither the subluxations nor the innate intelligence associated with chiropractic philosophy, because they do not exist." Attorney David Chapman-Smith, Secretary-General of the World Federation of Chiropractic, has stated that "Medical critics have asked how there can be a subluxation if it cannot be seen on x-ray. The answer is that the chiropractic subluxation is essentially a functional entity, not structural, and is therefore no more visible on static x-ray than a limp or headache or any other functional problem." The General Chiropractic Council, the statutory regulatory body for chiropractors in the United Kingdom, states that the chiropractic vertebral subluxation complex "is not supported by any clinical research evidence that would allow claims to be made that it is the cause of disease."

As of 2014, the National Board of Chiropractic Examiners states "The specific focus of chiropractic practice is known as the chiropractic subluxation or joint dysfunction. A subluxation is a health concern that manifests in the skeletal joints, and, through complex anatomical and physiological relationships, affects the nervous system and may lead to reduced function, disability or illness."

Scope of Practice

Chiropractors emphasize the conservative management of the neuromusculoskeletal system without the use of medicines or surgery, with special emphasis on the spine. Back and neck pain are the specialties of chiropractic but many chiropractors treat ailments other than musculoskeletal issues. There is a range of opinions among chiropractors: some believed that treatment should be confined to the spine, or back and neck pain; others disagreed. For example, while one 2009 survey of American chiropractors had found that 73% classified themselves as "back pain/musculoskeletal specialists", the label "back and neck pain specialists" was regarded by 47% of them as a *least* desirable description in a 2005 international survey. Chiropractic combines aspects from mainstream and alternative medicine, and there is no agreement about how to define the profession: although chiropractors have many attributes of primary care providers, chiropractic has more of the attributes of a medical specialty like dentistry or podiatry. It has been proposed that chiropractors specialize in nonsurgical spine care, instead of attempting to also treat other problems, but the more expansive view of chiropractic is still widespread. Mainstream health care and governmental organizations such as the World Health Organization consider chiropractic to be complementary and alternative medicine (CAM); and a 2008 study reported that 31% of surveyed chiropractors categorized chiropractic as CAM, 27% as integrated medicine, and 12% as mainstream medicine. Many chiropractors believe they are primary care providers, including US and UK chiropractors, but the length, breadth, and depth of chiropractic clinical training do not support the requirements to be considered primary care providers, so their role on primary care is limited and disputed.

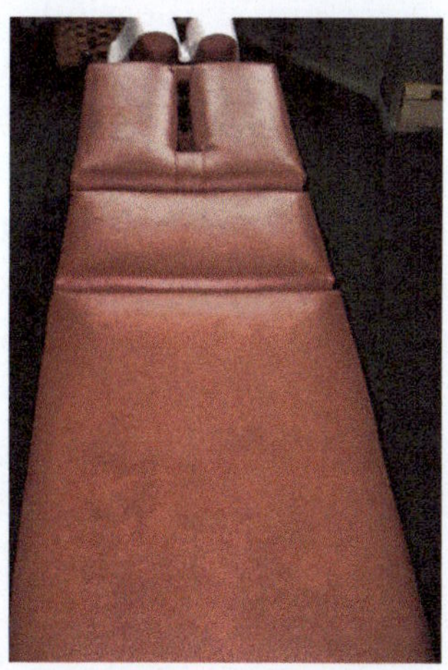

A treatment table at a chiropractic office

Chiropractic overlaps with several other forms of manual therapy, including massage therapy, osteopathy, physical therapy, and sports medicine. Chiropractic is autonomous from and competitive with mainstream medicine, and osteopathy outside the US remains primarily a manual medical system; physical therapists work alongside and cooperate with mainstream medicine, and osteopathic medicine in the U.S. has merged with the medical profession. Practitioners may distinguish these competing approaches through claims that, compared to other therapists, chiropractors heavily emphasize spinal manipulation, tend to use firmer manipulative techniques, and promote maintenance care; that osteopaths use a wider variety of treatment procedures; and that physical therapists emphasize machinery and exercise.

Chiropractic diagnosis may involve a range of methods including skeletal imaging, observational and tactile assessments, and orthopedic and neurological evaluation. A chiropractor may also refer a patient to an appropriate specialist, or co-manage with another health care provider. Common patient management involves spinal manipulation (SM) and other manual therapies to the joints and soft tissues, rehabilitative exercises, health promotion, electrical modalities, complementary procedures, and lifestyle advice.

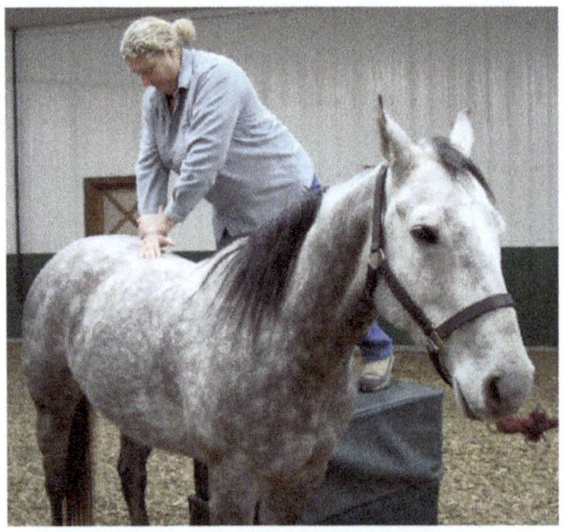

A chiropractic adjustment of a horse

Chiropractors are not normally licensed to write medical prescriptions or perform major surgery in the United States, (although New Mexico has become the first US state to allow "advanced practice" trained chiropractors to prescribe certain medications.). In the US, their scope of practice varies by state, based on inconsistent views of chiropractic care: some states, such as Iowa, broadly allow treatment of "human ailments"; some, such as Delaware, use vague concepts such as "transition of nerve energy" to define scope of practice; others, such as New Jersey, specify a severely narrowed scope. US states also differ over whether chiropractors may conduct laboratory tests or diagnostic procedures, dispense dietary supplements, or use other therapies such as homeopathy and acupuncture; in Oregon they can become certified to perform minor surgery and to deliver children via natural childbirth. A 2003 survey of North American chiropractors found that a slight majority favored allowing them to write prescriptions for over-the-counter drugs. A 2010 survey found 72% of Switzerland chiropractors judged the current allowance in Switzerland to prescribing nonprescription medication as an advantage for chiropractic treatment.

A related field, veterinary chiropractic, applies manual therapies to animals and is recognized in 40 US states, but is not recognized by the American Chiropractic Association as being chiropractic. It remains controversial within certain segments of the veterinary, and chiropractic profession.

No single profession "owns" spinal manipulation and there is little consensus as to which profession should administer SM, raising concerns by chiropractors that other medical physicians could "steal" SM procedures from chiropractors. A focus on evidence-based SM research has also raised concerns that the resulting practice guidelines could limit the scope of chiropractic practice to treating backs and necks. Two U.S. states (Washington and Arkansas) prohibit physical therapists from performing SM, some states allow them to do it only if they have completed advanced training in SM, and some states allow only chiropractors to perform SM, or only chiropractors and physicians. Bills to further prohibit non-chiropractors from performing SM are regularly introduced into state legislatures and are opposed by physical therapist organizations.

Treatments

Spinal manipulation, which chiropractors call "spinal adjustment" or "chiropractic adjustment", is the most common treatment used in chiropractic care. Spinal manipulation is a passive manual maneuver during which a three-joint complex is taken past the normal range of movement, but not so far as to dislocate or damage the joint. Its defining factor is a dynamic thrust, which is a sudden force that causes an audible release and attempts to increase a joint's range of motion. High-velocity, low-amplitude spinal manipulation (HVLA-SM) thrusts have physiological effects that signal neural discharge from paraspinal muscle tissues, depending on duration and amplitude of the thrust are factors of the degree in paraspinal muscle spindles activation. Clinical skill in employing HVLA-SM thrusts depends on the ability of the practitioner to handle the duration and magnitude of the load. More generally, spinal manipulative therapy (SMT) describes techniques where the hands are used to manipulate, massage, mobilize, adjust, stimulate, apply traction to, or otherwise influence the spine and related tissues.

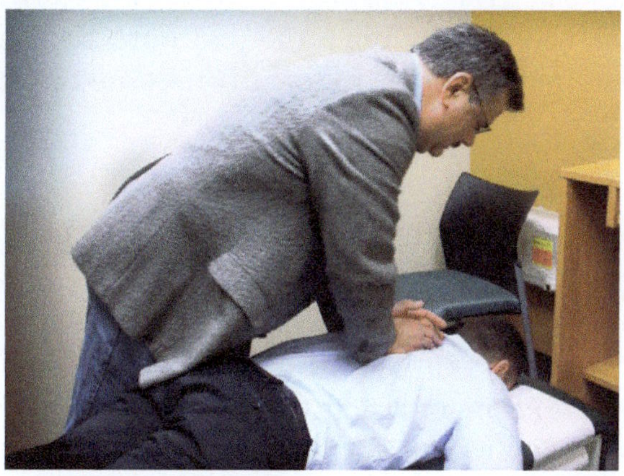

A chiropractor performs an adjustment on a patient.

There are several schools of chiropractic adjustive techniques, although most chiropractors mix techniques from several schools. The following adjustive procedures were received by more than 10% of patients of licensed U.S. chiropractors in a 2003 survey: Diversified technique (full-spine manipulation, employing various techniques), extremity adjusting, Activator technique (which uses a spring-loaded tool to deliver precise adjustments to the spine), Thompson Technique (which relies on a drop table and detailed procedural protocols), Gonstead (which emphasizes evaluating the spine along with specific adjustment that avoids rotational vectors), Cox/flexion-distraction (a gentle, low-force adjusting procedure which mixes chiropractic with osteopathic principles and utilizes specialized adjusting tables with movable parts), adjustive instrument, Sacro-Occipital Technique (which models the spine as a torsion bar), Nimmo Receptor-Tonus Technique, applied kinesiology (which emphasises "muscle testing" as a diagnostic tool), and cranial. Chiropractic biophysics technique uses inverse functions of rotations during spinal manipulation. Koren Specific Technique (KST) may use their hands, or they may use an electric device known as an "ArthroStim" for assessment and spinal manipulations. Insurers in the US and UK that cover other chiropractic techniques exclude KST from coverage because they consider it to be "experimental and investigational." Medicine-assisted manipulation, such as manipulation under anesthesia, involves sedation or local anesthetic and is done by a team that includes an anesthesiologist; a 2008 systematic review did not find enough evidence to make recommendations about its use for chronic low back pain.

Many other procedures are used by chiropractors for treating the spine, other joints and tissues, and general health issues. The following procedures were received by more than one-third of patients of licensed U.S. chiropractors in a 2003 survey: Diversified technique (full-spine manipulation; mentioned in previous paragraph), physical fitness/exercise promotion, corrective or therapeutic exercise, ergonomic/postural advice, self-care strategies, activities of daily living, changing risky/unhealthy behaviors, nutritional/dietary recommendations, relaxation/stress reduction recommendations, ice pack/cryotherapy, extremity adjusting (also mentioned in previous paragraph), trigger point therapy, and disease prevention/early screening advice.

A 2010 study describing Belgium chiropractors and their patients found chiropractors in Belgium mostly focus on neuromusculoskeletal complaints in adult patients, with emphasis on the spine. The diversified technique is the most often applied technique at 93%, followed by the Activator mechanical-assisted technique at 41%. A 2009 study assessing chiropractic students giving or receiving spinal manipulations while attending a U.S. chiropractic college found Diversified, Gonstead, and upper cervical manipulations are frequently used methods.

Practice Guidelines

Reviews of research studies within the chiropractic community have been used to generate practice guidelines outlining standards that specify which chiropractic treatments are "legitimate" (i.e. supported by evidence) and conceivably reimbursable under managed care health payment systems. Evidence-based guidelines are supported by one end of an ideological continuum among chiropractors; the other end employs antiscientific reasoning and makes unsubstantiated claims. Chiropractic remains at a crossroads, and that in order to progress it would need to embrace science; the promotion by some for it to be a cure-all was both "misguided and irrational". A 2007 survey of Alberta chiropractors found that they do not consistently apply research in practice, which may have resulted from a lack of research education and skills.

Effectiveness

There is no good evidence that chiropractic is effective for the treatment of any medical condition, except perhaps for certain kinds of back pain. Generally, the research carried out into the effectiveness of chiropractic has been of poor quality. Numerous controlled clinical studies of treatments used by chiropractors have been conducted, with conflicting results. Research published by chiropractors is distinctly biased. For reviews of SM for back pain chiropractic authors tend to have positive conclusions, while others did not show any effectiveness.

There is a wide range of ways to measure treatment outcomes. Chiropractic care, like all medical treatment, benefits from the placebo response. It is difficult to construct a trustworthy placebo for clinical trials of spinal manipulative therapy (SMT), as experts often disagree about whether a proposed placebo actually has no effect. The efficacy of maintenance care in chiropractic is unknown.

Available evidence covers the following conditions:

- Low back pain. A 2013 Cochrane review found very low to moderate evidence that SMT was no more effective than inert interventions, sham SMT or as an adjunct therapy for acute low back pain. The same review found that SMT appears to be no better than other recommended therapies. A 2012 overview of systematic reviews found that collectively, SM failed to show it is an effective intervention for pain. A 2011 Cochrane review found strong evidence that suggests there is no clinically meaningful difference between SMT and other treatments for reducing pain and improving function for chronic low back pain. A 2010 Cochrane review found no current evidence to support or refute a clinically significant difference between the effects of combined chiropractic interventions and other interventions for chronic or mixed duration low back pain. A 2010 systematic review found that most studies suggest SMT achieves equivalent or superior improvement in pain and function when compared with other commonly used interventions for short, intermediate, and long-term follow-up. Specific guidelines concerning the treatment of nonspecific (i.e. unknown cause) low back pain are inconsistent between countries.
- Radiculopathy. A 2013 systematic review and meta-analysis found a statistically significant improvement in overall recovery from sciatica following SM, when compared to usual care, and suggested that SM may be considered. There is moderate quality evidence to support the use of SM for the treatment of acute lumbar radiculopathy and acute lumbar disc herniation with associated radiculopathy. There is low or very low evidence supporting SM for chronic lumbar spine-related extremity symptoms and cervical spine-related extremity symptoms of any duration and no evidence exists for the treatment of thoracic radiculopathy.
- Whiplash and other neck pain. There is no consensus on the effectiveness of manual therapies for neck pain. A 2013 systematic review found that the data suggests that there are minimal short- and long-term treatment differences when comparing manipulation or mobilization of the cervical spine to physical therapy or exercise for neck pain improvement. A 2013 systematic review found that although there is insufficient evidence that thoracic SM is more effective than other treatments, it is a suitable intervention to treat some patients with non-specific neck pain. A 2011 systematic review found that thoracic SM may offer short-term improvement for the treatment of acute or subacute mechanical neck pain; although the body of literature is still weak. A 2010 Cochrane review found low quality evidence that suggests cervical manipulation may offer better short-term pain relief than a control for neck pain, and moderate evidence that cervical manipulation and mobilization produced similar effects on pain, function and patient satisfaction. A 2010 systematic review found low level evidence that suggests chiropractic care improves cervical range of motion and pain in the management of whiplash.
- Headache. A 2011 systematic review found evidence that suggests that chiropractic SMT might be as effective as propranolol or topiramate in the prevention of migraine headaches.

A 2011 systematic review found evidence that does not support the use of SM for the treatment of migraine headaches. A 2006 review found no rigorous evidence supporting SM or other manual therapies for tension headache. A 2005 review found that the evidence was weak for effectiveness of chiropractic manipulation for tension headache, and that it was probably more effective for tension headache than for migraine. A 2004 Cochrane review found evidence that suggests SM may be effective for migraine, tension headache and cervicogenic headache.

- Extremity conditions. A 2011 systematic review and meta-analysis concluded that the addition of manual mobilizations to an exercise program for the treatment of knee osteoarthritis resulted in better pain relief then a supervised exercise program alone and suggested that manual therapists consider adding manual mobilisation to optimise supervised active exercise programs. There is silver level evidence that manual therapy is more effective than exercise for the treatment of hip osteoarthritis, however this evidence could be considered to be inconclusive. A 2008 systematic review found that the addition of cervical spine mobilization to a treatment regimen for lateral epicondylosis (tennis elbow) resulted in significantly better pain relief and functional improvements in both the short and long-term. There is a small amount of research into the efficacy of chiropractic treatment for upper limbs, limited to low level evidence supporting chiropractic management of shoulder pain and limited or fair evidence supporting chiropractic management of leg conditions.

- Other. A 2012 systematic review found insufficient low bias evidence to support the use of spinal manipulation as a therapy for the treatment of hypertension. A 2011 systematic review found moderate evidence to support the use of manual therapy for cervicogenic dizziness. There is very weak evidence for chiropractic care for adult scoliosis (curved or rotated spine) and no scientific data for idiopathic adolescent scoliosis. A 2007 systematic review found that few studies of chiropractic care for nonmusculoskeletal conditions are available, and they are typically not of high quality; it also found that the entire clinical encounter of chiropractic care (as opposed to just SM) provides benefit to patients with cervicogenic dizziness, and that the evidence from reviews is negative, or too weak to draw conclusions, for a wide variety of other nonmusculoskeletal conditions, including ADHD/learning disabilities, dizziness, high blood pressure, and vision conditions. Other reviews have found no evidence of significant benefit for asthma, baby colic, bedwetting, carpal tunnel syndrome, fibromyalgia, gastrointestinal disorders, kinetic imbalance due to suboccipital strain (KISS) in infants, menstrual cramps, or pelvic and back pain during pregnancy.

Safety

There is not sufficient data to establish the safety of chiropractic manipulations. Manipulation is regarded as relatively safe but complications can arise, and it has known adverse effects, risks and contraindications. Absolute contraindications to spinal manipulative therapy are conditions that should not be manipulated; these contraindications include rheumatoid arthritis and conditions known to result in unstable joints. Relative contraindications are conditions where increased risk is acceptable in some situations and where low-force and soft-tissue techniques are treatments of choice; these contraindications include osteoporosis. Although most contraindications apply only to manipulation of the affected region, some neurological signs indicate referral to emergency medical services; these include sudden and severe headache or neck pain unlike that previously experienced. Indirect risks of chiropractic involve delayed or missed diagnoses through consulting a chiropractor.

Spinal manipulation is associated with frequent, mild and temporary adverse effects, including new or worsening pain or stiffness in the affected region. They have been estimated to occur in 33% to 61% of patients, and frequently occur within an hour of treatment and disappear within 24 to 48 hours; adverse reactions appear to be more common following manipulation than mobilization. Chiropractic is correlated with a very high incidence of minor adverse effects. Chiropractic are more commonly associated with serious related adverse effects than other professionals following manipulation. Rarely, spinal manipulation, particularly on the upper spine, can also result in complications that can lead to permanent disability or death; these can occur in adults and children. Estimates vary widely for the incidence of these complications, and the actual incidence is unknown, due to high levels of underreporting and to the difficulty of linking manipulation to adverse effects such as stroke, which is a particular concern. Adverse effects are poorly reported in recent studies investigating chiropractic manipulations. A 2016 systematic review concludes that the level of reporting is unsuitable and unacceptable. Reports of serious adverse events have occurred, resulting from spinal manipulation therapy of the lumbopelvic region. Estimates for serious adverse events vary from 5 strokes per 100,000 manipulations to 1.46 serious adverse events per 10 million manipulations and 2.68 deaths per 10 million manipulations, though it was determined that there was inadequate data to be conclusive. Several case reports show temporal associations between interventions and potentially serious complications. The published medical literature contains reports of 26 deaths since 1934 following chiropractic manipulations and many more seem to remain unpublished.

Vertebrobasilar artery stroke (VAS) is statistically associated with chiropractic services in persons under 45 years of age, but it is similarly associated with general practitioner services, suggesting that these associations are likely explained by preexisting conditions. Weak to moderately strong evidence supports causation (as opposed to statistical association) between cervical manipulative therapy (CMT) and VAS. There is insufficient evidence to support a strong association or no association between cervical manipulation and stroke. While the biomechanical evidence is not sufficient to support the statement that CMT causes cervical artery dissection (CD), clinical reports suggest that mechanical forces have a part in a substantial number of CDs and the majority of population controlled studies found an association between CMT and VAS in young people. It is strongly recommended that practitioners consider the plausibility of CD as a symptom, and people can be informed of the association between CD and CMT before administrating manipulation of the cervical spine. There is controversy regarding the degree of risk of stroke from cervical manipulation. Many chiropractors state that, the association between chiropractic therapy and vertebral arterial dissection is not proven. However, it has been suggested that the causality between chiropractic cervical manipulation beyond the normal range of motion and vascular accidents is probable or definite. There is very low evidence supporting a small association between internal carotid artery dissection and chiropractic neck manipulation. The incidence of internal carotid artery dissection following cervical spine manipulation is unknown. The literature infrequently reports helpful data to better understand the association between cervical manipulative therapy, cervical artery dissection and stroke. The limited evidence is inconclusive that chiropractic spinal manipulation therapy is not a cause of intracranial hypotension.

Chiropractors, like other primary care providers, sometimes employ diagnostic imaging techniques such as X-rays and CT scans that rely on ionizing radiation. Although there is no clear evidence for the practice, some chiropractors may still X-ray a patient several times a year. Practice guidelines aim to reduce unnecessary radiation exposure, which increases cancer risk in proportion to the amount of radiation received. Research suggests that radiology instruction given at chiropractic schools worldwide seem to be evidence-based. Although, there seems to be a disparity between some schools and available evidence regarding the aspect of radiography for patients with acute low back pain without an indication of a serious disease, which may contribute to chiropractic overuse of radiography for low back pain.

Risk-benefit

A 2012 systematic review concluded that no accurate assessment of risk-benefit exists for cervical manipulation. A 2010 systematic review stated that there is no good evidence to assume that neck manipulation is an effective treatment for any medical condition and suggested a precautionary principle in healthcare for chiropractic intervention even if a causality with vertebral artery dissection after neck manipulation were merely a remote possibility. The same review concluded that the risk of death from manipulations to the neck outweighs the benefits. Chiropractors have criticized this conclusion, claiming that the author did not evaluate the potential benefits of spinal manipulation. Edzard Ernst stated "This detail was not the subject of my review. I do, however, refer to such evaluations and should add that a report recently commissioned by the General Chiropractic Council did not support many of the outlandish claims made by many chiropractors across the world."

A 2009 review evaluating maintenance chiropractic care found that spinal manipulation is routinely associated with considerable harm and no compelling evidence exists to indicate that it adequately prevents symptoms or diseases, thus the risk-benefit is not evidently favorable.

Cost-effectiveness

A 2012 systematic review suggested that the use of spine manipulation in clinical practice is a cost-effective treatment when used alone or in combination with other treatment approaches. A 2011 systematic review found evidence supporting the cost-effectiveness of using spinal manipulation for the treatment of sub-acute or chronic low back pain; the results for acute low back pain were insufficient.

A 2006 systematic cost-effectiveness review found that the reported cost-effectiveness of spinal manipulation in the United Kingdom compared favorably with other treatments for back pain, but that reports were based on data from clinical trials without sham controls and that the specific cost-effectiveness of the treatment (as opposed to non-specific effects) remains uncertain. A 2005 American systematic review of economic evaluations of conservative treatments for low back pain found that significant quality problems in available studies meant that definite conclusions could not be drawn about the most cost-effective intervention. The cost-effectiveness of maintenance chiropractic care is unknown.

Analysis of a clinical and cost utilization data from the years 2003 to 2005 by an integrative medicine independent physician association (IPA) which looked the chiropractic services utilization found that the clinical and cost utilization of chiropractic services based on 70,274 member-months over a 7-year period decreased patient costs associate with the following use of services by 60.2% for in-hospital admissions, 59.0% for hospital days, 62.0% for outpatient surgeries and procedures, and 85% for pharmaceutical costs when compared with conventional medicine (visit to a medical doctor primary care provider) IPA performance for the same health maintenance organization product in the same geography and time frame.

Education, Licensing, and Regulation

Requirements vary between countries. In the U.S. chiropractors obtain a first professional degree in the field of chiropractic. Chiropractic education in the U.S. have been criticized for failing to meet generally accepted standards of evidence-based medicine. The curriculum content of North American chiropractic and medical colleges with regard to basic and clinical sciences has been more similar than not, both in the kinds of subjects offered and in the time assigned to each subject. Accredited chiropractic programs in the U.S. require that applicants have 90 semester hours of undergraduate education with a grade point average of at least 3.0 on a 4.0 scale. Many programs require at least three years of undergraduate education, and more are requiring a bachelor's degree. Canada requires a minimum three years of undergraduate education for applicants, and at least 4200 instructional hours (or the equivalent) of full□time chiropractic education for matriculation through an accredited chiropractic program. Graduates of the Canadian Memorial Chiropractic College (CMCC) are formally recognized to have at least 7–8 years of university level education. The World Health Organization (WHO) guidelines suggest three major full-time educational paths culminating in either a DC, DCM, BSc, or MSc degree. Besides the full-time paths, they also suggest a conversion program for people with other health care education and limited training programs for regions where no legislation governs chiropractic.

Upon graduation, there may be a requirement to pass national, state, or provincial board examinations before being licensed to practice in a particular jurisdiction. Depending on the location, continuing education may be required to renew these licenses. Specialty training is available through part-time postgraduate education programs such as chiropractic orthopedics and sports chiropractic, and through full-time residency programs such as radiology or orthopedics.

In the U.S., chiropractic schools are accredited through the Council on Chiropractic Education (CCE) while the General Chiropractic Council (GCC) is the statutory governmental body responsible for the regulation of chiropractic in the UK. The U.S. CCE requires a mixing curriculum, which means a straight-educated chiropractor may not be eligible for licensing in states requiring CCE accreditation. CCEs in the U.S., Canada, Australia and Europe have joined to form CCE-International (CCE-I) as a model of accreditation standards with the goal of having credentials portable internationally. Today, there are 18 accredited Doctor of Chiropractic programs in the U.S., 2 in Canada, 6 in Australasia, and 5 in Europe. All but one of the chiropractic colleges in the U.S. are privately funded, but in several other countries they are in government-sponsored universities and colleges. Of the two chiropractic colleges in Canada, one is publicly funded (UQTR) and one is privately funded (CMCC). In 2005, CMCC was granted the privilege of offering a professional health care degree under the Post-secondary Education Choice and Excellence Act, which sets the program within the hierarchy of education in Canada as comparable to that of other primary contact health care professions such as medicine, dentistry and optometry.

Regulatory colleges and chiropractic boards in the U.S., Canada, Mexico, and Australia are responsible for protecting the public, standards of practice, disciplinary issues, quality assurance and maintenance of competency. There are an estimated 49,000 chiropractors in the U.S. (2008), 6,500 in Canada (2010), 2,500 in Australia (2000), and 1,500 in the UK (2000).

Chiropractors often argue that this education is as good as or better than medical physicians', but most chiropractic training is confined to classrooms with much time spent learning theory, adjustment, and marketing. The fourth year of chiropractic education persistently showed the highest stress levels. Every student, irrespective of year, experienced different ranges of stress when studying. The chiropractic leaders and colleges have had internal struggles. Rather than cooperation, there has been infighting between different factions. A number of actions were posturing due to the confidential nature of the chiropractic colleges in an attempt to enroll students.

Ethics

The chiropractic oath is a modern variation of the classical Hippocratic Oath historically taken by physicians and other healthcare professionals swearing to practice their professions ethically. The American Chiropractic Association (ACA) has an ethical code "based upon the acknowledgement that the social contract dictates the profession's responsibilities to the patient, the public, and the profession; and upholds the fundamental principle that the paramount purpose of the chiropractic doctor's professional services shall be to benefit the patient." The International Chiropractor's Association (ICA) also has a set of professional canons.

A 2008 commentary proposed that the chiropractic profession actively regulate itself to combat abuse, fraud, and quackery, which are more prevalent in chiropractic than in other health care professions, violating the social contract between patients and physicians. According to a 2015 Gallup poll of U.S. adults, the perception of chiropractors is generally favourable; two-thirds of American adults agree that chiropractors have their patient's best interest in mind and more than half also agree that most chiropractors are trustworthy. Less than 10% of US adults disagreed with the statement that chiropractors were trustworthy.

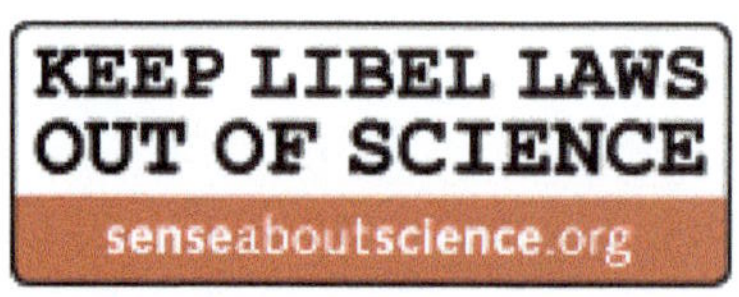

The charity Sense About Science launched a campaign to draw attention to this particular legal case against science writer Simon Singh. In 2009, a number of organizations and public figures signed a statement entitled "The law has no place in scientific disputes".

Chiropractors, especially in America, have a reputation for unnecessarily treating patients. In many circumstances the focus seems to be put on economics instead of health care. Sustained chiropractic care is promoted as a preventative tool, but unnecessary manipulation could possibly present a risk to patients. Some chiropractors are concerned by the routine unjustified claims chiropractors have made. A 2010 analysis of chiropractic websites found the majority of chiropractors and their associations made claims of effectiveness not supported by scientific evidence, while 28% of chiropractor websites advocate lower back pain care, which has some sound evidence.

In 2009, a backlash to the libel suit filed by the British Chiropractic Association (BCA) against Simon Singh, has inspired the filing of formal complaints of false advertising against more than 500 individual chiropractors within one 24-hour period, prompting the McTimoney Chiropractic Association to write to its members advising them to remove leaflets that make claims about whiplash and colic from their practice, to be wary of new patients and telephone inquiries, and telling their members: "If you have a website, take it down NOW." and "Finally, we strongly suggest you do NOT discuss this with others, especially patients." An editorial in *Nature* has suggested that the BCA may be trying to suppress debate and that this use of British libel law is a burden on the right to freedom of expression, which is protected by the European Convention on Human Rights. The libel case ended with the BCA withdrawing its suit in 2010.

Reception

Chiropractic is established in the US, Canada, and Australia, and is present to a lesser extent in many other countries. It is viewed as a marginal complementary and alternative medicine health care profession.

Australia

In Australia, most private health insurance funds cover chiropractic care, and the federal government funds chiropractic care when the patient is referred by a medical practitioner.

United Kingdom

In the United Kingdom chiropractic is available on the National Health Service in some areas, such as Cornwall where the treatment is only available for neck or back pain.

A 2010 study by questionnaire presented to UK chiropractors indicated only 45% of chiropractors disclosed with patients the serious risk associated with manipulation of the cervical spine and that 46% believed there was possibility of patient would refuse treatment if risk correctly explained. However 80% acknowledged the ethical/moral responsibility to disclose risk to patient.

United States and Canada

The percentage of the population that utilizes chiropractic care at any given time generally falls into a range from 6% to 12% in the U.S. and Canada, with a global high of 20% in Alberta in 2006. In 2008, chiropractors were reported to be the most common CAM providers for children and adolescents, consuming up to 14% of all visits to chiropractors. In 2002–03, the majority of those who sought chiropractic did so for relief from back and neck pain and other neuromusculoskeletal complaints; most do so specifically for low back pain. The majority of U.S. chiropractors participate in some form of managed care. Although the majority of U.S. chiropractors view themselves as specialists in neuroleptic malignant syndrome conditions, many also consider chiropractic as a type of primary care. In the majority of cases, the care that chiropractors and physicians provide divides the market, however for some, their care is complementary.

In the U.S., chiropractors perform over 90% of all manipulative treatments. Satisfaction rates are typically higher for chiropractic care compared to medical care, with a 1998 U.S. survey reporting

83% of respondents satisfied or very satisfied with their care; quality of communication seems to be a consistent predictor of patient satisfaction with chiropractors.

Utilization of chiropractic care is sensitive to the costs incurred by the co-payment by the patient. The use of chiropractic declined from 9.9% of U.S. adults in 1997 to 7.4% in 2002; this was the largest relative decrease among CAM professions, which overall had a stable use rate. As of 2007 7% of the U.S. population is being reached by chiropractic. Employment of U.S. chiropractors is expected to increase 14% between 2006 and 2016, faster than the average for all occupations.

In the U.S., most states require insurers to cover chiropractic care, and most HMOs cover these services.

History

Early chiropractors believed that all disease was caused by interruptions in the flow of innate intelligence, a vitalistic nervous energy or life force that represented God's presence in man; chiropractic leaders often invoked religious imagery and moral traditions. D.D. and B.J. both seriously considered declaring chiropractic a religion, which might have provided legal protection under the U.S. constitution, but decided against it partly to avoid confusion with Christian Science. Early chiropractors also tapped into the Populist movement, emphasizing craft, hard work, competition, and advertisement, aligning themselves with the common man against intellectuals and trusts, among which they included the American Medical Association (AMA).

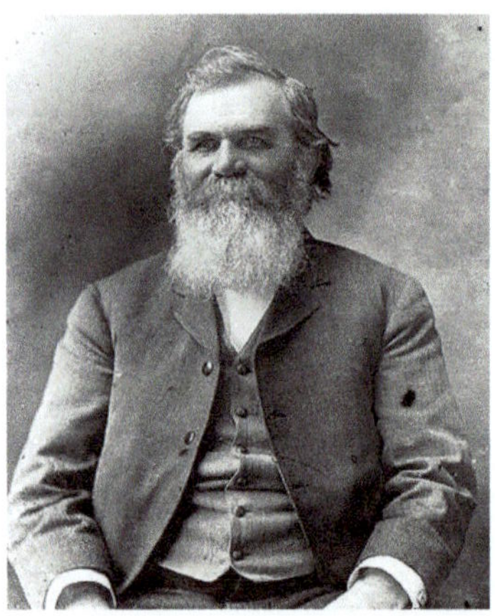

D.D. Palmer, founder of chiropractic

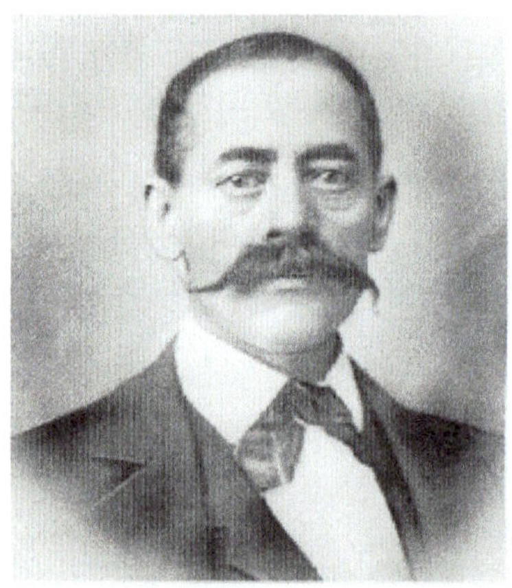

Harvey Lillard, first chiropractic patient

Chiropractic has seen considerable controversy and criticism. Although D.D. and B.J. were "straight" and disdained the use of instruments, some early chiropractors, whom B.J. scornfully called "mixers", advocated the use of instruments. In 1910 B.J. changed course and endorsed X-rays as necessary for diagnosis; this resulted in a significant exodus from the Palmer School of the more conservative faculty and students. The mixer camp grew until by 1924 B.J. estimated that only 3,000 of the U.S.'s 25,000 chiropractors remained straight. That year, B.J.'s invention and promotion of the neurocalometer, a temperature-sensing device, was highly controversial among B.J.'s fellow straights. By the 1930s chiropractic was the largest alternative healing profession in the U.S.

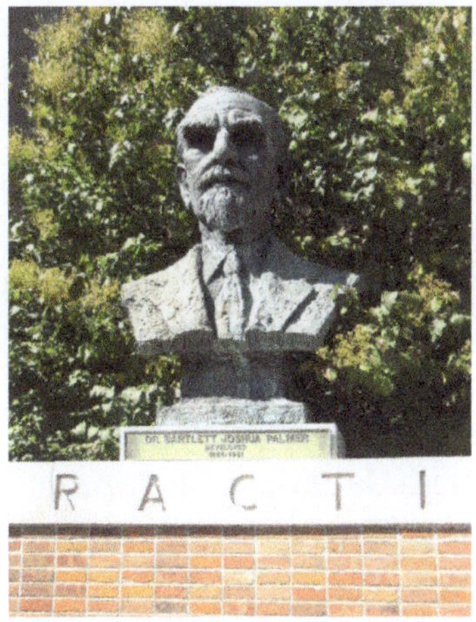

B. J. Palmer, early developer of chiropractic

Chiropractors faced heavy opposition from organized medicine. Thousands of chiropractors were prosecuted for practicing medicine without a license, and D.D. and many other chiropractors were jailed. To defend against medical statutes B.J. argued that chiropractic was separate and distinct from medicine, asserting that chiropractors "analyzed" rather than "diagnosed", and "adjusted" subluxations rather than "treated" disease. B.J. cofounded the Universal Chiropractors' Association (UCA) to provide legal services to arrested chiropractors. Although the UCA won their first test case in Wisconsin in 1907, prosecutions instigated by state medical boards became increasingly common and in many cases were successful. In response, chiropractors conducted political campaigns to secure separate licensing statutes, eventually succeeding in all fifty states, from Kansas in 1913 through Louisiana in 1974. The longstanding feud between chiropractors and medical doctors continued for decades. The AMA labeled chiropractic an "unscientific cult" in 1966, and until 1980 advised its members that it was unethical for medical doctors to associate with "unscientific practitioners". This culminated in a landmark 1987 decision, *Wilk v. AMA*, in which the court found that the AMA had engaged in unreasonable restraint of trade and conspiracy, and which ended the AMA's de facto boycott of chiropractic.

Serious research to test chiropractic theories did not begin until the 1970s, and is continuing to be hampered by antiscientific and pseudoscientific ideas that sustained the profession in its long battle with organized medicine. By the mid 1990s there was a growing scholarly interest in chiropractic, which helped efforts to improve service quality and establish clinical guidelines that recommended manual therapies for acute low back pain. In recent decades chiropractic gained legitimacy and greater acceptance by medical physicians and health plans, and enjoyed a strong political base and sustained demand for services. However, its future seemed uncertain: as the number of practitioners grew, evidence-based medicine insisted on treatments with demonstrated value, managed care restricted payment, and competition grew from massage therapists and other health professions. The profession responded by marketing natural products and devices more aggressively, and by reaching deeper into alternative medicine and primary care.

Public Health

Some chiropractors oppose vaccination and water fluoridation, which are common public health practices. Within the chiropractic community there are significant disagreements about vaccination, one of the most cost-effective public health interventions available. Most chiropractic writings on vaccination focus on its negative aspects, claiming that it is hazardous, ineffective, and unnecessary. Some chiropractors have embraced vaccination, but a significant portion of the profession rejects it, as original chiropractic philosophy traces diseases to causes in the spine and states that vaccines interfere with healing. The extent to which anti-vaccination views perpetuate the current chiropractic profession is uncertain. The American Chiropractic Association and the International Chiropractors Association support individual exemptions to compulsory vaccination laws, and a 1995 survey of U.S. chiropractors found that about a third believed there was no scientific proof that immunization prevents disease. The Canadian Chiropractic Association supports vaccination; a survey in Alberta in 2002 found that 25% of chiropractors advised patients for, and 27% against, vaccinating themselves or their children.

Early opposition to water fluoridation included chiropractors, some of whom continue to oppose it as being incompatible with chiropractic philosophy and an infringement of personal freedom. Other chiropractors have actively promoted fluoridation, and several chiropractic organizations have endorsed scientific principles of public health. In addition to traditional chiropractic opposition to water fluoridation and vaccination, chiropractors' attempts to establish a positive reputation for their public health role are also compromised by their reputation for recommending repetitive lifelong chiropractic treatment.

Controversy

Throughout its history chiropractic has been the subject of internal and external controversy and criticism. According to Daniel D. Palmer, the founder of chiropractic, subluxation is the sole cause of disease and manipulation is the cure for all diseases of the human race. A 2003 profession-wide survey found "most chiropractors (whether "straights" or "mixers") still hold views of Innate Intelligence and of the cause and cure of disease (not just back pain) consistent with those of the Palmers." A critical evaluation stated "Chiropractic is rooted in mystical concepts. This led to an internal conflict within the chiropractic profession, which continues today." Chiropractors, including D.D. Palmer, were jailed for practicing medicine without a license. For most of its existence, chiropractic has battled with mainstream medicine, sustained by antiscientific and pseudoscientific ideas such as subluxation. Collectively, systematic reviews have not demonstrated that spinal manipulation, the main treatment method employed by chiropractors, is effective for any medical condition, with the possible exception of treatment for back pain. Chiropractic remains controversial, though to a lesser extent than in past years.

Chiropractic Treatment Techniques

Chiropractors primarily use manipulation ("adjustment") of the spine as a treatment. Such treatments trace back to ancient China, Greece and Egypt. It gained popularity in the late 19th century, with the development of osteopathic and chiropractic medicine in North America.

Spinal manipulation (*SMT*) became more popular in the 1980s. It includes manipulation and massage to "adjust" the spine and related tissues, and is a primary basis of chiropractic. Systematic reviews have not found evidence that chiropractic manipulation is effective for any medical condition, with the possible exception of treatment for lower back pain. The safety of manipulation, particularly on the cervical spine has been debated. Adverse results, including death, are rare. Chiropractors may use exercise and other treatments and advice.

Interventions

Skilled, specific hands-on techniques, including manipulation and mobilization, are used to diagnose and treat soft tissues and joint structures, to reduce pain and to increase range of motion and general health.

The approach is generally conservative, and treatment may include:

- manual procedures, including spinal or joint manipulation or mobilization, soft-tissue and reflex techniques;
- exercise, and other active care;
- psychosocial aspects of patient management;
- patient education on spinal health, posture, nutrition and lifestyle modifications;
- emergency treatment and acute pain management;
- other supportive measures, including the use of back supports and orthotics;
- recognition of the limitations of chiropractic care, and of the need for referral to other health professionals.

Chiropractors may also use exercise and other conservative treatments and advice.

Manual and Manipulative Therapy

The Chinese used such techniques more than 3000 years ago. Hippocrates also used such techniques as did the ancient Egyptians and other cultures.

In the late 19th century in North America, therapies including osteopathy and chiropractic became popular. Spinal manipulation gained mainstream recognition during the 1980s.

In this system, hands are used to manipulate, massage or otherwise influence the spine and related tissues. It is the most common and primary intervention used in chiropractic care.

Effectiveness

Neuromusculoskeletal Disorders

Treatment is usually for neck or low back pain and related disorders.

For acute low back pain, low quality evidence has suggested no difference between real and sham spine manipulation, and moderate quality evidence has suggested no difference between spine manipulation and other commonly used treatments, such as medication and physical therapy.

National guidelines vary; some recommend the therapy for those who do not improve with other treatment. It may be effective for lumbar disc herniation with radiculopathy, as effective as mobilization for neck pain, some forms of headache, and some extremity joint conditions. A 2011 Cochrane review found strong evidence that suggests there is no clinically meaningful difference between spinal manipulation therapy and other treatments for reducing pain and improving function for chronic low back pain. A 2008 review found that with the possible exception of back pain, chiropractic manipulation has not been shown to be effective for any medical condition.

Non-musculoskeletal Disorders

The use of spinal manipulation for non-musculoskeletal is controversial. It has not been shown to be effective for asthma, headache, hypertension, or dysmenorrhea. There is no scientific data that supports the use of SMT for idiopathic adolescent scoliosis.

Cost-effectiveness

Spinal manipulation is generally regarded as cost-effective treatment of musculoskeletal conditions when used alone or in combination with other treatment approaches. Evidence supports the cost-effectiveness of using spinal manipulation for the treatment of sub-acute or chronic low back pain whereas the results for acute low back pain were inconsistent.

Safety

All treatments need a thorough medical history, diagnosis and plan of management. Chiropractors, must rule out contraindications to any treatments, including adverse events.

Relative contraindications, such as osteoporosis are conditions where increased risk is acceptable in some situations and where mobilization and soft-tissue techniques may be treatments of choice. Most contraindications apply to the manipulation of the affected region.

While safety has been debated, and serious injuries and deaths can occur and may be under-reported, these are generally rare and spinal manipulation is relatively safe when employed skillfully and appropriately.

Adverse events are believed to be under-reported and appear to be more common following high velocity/ low amplitude manipulation than mobilization. Mild, frequent and temporary adverse events occur in SMT which include temporary increase in pain, tenderness and stiffness. These effects generally are reduced within 24–48 hours Serious injuries and fatal consequences, especially to SM in the upper cervical region, can occur. but are regarded as rare when spinal manipulation is employed skillfully and appropriately.

The relationship to stroke has been debated. Stroke is statistically associated with both general practitioner and chiropractic services in persons under 45 years of age, and these associations may be related to preexisting conditions. Weak to moderately strong evidence supports causation (as opposed to statistical association) between cervical manipulative therapy and vertebrobasilar artery stroke. A 2012 review found that there is not enough evidence to support a strong association or no association between cervical manipulation and stroke. A 2008 review found chiropractic are more commonly associated with serious related adverse effects than other professionals following manipulation and concluded that the risk of death from manipulations to the neck outweighs the benefits.

Techniques

According to the American Chiropractic Association the most frequently used techniques by chiropractors are Diversified technique 95.9%, Extremity manipulating/adjusting 95.5%, Activator Methods 62.8%, Gonstead technique 58.5%, Cox Flexion/Distraction 58.0%, Thompson 55.9%, Sacro Occipital Technique [SOT] 41.3%, Applied Kinesiology 43.2%, NIMMO/Receptor Tonus 40.0%, Cranial 37.3%, Manipulative/Adjustive Instruments 34.5%, Palmer upper cervical [HIO] 28.8%, Logan Basic 28.7%, Meric 19.9%, and Pierce-Stillwagon 17.1%. Koren Specific Technique (KST) is a chiropractic technique was created around 2004. There are about 200 chiropractic technique, but there is a mostly overlap between them, and many techniques involve slight changes of other techniques.

Diversified Technique

Diversified technique is a non-proprietary and eclectic approach to spinal manipulation that is commonly used by chiropractors. The technique, as it is applied today, is largely attributed to the work of Joe Janse, D.C. Diversified is the most common spine manipulation technique used by chiropractors, with approximately 96% of chiropractors using it for approximately 70% of their patients. Diversified is also the technique most preferred for use during future practice by chiropractic students. Diversified is the only spine manipulation technique taught in Canadian chiropractic programs. Like many chiropractic and osteopathic manipulative techniques, Diversified is characterized by a high-velocity, low-amplitude thrust. is considered the most generic chiropractic manipulative technique and is differentiated from other techniques in that its objective is to restore proper movement and alignment of spine and joint dysfunction.

Atlas Orthogonal Technique

Atlas Orthogonal Technique is an upper cervical chiropractic treatment technique created by Roy Sweat, DC. It is a technique which uses a percussion instrument in attempts to adjust what is perceived to be a subluxation of the atlas vertebra, the top vertebra in the cervical spine. It is based on the teachings of B. J. Palmer, who advocated the Hole-In-One version of spinal adjustment. It is primarily used by straight chiropractors. Referring to the origins of upper cervical techniques, Dan Murphy, DC, DABCO, wrote: "Over the past 100 years, the practice of chiropractic has branched into dozens of specialty techniques. However, historically, for a third of this time, from the 1930s into the 1960s, the predominant practice of chiropractic involved primarily the upper cervical spine."

Extremity Manipulating/Adjusting

Activator Methods

The Activator Method Chiropractic Technique (AMCT) is a chiropractic treatment method and device created by Arlan Fuhr as an alternative to manual manipulation of the spine or extremity joints. The device is categorized as a mechanical force manual assisted (MFMA) instrument which is generally regarded as a softer chiropractic treatment technique.

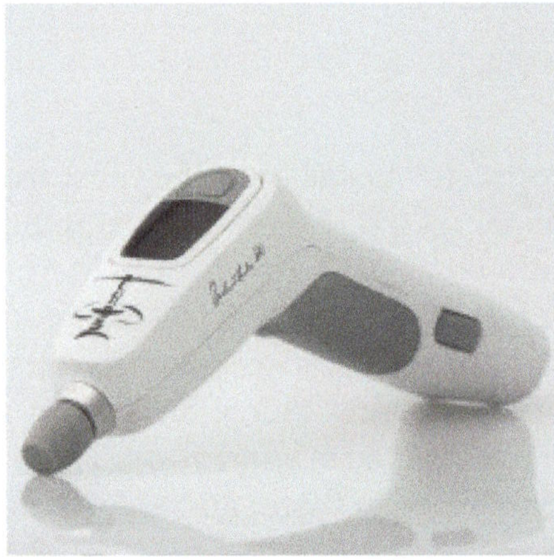

Activator V Chiropractic Adjusting Instrument

The activator is a small handheld spring-loaded instrument which delivers a small impulse to the spine. It was found to give off no more than 0.3 J of kinetic energy in a 3-millisecond pulse. The aim is to produce enough force to move the vertebrae but not enough to cause injury.

The AMCT involves having the patient lie in a prone position and comparing the functional leg lengths. Often one leg will seem to be shorter than the other. The chiropractor then carries out a series of muscle tests such as having the patient move their arms in a certain position in order to activate the muscles attached to specific vertebrae. If the leg lengths are not the same, that is taken as a sign that the problem is located at that vertebra. The chiropractor treats problems found in this way moving progressively along the spine in the direction from the feet towards the head.

Although prone "functional leg length" is a widely used chiropractic tool, it is not a recognized anthropometric technique, since legs are often of unequal length, and measurements in the prone position are not entirely valid estimates of standing X-ray differences. Measurements in the standing position are far more reliable. Another confounding factor is that simply moving the two legs held together and leaning them imperceptibly to one side or the other produces different results. Fuhr claims that properly trained doctors show good interexaminer reliability.

In 2003, the National Board of Chiropractic Examiners found that 69.9% of chiropractors used the technique, and 23.9% of patients received it. The majority of U.S. chiropractic schools and some schools in other countries teach the AMCT method, and an estimated 45,000 chiropractors worldwide use AMCT or some part of the technique.

There have been a number of studies of AMCT, including case reports, clinical studies and randomized controlled trials, but there are still unanswered questions. A few studies suggest that the activator may be as effective as manual adjustment in treatment of back pain.

Graston Technique

Graston Technique (GT) is a trademarked therapeutic method for diagnosing and treating disorders of the skeletal muscles and related connective tissue. The method employs a collection of six stainless steel instruments of particular shape and size, which are used by practitioners to rub patients' muscles in order to detect and resolve adhesions in the muscles and tendons. Practitioners must be licensed by the parent corporation (Graston Technique, LLC.) in order to use the Graston Technique trademark or the patented instruments.

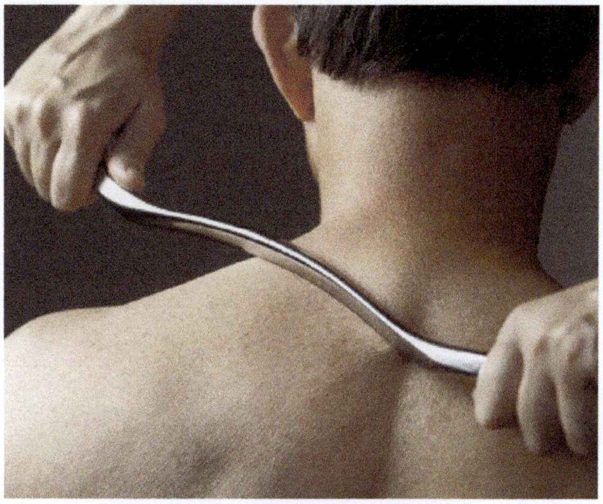

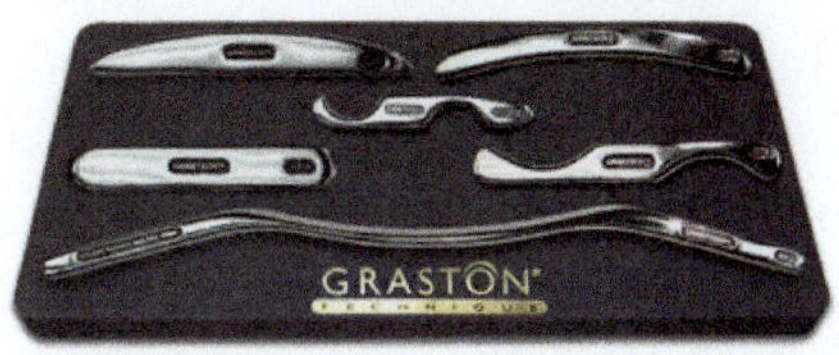

Several examples of Graston treatment have been used in contact sports where scars and contusions are common. However, the Graston Technique has not been rigorously scientifically tested and its evidence basis and assumptions are considered questionable at best. There are no high quality clinical trials that validate the efficacy of the Graston Techniques.

Koren Specific Technique

Koren specific technique (KST) is a technique developed by Tedd Koren. While the technique is associated with chiropractic techniques, Koren has variously described it as an "analysis protocol" or "healthcare protocol". KST may use their hands, or they may use an electric device known as an "ArthroStim" for assessment and adjustments. KST can use different postures. The insurers Aetna, NHS Leeds West CCG, North Dakota Department of Human Services, and The Ohio State University cover other chiropractic techniques but exclude KST from coverage because they consider it to be "experimental and investigational." Aetna's policy states there is a lack of efficacy regarding this method.

Cox Flexion/Distraction

Gonstead Technique

The Gonstead technique is chiropractic method that had been developed by Clarence Gonstead since 1923. The technique focuses on hands-on adjustment and is claimed to expand "*standard diversified technique*" by implementing additional instrumentation including X-rays, Gonstead

Radiographic Parallel, a measuring device, and the development of Nervo-Scope, a device said to detect the level of neurophysiologic activity due to the existence of vertebral subluxation based on changes in skin temperature. Heat detector devices are unreliable and lack scientific evidence. The technique gained popularity in the 1960s. About 28.9% of patients have been treated with the Gonstead technique.

Trigenics Technique

Trigenics is a neurological-based manual or instrument-assisted assessment and treatment system developed and patented by Allan Oolo Austin, DC, DO, CCSP, CCRD. The technique originally began as a chiropractic technique, but is now practiced by osteopaths, physiotherapists and massage therapists. The technique is relatively infrequently used by chiropractors compared to other chiropractic techniques such as Diversified, Trigger point therapy and Activator.

Chiropractic Controversy and Criticism

Throughout its history chiropractic has been the subject of internal and external controversy and criticism. According to magnetic healer Daniel D. Palmer, the founder of chiropractic, "vertebral subluxation" was the sole cause of all diseases and manipulation was the cure for all diseases of the human race. A 2003 profession-wide survey found "most chiropractors (whether 'straights' or 'mixers') still hold views of Innate Intelligence and of the cause and cure of disease (not just back pain) consistent with those of the Palmers." A critical evaluation stated "Chiropractic is rooted in mystical concepts. This led to an internal conflict within the chiropractic profession, which continues today." Chiropractors, including D.D. Palmer, were jailed for practicing medicine without a license. D.D. Palmer considered establishing chiropractic as a religion to resolve this problem. For most of its existence, chiropractic has battled with mainstream medicine, sustained by antiscientific and pseudoscientific ideas such as subluxation.

Chiropractic researchers have documented that fraud, abuse and quackery are more prevalent in chiropractic than in other health care professions. Unsubstantiated claims about the efficacy of chiropractic have continued to be made by individual chiropractors and chiropractic associations. The core concept of traditional chiropractic, vertebral subluxation, is not based on sound science. Collectively, systematic reviews have not demonstrated that spinal manipulation, the main treatment method employed by chiropractors, was effective for any medical condition, with the possible exception of treatment for back pain. Although rare, spinal manipulation, particularly of the upper spine, can also result in complications that can lead to permanent disability or death; these can occur in adults and children.

In 2008, Simon Singh was sued for libel by the British Chiropractic Association (BCA) for criticizing their activities in a column in *The Guardian*. A preliminary hearing took place at the Royal Courts of Justice in front of judge David Eady. The judge held that merely using the phrase "happily promotes bogus treatments" meant that he was stating, as a matter of fact, that the British Chiropractic Association was being consciously dishonest in promoting chiropractic for treating the children's ailments in question. An editorial in *Nature* has suggested that the BCA may be trying to suppress debate and that this use of British libel law is a burden on the right to freedom of expression, which is protected by the European Convention on Human Rights. The libel case ended with the BCA withdrawing its suit in 2010.

Chiropractors historically were strongly opposed to vaccination based on their belief that all diseases were traceable to causes in the spine, and therefore could not be affected by vaccines. Some chiropractors continue to be opposed to vaccination. Early opposition to water fluoridation included chiropractors in the U.S. Some chiropractors opposed water fluoridation as being incompatible with chiropractic philosophy and an infringement of personal freedom. Recently, other chiropractors have actively promoted fluoridation, and several chiropractic organizations have endorsed scientific principles of public health.

Historical Controversy and Critical Elements

The birth of chiropractic was on September 18, 1895. There is controversy over what happened with several different accounts. Daniel D. Palmer later claimed that on that day he manipulated the spine of Harvey Lillard, a man who was nearly deaf, allegedly curing him of deafness. Palmer said *"there was nothing accidental about this, as it was accomplished with an object in view, and the expected result was obtained. There was nothing 'crude' about this adjustment; it was specific so much so that no chiropractor has equaled it."*

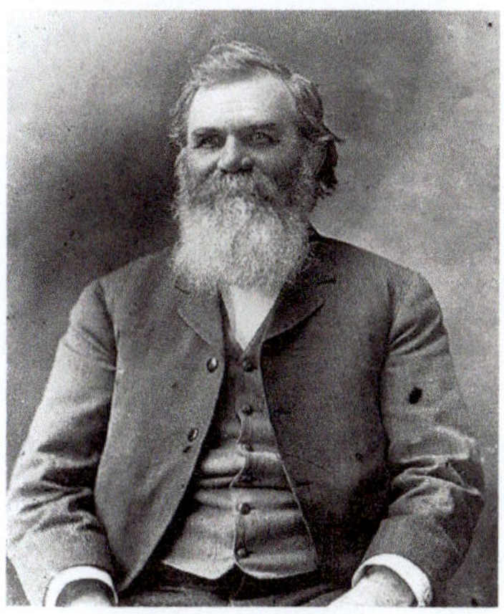

D.D. Palmer

However, this version was disputed by Lillard's daughter, Valdeenia Lillard Simons. She said that her father told her that he was telling jokes to a friend in the hall outside Palmer's office and Palmer, who had been reading, joined them. When Lillard reached the punch line, Palmer, laughing heartily, slapped Lillard on the back with the hand holding the heavy book he had been reading. A few days later, Lillard told Palmer that his hearing seemed better. Palmer then decided to explore manipulation as an expansion of his magnetic healing practice. Simons said "the compact was that if they can make [something of] it, then they both would share. But, it didn't happen."

In spite of the fact that Lillard could hear well enough to tell jokes, B.J. Palmer claimed under sworn testimony that Lillard had been "thoroughly deaf". Since 1895, the story of Palmer's curing a man of deafness has been a part of chiropractic tradition. Palmer's account differs significantly from what actually happened, in that, according to Lillard's daughter, his improved hearing was likely caused by an accidentally fortuitous jarring of Lillard's body and not, as claimed by D.D. Palmer, caused by a "specific" adjustment. It was after this event that Palmer began to experiment with manipulation. He also claimed that his second patient, a man with heart disease, was also cured by spinal manipulation.

Chiropractic included vitalistic ideas of Innate Intelligence with religious attributes of Universal Intelligence as substitutes for science. Evidence suggests that D.D. Palmer had acquired knowledge of manipulative techniques from Andrew Taylor Still, the founder of osteopathy. Although D.D. Palmer combined bonesetting to give chiropractic its method, and "magnetic healing" for the theory, he acknowledged a special relation to magnetic healing when he wrote, "chiropractic was not evolved from medicine or any other method, except that of magnetic." He also "claimed that his profession had nothing to do with medicine, that he healed by the laying on of hands;... He also said that he had a diploma from no earthly school but from High Heaven."

According to D.D. Palmer, subluxation was the sole cause of all diseases and manipulation was the cure for all diseases of the human race. A 2003 profession-wide survey found "most chiropractors (whether "straights" or "mixers") still hold views of Innate and of the cause and cure of disease (not just back pain) consistent with those of the Palmers. On the one hand, modern promotional brochures make a bid for medical legitimacy by describing Innate and adjustments using more scientific-sounding terms such as "inherent" and "nerve force.""

Chiropractic has had a strong salesmanship element since it was started by D.D. Palmer. His son, B.J. Palmer, asserted that their chiropractic school was founded on "...a business, not a professional basis. We manufacture chiropractors. We teach them the idea and then we show them how to sell it". D.D. Palmer established a magnetic healing facility in Davenport, Iowa, styling himself 'doctor'. Not everyone was convinced, as a local paper in 1894 wrote about him:

> "A crank on magnetism has a crazy notion that he can cure the sick and crippled with his magnetic hands. His victims are the weak-minded, ignorant and superstitious, those foolish people who have been sick for years and have become tired of the regular physician and want health by the short-cut method...he has certainly profited by the ignorance of his victims...His increase in business shows what can be done in Davenport, even by a quack."

Before adopting the term "chiropractic" in about 1896, his advertising used the term "magnetic". In 1891-92, a city business directory stated: "Dr. Palmer can cure with his Magnetic Hands Diseases of the Head, Throat, Heart, Lungs, Stomach, Liver, Spleen, Kidneys, Nerves, and Muscles, ten times quicker than any one can with medicines."

The following remark by D.D. Palmer implied that naivety is required to accept the implausibility of the chiropractic concepts.:

> "Give me a simple mind that thinks along single tracts, give me 30 days to instruct him, and that individual can go forth on the highways and byways and get more sick people well than the best, most complete, all around, unlimited medical education of any medical man who ever lived."

Chiropractic was rooted in mystical concepts, leading to internal conflicts between straights and mixers which continue to this day. It has two main groups: "straights", now the minority, emphasize vitalism, innate intelligence and spinal adjustments, and consider subluxations to be the leading cause of all disease; "mixers" are more open to mainstream and alternative medical techniques such as exercise, massage, nutritional supplements, and acupuncture. The straights adhere religiously to the gospel of its founders while mixers are more open. There is a lack of uniformity and consensus among chiropractors in regard to their role. Depending upon whose point of view, chiropractors are, for example, subluxation-correctors, primary care physicians, neuromusculoskeletal specialists, or holistic health specialists. Straights have claimed mixers are not real chiropractors because they do not acknowledge Palmer's foundation of chiropractic therapy.

In 1906, D.D. Palmer was the first of hundreds of chiropractors who went to jail. Chiropractors were jailed for practicing medicine without a license. In the 1920s hundreds of unlicensed chiropractors chose jail rather than fines. Herbert Reaver was the most jailed chiropractor in the U.S. Chiropractors were charged with not complying with the medical practice act. California chiropractors adopted the motto, "Go to jail for chiropractic." 450 chiropractors were jailed in a single year at the peak of the controversy. Many chiropractors treated fellow prisoners and visiting patients while in jail.

D.D. Palmer defined chiropractic as "a science of healing without drugs" and considered establishing chiropractic as a religion as a means to use religious "exemption clauses" to resolve legal difficulties presented by restrictive "chiro laws". In 1911, he stated:

> "You ask, what I think will be the final outcome of our law getting. It will be that we will have to build a boat similar to Christian Science and hoist a religious flag. I have received chiropractic from the other world, similar as did Mrs. Eddy. No other one has lad claim to that, NOT EVEN B.J.
>
> "Exemption clauses instead of chiro laws by all means, and LET THAT EXEMPTION BE THE RIGHT TO PRACTICE OUR RELIGION. But we must have a religious head, one who is the founder, as did Christ, Mohamed, Jo. Smith, Mrs. Eddy, Martin Luther and other who have founded religions. I am the fountain head. I am the founder of chiropractic in its science, in its art, in its philosophy and in its religious phase. Now, if chiorpractors desire to claim me as their head, their leader, the way is clear. My writings have been gradually steering in that direction until now it is time to assume that we have the same right to as has Christian Scientists."

Chiropractors have struggled with survival and identity during its formative years, including internal struggles between its leaders and colleges. For much of the history of the chiropractic profession chiropractors showed little interest in scientific research and regarded their principles and practices as valid. Despite heavy opposition by mainstream medicine, by the 1930s chiropractic was the largest alternative healing profession in the U.S. Long-standing American Medical Association (AMA) policies against chiropractic contributed to a lack of acceptance within mainstream public health. The AMA created the Committee on Quackery "to contain and eliminate chiropractic." Using the Committee on Quackery, efforts were made to prevent the participation of chiropractic in organized health care. In 1966 a policy passed by the AMA House of Delegates stating: "It is the position of the medical profession that chiropractic is an unscientific cult whose practitioners lack the necessary training and background to diagnose and treat human disease. Chiropractic constitutes a hazard to rational health care in the United States because of its substandard and unscientific education of its practitioners and their rigid adherence to an irrational, unscientific approach to disease causation." The longstanding feud between chiropractors and medical doctors continued for decades. The AMA labeled chiropractic an "unscientific cult" in 1966, and until 1980 held that it was unethical for medical doctors to associate with "unscientific practitioners". This culminated in a landmark 1987 decision, *Wilk v. AMA*, in which the court found that the AMA had engaged in unreasonable restraint of trade and conspiracy, and which ended the AMA's de facto boycott of chiropractic. The rivalry was not solely with conventional medicine; many osteopaths proclaimed that chiropractic was a bastardized form of osteopathy.

Serious research to test chiropractic theories did not begin until the 1970s, and is continuing to be hampered by antiscientific and pseudoscientific ideas that sustained the profession in its long battle with organized medicine. By the mid-1990s there was a growing scholarly interest in chiropractic, which helped efforts to improve service quality and establish clinical guidelines that recommended manual therapies for acute low back pain. Some people believe chiropractic has little more than a placebo effect, while some randomized trials of spinal manipulation have verified its effectiveness for the treatment of (specifically) low back pain. There are several barriers between primary care physicians and chiropractors for having positive referral relationships which includes a lack of good communication. The medical establishment has not entirely accepted chiropractic care as mainstream. After 100 years, the chiropractic profession has failed to define a message that is understandable, credible, and scientifically valid. The future of chiropractic is uncertain due to the economic struggles and restrictions of the science and methods in chiropractic.

Chiropractic has seen considerable controversy within the profession over its philosophy. In connection with a controversial and divisive 2015 organizational split in the Australian chiropractic community, an article described the profession's long standing and current problems:

> "The chiropractic profession is notorious for its infighting, with quarrels over the value of vaccination, the evidence or lack thereof to support the theory of subluxation and whether spinal adjustments should be performed on children."

Allegations of Patricide Connected With The Death Of D.D. Palmer

The 2008 book *Trick or Treatment* states that in 1913 B.J. Palmer ran over his father, D.D. Palmer, at a homecoming parade during the Palmer School of Chiropractic. Weeks later D.D. Palmer died. The official cause of death was recorded as typhoid. The book *Trick or Treatment* indicated "it seems more likely that his death was a direct result of injuries caused by his son. Indeed there is speculation that this was not an accident, but rather a case of patricide." A 1999 documentary study suggests D.D. Palmer's widow may have also played a role in the patricide controversy. D.D. Palmer's attending physicians were persuaded to change their opinions about the main cause of death. Chiropractic historian Joseph C. Keating, Jr. has described the attempted patricide of D.D. Palmer as a "myth" and "absurd on its face" and cites an eyewitness who recalled that D.D. was not struck by B.J.'s car, but rather, had stumbled. He also says that "Joy Loban, DC, executor of D.D.'s estate, voluntarily withdrew a civil suit claiming damages against B.J. Palmer, and that several grand juries repeatedly refused to bring criminal charges against the son." A 1969 article stated that in July 1913 at the Palmer School of Chiropractic B.J. Palmer "insisted on leading the alumni procession, but was prohibited from doing so by the marshal of the parade, who was a student at the school. An altercation ensued. B.J. drove up in his automobile. Words passed between father and son. What happened after that depends on whom you believe. Daniel David claimed that B.J. struck him with his automobile, and D.D's friends and allies later produced affidavits of witnesses to prove it. B.J. flatly denied it, and produced many more affidavits to this effect than D.D.'s cohorts were able to muster."

Ethics and Claims

A study of California disciplinary statistics during 1997–2000 reported 4.5 disciplinary actions per 1000 chiropractors per year, compared to 2.27 for medical doctors, and the incident rate for fraud was 9 times greater among chiropractors (1.99 per 1000 chiropractors per year) than among medical doctors (0.20). According to a 2006 Gallup Poll of U.S. adults, when asked how they would "rate the honesty and ethical standards of people in these different fields", chiropractic compared unfavorably with mainstream medicine. When chiropractic was rated, it "rated dead last amongst healthcare professions". While 84% of respondents considered nurses' ethics "very high" or "high," only 36% felt that way about chiropractors. Other healthcare professions ranged from 38% for psychiatrists, to 62% for dentists, 69% for medical doctors, 71% for veterinarians, and 73% for druggists or pharmacists. Similar results were found in the 2003 Gallup Poll. Chiropractic authors have placed these results in perspective in articles, with one writing that "we were the least trusted and least believed health care discipline", and another writing that chiropractors who use unethical marketing methods "poison the well" for others in the profession, and that they "might be responsible for the negative opinion people have about the ethics of the chiropractic profession." Many chiropractors have sought to address their minor status within the U.S. medical community by attending practice-building seminars to assist chiropractors to persuade their patients of the efficacy of their treatments, increase their revenue, and boost their morale as unorthodox medical practitioners.

Historically the profession has often been accused of quackery, with the profession often responding negatively to such accusations. In its early days, the accusation of quackery was voiced in a 1913 editorial in the *Journal of the American Medical Association*:

> "Chiropractic is a freak offshoot from osteopathy. Disease, say the chiropractors, is due to pressure on the spinal nerves; ergo it can be cured by "adjusting" the spinal column. It is the sheerest quackery, and those who profess to teach it make their appeal to the cupidity of the ignorant. Its practice is in no sense a profession but a trade - and a trade that is potent for great harm. It is carried on almost exclusively by those of no education, ignorant of anatomy, ignorant even of the fundamental sciences on which the treatment of disease depends." (p. 29)

The view that chiropractic was a trade, rather than a profession, was stated clearly by B.J. Palmer, who asserted that chiropractic was founded on "...a business, not a professional basis. We manufacture chiropractors. We teach them the idea and then we show them how to sell it".

In more modern times (1991), when the president of the ACA called accusations of quackery a "myth", chiropractic historian, Joseph C. Keating, Jr. responded by calling his comments "absurd" and stated:

> "The so-called 'quackery myth about chiropractic' is no myth.....the kernels of quackery (i.e., unsubstantiated and untested health remedies offered as "proven") are ubiquitous in this profession. I dare say that health misinformation (if not quackery) can be found in

> just about any issue of any chiropractic trade publication and much of the promotional materials chiropractors disseminate to patients. The recent unsubstantiated claims of the ACA are exemplary *[examples provided]*...It escapes me entirely how Dr. Downing, the ACA, MPI, and Dynamic Chiropractic can suggest that there is no quackery in chiropractic. Either these groups and individuals do not read the chiropractic literature or have no crap-detectors. I urge a reconsideration of advertising and promotion policies in chiropractic."

In an article on quackery, W.T. Jarvis has stated that "Non-scientific health care (e.g., acupuncture, ayurvedic medicine, chiropractic, homeopathy, naturopathy) is licensed by individual states. Practitioners use unscientific practices and deception on a public who, lacking complex healthcare knowledge, must rely upon the trustworthiness of providers. Quackery not only harms people, it undermines the scientific enterprise and should be actively opposed by every scientist."

In a 2008 commentary, the chiropractic authors proposed that "the chiropractic profession has an obligation to actively divorce itself from metaphysical explanations of health and disease as well as to actively regulate itself in refusing to tolerate fraud, abuse and quackery, which are more rampant in our profession than in other healthcare professions," a situation which violates the social contract between patients and physicians. Such self-regulation "will dramatically increase the level of trust in and respect for the profession from society at large." Another chiropractic study documented that the largest chiropractic associations in the U.S. and Canada distributed patient brochures which contained unsubstantiated claims. Chiropractors, especially in America, have a reputation for unnecessarily treating patients. Sustained chiropractic care is promoted as a preventative tool but unnecessary manipulation could possibly present a risk to patients. Some chiropractors are concerned by the routine unjustified claims chiropractors have made. In English speaking countries the majority of chiropractors and their associations appear to make efficacy claims that are unsupported by scientific evidence. Claims not supported by solid evidence were made about asthma, ear infection, earache, otitis media, and neck pain.

A 2009 chiropractic spinal manipulation review for infant colic stated "Some chiropractors claim that spinal manipulation is an effective treatment for infant colic but the "evidence fails to demonstrate the effectiveness of this treatment. It is concluded that the above claim is not based on convincing data from rigorous clinical trials."

Some New Zealand chiropractors appeared to have used the title 'Doctor' in a New Zealand Yellow pages telephone directory in a way that implied they are registered medical practitioners, when no evidence was presented it was true. In New Zealand, chiropractors are allowed to use the title 'doctor' when it is qualified to show that the title refers to their chiropractic role. A representative from the NZ Chiropractic Board states that entries in the Yellow Pages under the heading of 'Chiropractors' fulfills this obligation when suitably qualified. If a chiropractor is not a registered medical practitioner, then the misuse of the title 'Doctor' while working in healthcare will not comply with the Health Practitioners Competence Assurance Act 2003.

UK chiropractic organizations and their members make numerous claims which are not supported by scientific evidence. Many chiropractors adhere to ideas which are against science and most seemingly violate important principles of ethical behaviour on a regular basis. The advice chiropractors gave to their patients is often misleading and dangerous. This situation, coupled with a backlash to the libel suit filed against Simon Singh, has inspired the filing of formal complaints of false advertising against more than 500 individual chiropractors within one 24-hour period, prompting the McTimoney Chiropractic Association to write to its members advising them to remove leaflets that make claims about whiplash and colic from their practice, to be wary of new patients and telephone inquiries, and telling their members: "If you have a website, take it down NOW." and "Finally, we strongly suggest you do NOT discuss this with others, especially patients."

On 19 April 2008, Simon Singh wrote a cautionary article about chiropractic therapies in *The Guardian* which resulted in him being sued for libel by the British Chiropractic Association. Singh wrote in *The Guardian* criticising the claims made by chiropractors about the efficacy of spinal manipulation in treating childhood ailments, among other things. He suggested there was "not a jot" of evidence to support such interventions for these ailments, and argued that the British Chiropractic Association "happily promotes bogus treatments". Singh stated that he would "contest the action vigorously... There is an important issue of freedom of speech at stake." The article developed the theme of Singh's recently published book *Trick or Treatment? Alternative Medicine on Trial*, making various claims about the usefulness of chiropractic. Commentators suggested this ruling could set a precedent to restrict freedom of speech to criticise alternative medicine. The charity Sense About Science launched a campaign to draw attention to this particular case. They issued a statement entitled "The law has no place in scientific disputes", which was signed by myriad signers representing science, journalism, publishing, arts, humanities, entertainment, skeptics, campaign groups and law. As of April 16, 2010, over 50,000 had signed. On 1 April 2010, Simon Singh won his court appeal for the right to rely on the defence of fair comment. On 15 April 2010, the BCA officially withdrew its lawsuit, thus ending the case.

Efficacy

Not all criticism originated from critics in the medical profession. Some chiropractors are cautiously calling for reform. Evidence-based guidelines are supported by one end of an ideological continuum among chiropractors; the other end employs antiscientific reasoning and unsubstantiated claims, that are ethically suspect when they let practitioners maintain their beliefs to patients' detriment. Samuel Homola writes that the bottom line is "A good chiropractor can do a lot to help you when you have mechanical-type back pain and other musculoskeletal problems. But until the chiropractic profession cleans up its act, and its colleges uniformly graduate properly limited chiropractors who specialize in neuromusculoskeletal problems, you'll have to exercise caution and informed judgment when seeking chiropractic care."

Vertebral subluxation, the core concept of chiropractic, is not based on solid science. A 2008 review found that with the possible exception of back pain, chiropractic manipulation has not been shown to be effective for any medical condition. Commenting on a famous 'systematic' review by Bronfort et al., Edzard Ernst stated that it was a notorious example of a pseudo-systematic review that omitted evidence, for instance, of negative primary studies. The concept of subluxation remains unsubstantiated and largely untested, and has been debated about whether to keep it in the chiropractic paradigm for decades. The dogma of subluxation is the biggest single barrier to professional development for chiropractors. Vertebral subluxation skews the practice of legitimacy in ways that bring ridicule from the scientific community and uncertainty among the general public. Commitment to the subluxation dogma undermines the desire for scientific investigation of subluxation as hypothesis, and further perpetuates a cycle of a marketing tradition, inevitably bringing charges of quackery. The cost, effectiveness, and safety, of spinal manipulation are uncertain. Edzard Ernst stated "the best evidence available to date fails to demonstrate clinically relevant benefits of chiropractic for paediatric patients, and some evidence even suggests that chiropractors can cause serious harm to children". A 2007 survey of Alberta chiropractors found that they do not consistently apply research in practice, which may have resulted from a lack of research education and skills though the chiropractic profession has research-focused professional training encouraged by professional association incentives which provide time and support for research. According to David Colquhoun, chiropractic is no more effective than conventional treatment at its best, and has a disadvantage of being "surrounded by gobbledygook about 'subluxations'", and, more seriously, it does kill patients occasionally. Neck spinal manipulation has a risk of stroke or death. Although rare, spinal manipulation, particularly of the upper spine, can also result in complications that can lead to permanent disability or death; these can occur in adults and children. Most of the adverse events were benign, however, there are complications that were life-threatening. A 2010 systematic review found that numerous deaths since 1934 have been recorded after chiropractic neck manipulation typically associated with vertebral artery dissection. Some chiropractic proponents seem to think that a critical evaluation of the research is tantamount to a 'scare story' or to 'puffing up (the evidence) out of all proportion'. A reasonable approach to serious risk from chiropractic therapy, however, requires an open examination.

The 2008 book *Trick or Treatment* states that "chiropractors may X-ray the same patient several times a year, even though there is no clear evidence that X-rays will help the therapist treat the patient. X-rays can reveal neither the subluxations nor the innate intelligence associated with chiropractic philosophy, because they do not exist. There is no conceivable reason at all why X-raying the spine should help a straight chiropractor treat an ear infection, asthma or period pains. Most worrying of all, chiropractors generally require a full spine X-ray, which delivers a significant higher radiation dose than most other X-ray procedures". Practice guidelines aim to reduce unnecessary radiation exposure, which increases cancer risk in proportion to the amount of radiation received. Research suggests that radiology instruction given at chiropractic schools worldwide seem to be evidence-based. Although, there seems to be a disparity between some schools and available evidence regarding the aspect of radiography for patients with acute low back pain without an indication of a serious disease, which may contribute to chiropractic overuse of radiography for low back pain.

Quackwatch is critical of chiropractic; its founder, Stephen Barrett, has written that it is "absurd" to think that chiropractors are qualified to be primary care providers and considers applied kinesiology to be a "term most commonly used to identify a pseudoscientific system of muscle-testing and therapy".

A 2009 perspective stated there is consistent evidence that manual therapies such as chiropractic manipulations are "helpful and generally produce moderate but significant and sustained improvement for back pain in populations" and writes that the suggestion that chiropractic does more harm than good as "specious". The author went on to write that the more serious suggestion is that chiropractic treatment can kill people, and it is often claimed that chiropractic manipulation causes strokes.

Lon Morgan, DC, a reform chiropractor, expressed his view of Innate Intelligence this way: "Innate Intelligence clearly has its origins in borrowed mystical and occult practices of a bygone era. It remains untestable and unverifiable and has an unacceptably high penalty/benefit ratio for the chiropractic profession. The chiropractic concept of Innate Intelligence is an anachronistic holdover from a time when insufficient scientific understanding existed to explain human physiological processes. It is clearly religious in nature and must be considered harmful to normal scientific activity."

Chiropractic historian Joseph C. Keating, Jr. articulated that "So long as we propound the "One cause, one cure" rhetoric of Innate, we should expect to be met by ridicule from the wider health science community. Chiropractors can't have it both ways. Our theories cannot be both dogmatically held vitalistic constructs and be scientific at the same time. The purposiveness, consciousness and rigidity of the Palmers' Innate should be rejected."

William T. Jarvis, Ph.D. has stated: "Chiropractic is a controversial health-care system that has been legalized throughout the United States and in several other countries. In the United States in 1984, roughly 10.7 million people made 163 million office visits to 30,000 chiropractors. More than three fourths of the states require insurance companies to include chiropractic services in health and accident policies. The federal government pays for limited chiropractic services under Medicare, Medicaid, and its vocational rehabilitation program, and the Internal Revenue Service allows a medical deduction for chiropractic services. Chiropractors cite such facts as evidence of "recognition." However, these are merely business statistics and legal arrangements that have nothing to do with chiropractic's scientific validity."

Vaccination and Water Fluoridation

Many forms of alternative medicine are based on philosophies that oppose vaccination and have practitioners who voice their opposition. These include some elements of the chiropractic community. The reasons for this negative vaccination view are complicated and rest, at least in part, on the early philosophies which shape the foundation of these professions. Chiropractors historically were strongly opposed to vaccination based on their belief that all diseases were traceable to causes in the spine, and therefore could not be affected by vaccines; D.D. Palmer wrote, "It is the very height of absurdity to strive to 'protect' any person from smallpox or any other malady by inoculating them with a filthy animal poison." Some chiropractors continue to be opposed to vaccination, one of the most effective public health measures in history.

Some chiropractic groups still oppose attempts to limit or eliminate nonmedical exemptions to vaccination. In March 2015, the Oregon Chiropractic Association invited Andrew Wakefield, chief author of a fraudulent research paper, to testify against Senate Bill 442, "a bill that would eliminate nonmedical exemptions from Oregon's school immunization law." The California Chiropractic Association lobbied against a 2015 bill ending belief exemptions for vaccines. They had also opposed a 2012 bill related to vaccination exemptions. On April 24, 2015, Wakefield received two standing ovations from the students at Life Chiropractic College West when he told them to oppose Senate Bill SB277, a bill which proposes limits on non-medical vaccine exemptions. Responding to his critics, he stated that "[i]t doesn't matter if I go to the grave discredited. I don't care what they say about me. In fact, I have nothing to lose now. This is such an important issue." Wakefield had previously been a featured speaker at a 2014 "California Jam" gathering of chiropractors, as well as a 2015 "California Jam" seminar, with continuing education credits, sponsored by Life Chiropractic College West.

In response to threatening activities by anti-vaccination activists, the California Medical Association (CMA) sent a warning letter to California Chiropractic Association President Brian Stenzler, whom they could document had encouraged the stalking of lobbyists who supported Senate Bill SB277. The CMA also filed a police report.

Early opposition to water fluoridation included chiropractors in the U.S. Some chiropractors oppose water fluoridation as being incompatible with chiropractic philosophy and an infringement of personal freedom. Recently, other chiropractors have actively promoted fluoridation, and several chiropractic organizations have endorsed scientific principles of public health.

Ownership of Spinal Manipulation

While no single profession "owns" spinal manipulation (SM), and there is little consensus as to which profession should administer SM, chiropractors have expressed concern that orthodox medical physicians and physical therapists could "steal" SM procedures from chiropractors. Chiropractors regularly introduce bills into state legislatures to further prohibit non-chiropractors from performing SM, and they are opposed by physical therapist organizations. Two U.S. states (Washington and Arkansas) prohibit physical therapists from performing SM, some states allow them to do it only if they have completed advanced training in SM. In the most restrictive states, SM is limited to chiropractors and medical physicians.

A focus on evidence-based SM research has also raised concerns that the resulting tighter practice guidelines could limit the scope of chiropractic practice to treating backs and necks.

Chiropractic Professional Ethics

Various organizations of practicing chiropractors have outlined formal codes of professional ethics. Actual practice has revealed a wide range of behaviors which may or may not conform to these standards.

Official Positions

The American Chiropractic Association (ACA) has a "Code of Ethics" "based upon the acknowledgement that the social contract dictates the profession's responsibilities to the patient, the public, and the profession; and upholds the fundamental principle that the paramount purpose of the chiropractic doctor's professional services shall be to benefit the patient." The smaller International Chiropractor's Association (ICA) also has a detailed set of professional canons.

Reports of Actual Practice

Various situations have occurred in which the ethics of chiropractors and chiropractic organizations have been called into question.

A 2008 commentary proposed that the chiropractic profession actively regulate itself to combat abuse, fraud, and quackery, which are more prevalent in chiropractic than in other health care professions, violating the social contract between patients and physicians.

Gleberzon *et al.* identify "deliberate fraud" as a notably harmful element of the chiropractic profession, finding that dubious practice techniques can translate into "outlandish billing and utilization rates". Those at the "fringe of ethical behavior" present the profession with a challenge, they believe, and must be weeded out.

A study of California disciplinary statistics during 1997–2000 reported 4.5 disciplinary actions per 1000 chiropractors per year, compared to 2.27 for medical doctors, and the incident rate for fraud was nine times greater among chiropractors (1.99 per 1000 chiropractors per year) than among medical doctors (0.20). According to a 2006 Gallup poll of U.S. adults, when asked how they would "rate the honesty and ethical standards of people in these different fields", chiropractic compared unfavorably with mainstream medicine. When chiropractic was rated, it "rated dead last amongst healthcare professions". While 84% of respondents considered nurses' ethics "very high" or "high," only 36% felt that way about chiropractors. Other healthcare professions ranged from 38% for psychiatrists, to 62% for dentists, 69% for medical doctors, 71% for veterinarians, and 73% for druggists or pharmacists. Similar results were found in the 2003 Gallup Poll.

In 2001, the largest chiropractic associations in the U.S. and Canada were reported to have distributed patient brochures which contained unsubstantiated claims. Chiropractors, especially in America, have a reputation for unnecessarily treating patients. In many circumstances the focus seems to be put on economics instead of health care. Sustained chiropractic care is promoted as a preventative tool, but unnecessary manipulation could possibly present a risk to patients. Some chiropractors are concerned by the routine unjustified claims chiropractors have made. A 2010 analysis of chiropractic websites found the majority of chiropractors and their associations made claims of effectiveness not supported by scientific evidence, while 28% of chiropractic websites advocate lower back pain care, which has some sound evidence.

Although in the vast majority of US States chiropractors are considered physicians pursuant to statute (exceptions are *inter alia*, New York and California). The Joint Commission recognizes chiropractors as physicians as well. In some jurisdictions, like New Zealand, chiropractors appeared to have used the title 'doctor' in a New Zealand yellow pages telephone directory in a way that implied they are registered medical practitioners, when no evidence was presented it was true. In New Zealand, chiropractors are allowed to use the title 'doctor' when it is qualified to show that the title refers to their chiropractic role. A representative from the NZ Chiropractic Board states that entries in the yellow pages under the heading of 'Chiropractors' fulfills this obligation when suitably qualified. If a chiropractor is not a registered medical practitioner, then the misuse of the title 'doctor' while working in healthcare will not comply with the Health Practitioners Competence Assurance Act 2003.

UK chiropractic organizations and their members make numerous claims which are not supported by scientific evidence. Many chiropractors adhere to ideas which are against science and most seemingly violate important principles of ethical behaviour on a regular basis. The advice chiropractors gave to their patients is often misleading and dangerous. In 2009, a backlash to the libel suit filed by the British Chiropractic Association (BCA) against Simon Singh, has inspired the filing of formal complaints of false advertising against more than 500 individual chiropractors within one 24-hour period, prompting the McTimoney Chiropractic Association to write to its members advising them to remove leaflets that make claims about whiplash and colic from their practice, to be wary of new patients and telephone inquiries, and telling their members: "If you have a website, take it down NOW." and "Finally, we strongly suggest you do NOT discuss this with others, especially patients." An editorial in *Nature* has suggested that the BCA may be trying to suppress debate and that this use of British libel law is a burden on the right to freedom of expression, which is protected by the European Convention on Human Rights. The libel case ended with the BCA withdrawing its suit in 2010.

Tenets

- ACA's Page on Ethical Practice
- ICA Ethics.

Spinal Adjustment

Spinal adjustment and chiropractic adjustment are terms used by chiropractors to describe their approaches to spinal manipulation, as well as some osteopaths, who use the term adjustment.

Spinal adjustments were among many chiropractic techniques invented in the 19th century by Daniel David Palmer, the founder of Chiropractic. Claims made for the benefits of spinal adjustments range from temporary, palliative (pain relieving) effects to long term wellness and preventive care. Despite anecdotal success, there is not yet scientific evidence that spinal adjustment is effective against disease.

Adjustment/Manipulation

In a section titled "Spinal Manipulation: The Chiropractic Adjustment", chiropractic authors and researchers Meeker and Haldeman write that the core clinical method that all chiropractors agree upon is spinal manipulation, although chiropractors much prefer to use the term spinal "adjustment", a term which reflects "their belief in the therapeutic and health-enhancing effect of correcting spinal joint abnormalities." (p. 218)

Defined as Unique to Chiropractic

The International Chiropractor's Association (ICA) states that the "chiropractic spinal adjustment is unique and singular to the chiropractic profession", and that it "is characterized by a specific thrust applied to the vertebra utilizing parts of the vertebra and contiguous structures as levers to directionally correct articular malposition. Adjustment shall be differentiated from spinal manipulation in that the adjustment can only be applied to a vertebral malposition with the express intent to improve or correct the subluxation, whereas any joint, subluxated or not, may be manipulated to mobilize the joint or to put the joint through its range of motion... Chiropractic is a specialized field in the healing arts, and by prior rights, the spinal adjustment is distinct and singular to the chiropractic profession." One author claims that this concept is now repudiated by mainstream chiropractic. The definition of this procedure describes the use of a load (force) to specific body tissues with therapeutic intent. This 'load' is traditionally supplied by hand, and can vary in its velocity, amplitude, duration, frequency, and body location (p. 218) and is usually abbreviated HVLA (high velocity low amplitude) thrust.

Intention: To Correct Vertebral Subluxations

The intention of a chiropractic adjustment is to affect or correct the alignment, motion and/or function of a vertebral joint. Specifically, they are intended to correct "vertebral subluxations", the term given to the signs and symptoms that are said by chiropractors to result from abnormal alignment of vertebrae. (p. 218) This intention forms the legal and philosophical foundation of the profession, and US Medicare law formulates it in this manner:

> "Coverage of chiropractic services is specifically limited to manual manipulation of the spine to correct a subluxation... Medicare will not pay for treatment unless it is 'manual manipulation of the spine to correct a subluxation'."

Adjustment Methods

As the chiropractic profession grew, individual practitioners and institutions proposed and developed various proprietary techniques and methods. While many of these techniques did not endure, hundreds of different approaches remain in chiropractic practice today. Not all of them involve HVLA thrust manipulation. Most cite case studies, anecdotal evidence, and patient testimonials as evidence for effectiveness. These techniques include:

- Toggle Drop – this is when the chiropractor, using crossed hands, presses down firmly on a particular area of the spine. Then, with a quick and precise thrust, the chiropractor adjusts the spine. This is done to improve mobility in the vertebral joints.
- Lumbar Roll (aka side posture) – the chiropractor positions the patient on his or her side, then applies a quick and precise manipulative thrust to the misaligned vertebra, returning it to its proper position.
- Release Work – the chiropractor applies gentle pressure using his or her fingertips to separate the vertebrae.
- Table adjustments – The patient lies on a special table with sections that drop down. The chiropractor applies a quick thrust at the same time the section drops. The dropping of the table allows for a lighter adjustment without the twisting positions that can accompany other techniques.
- Instrument adjustments – often the gentlest methods of adjusting the spine. The patient lies on the table face down while the chiropractor uses a spring-loaded activator instrument to perform the adjustment. This technique is often used to perform adjustments on animals as well.
- Manipulation under anesthesia (MUA) – this is performed by a chiropractor certified in this technique in a hospital outpatient setting when the patient is unresponsive to traditional adjustments.

Techniques

There are many techniques which chiropractors can specialize in and employ in spinal adjustments. Some of the most notable techniques include:

- Activator Methods – uses the Activator Adjusting Instrument instead of by-hand adjustments to give consistent mechanical low-force, high-speed impulses to the body. Utilizes a leg-length analysis to determine segmental aberration.
- Active Release Techniques – soft tissue system/movement based technique that treats

problems with muscles, tendons, ligaments, fascia and nerves.

- Bio-Geometric Integration – a framework for understanding the body's response to force dynamics. Can be utilized with many techniques. Focuses on the body's full integration of forces and on assessment for choosing the most appropriate adjustive force application, ranging from light pressure to traditional joint cavitation, for each particular case presentation.
- Blair Upper Cervical Technique – an objective upper cervical technique focusing primarily on misalignments in the first bone of the spine (Atlas) as it comes into contact with the head (Occiput).
- Chiropractic Biophysics (CBP) - a research and evidence based technique which aims to correct improper curvatures of the spine with traditional chiropractic manipulation (SMT), focused rehabilitation exercises, and a unique form of spinal traction which utilizes mechanically assisted and focused stretching to stretch and remodel the ligaments and related tissues of the spine.
- Cox Flexion-Distraction – a decompression focused procedure which utilizes specialized adjusting tables with movable parts; these tables stretch and decompress the facets and ligaments of the spine in a gentle rocking motion.
- Directional Non-Force Technique – utilizes a diagnostic system for subluxation analysis consisting of gentle challenging and a unique leg check allowing the body to indicate the directions of misalignment of structures that are producing nerve interference. A gentle but directionally specific thumb impulse provides a long lasting correction to bony and soft tissue structures.
- Diversified – the classic chiropractic technique, developed by D.D. Palmer, DC. Uses specific manual thrusts focused on restoring normal biomechanical function. Has been developed to adjust extremity joints as well.
- Gonstead Technique – Developed by an automotive engineer turned chiropractor, this technique uses a very specific method of analysis by the use of nervoscopes, full spine x-rays and precise adjusting techniques that condemns "torquing" of the spine, which may harm the Intervertebral disc.
- Hole-in-one Technique/Toggle Recoil Technique – Synonyms for the upper cervical technique developed by B.J. Palmer which utilizes a quick thrust and release, and later incorporated a drop table as seen in modern practice.
- Kale Technique (Specific Chiropractic) – gentle technique which utilizes a special adjusting table that helps adjust and stabilize the upper cervical region surrounding the brain stem.
- Logan Basic Technique – a light touch technique that works to "level the foundation" or sacrum. Its concept employs the use of heel lifts and specific contacts.
- NUCCA Technique – manual method of adjusting the atlas subluxation complex based on 3D x-ray studies which determine the correct line of drive or vector of force.
- Orthospinology Procedure – is a method of analyzing and correcting the chiropractic upper cervical subluxation complex based on vertebral alignment measurements on neck x-rays

taken from three different directions. The adjustment can be delivered by hand, hand-held or table mounted instruments along a pre-calculated vector using approximately 1 to 7 pounds of force. The patient is in a side-lying posture with a solid mastoid support. The procedure is based on the work of the late John F. Grostic, D.C.

- Thompson Terminal Point Technique (Thompson Drop-Table Technique) – uses a precision adjusting table with a weighing mechanism which adds only enough tension to hold the patient in the "up" position before the thrust is given.

Over the years, many variations of these techniques have been delivered, most as proprietary techniques developed by individual practitioners. WebMD has made a partial list:

• Activator technique	• Blair	• Craniosacral Therapy	• Manual Adjusting	• Pettibon	• Thompson
• Advanced BioStructural Correction	• Body Restoration Technique	• Directional Non-Force	• Meric	• Pierce	• Thompson Terminal Point
• Applied Kinesiology	• Carver Technique	• Diversified technique	• Motion Palpation	• Pierce Stillwagon	• Toftness
• Atlas Orthogonal	• Cervical Care	• Flexion-Distraction	• Network	• Pro-Adjuster	• Toggle Recoil
• Auricular	• Cervical Drop	• Gonstead	• Neural Organization Technique	• Receptor Tonus	• Torque Release
• Barge Analysis	• Chiropractic Biophysics (CBP)	• Grostic	• Neuro Emotional Technique	• Sacral Occipital Technique (SOT)	• Total Body Modification
• Bio Magnetic	• Clinical Kinesiology	• Hole in one [HIO]	• Neuro Muscular Technique	• Soft Tissue Orthopedics	• Traction
• Bio-Energetic Synchronization	• Concept Therapy	• Kale	• Neuro Vascular Technique	• Spinal Biomechanics	• Upper Cervical
• Bio-Geometric Integration	• Contact Reflex Analysis	• Leander	• Nimmo	• Spinal Biomedical Engineering	• Vector Point Therapy
• Biomechanics	• Cox	• Logan Basic	• Nutrition Response Testing	• Spinal Biophysics	• Versendaal
			• Palmer Package		

Effects

The effects of spinal adjustment vary depending on the method performed. All techniques claim effects similar to other manual therapies, ranging from decreased muscle tension to reduced stress. Studies show that most patients go to chiropractors for musculoskeletal problems: 60% with low back pain, and the rest with head, neck and extremity symptoms. (p. 219) Also the article "Chiropractic: A Profession at the Crossroads of Mainstream and Alternative Medicine" states that, "chiropractic was to be a revolutionary system of healing based on the premise that neurologic dysfunction caused by 'impinged' nerves at the spinal level was the cause of most disease". (p. 218) The mechanisms that are claimed to alter nervous system function and affect overall health are seen as speculative in nature, however, clinical trials have been conducted that include "placebo-controlled comparisons [and] comparisons with other treatments". (p. 220) The American Chiropractic Association promotes chiropractic care of infants and children under the theory that "poor posture and physical injury, including birth trauma, may be common primary causes of illness in children and can have a direct and significant impact not only on spinal mechanics, but on other bodily functions".

The effects of spinal manipulation have been shown to include: temporary relief of musculoskeletal pain, increased range of joint motion, changes in facet joint kinematics, increased pain tolerance and increased muscle strength. (p. 222) Common side effects of spinal manipulative therapy (SMT) are characterized as mild to moderate and may include: local discomfort, headache, tiredness, or radiating discomfort. (p. 222)

Safety

The World Health Organization states that when "employed skillfully and appropriately, chiropractic care is safe and effective for the prevention and management of a number of health problems." As with all interventions, there are risks associated with spinal manipulative therapy (SMT). Common, but nonserious side effects include: discomfort, headache, and fatigue which will go away after 24 to 48 hours. Extremely rare, but potentially serious side effects include: strokes, spinal disc herniation, vertebral and rib fractures and cauda equina syndrome. (p. 222).

Vertebral Subluxation

In chiropractic, vertebral subluxation is a supposed misalignment of the spinal column leading to a set of set of signs and symptoms sometimes termed vertebral subluxation complex. It has no biomedical basis and is categorized as pseudoscientific by leading authorities. Traditionally, the "specific focus of chiropractic practice" is the chiropractic subluxation and historical chiropractic practice assumes that a vertebral subluxation or spinal joint dysfunction interferes with the body's function and its innate intelligence, as promulgated by D. D. Palmer, the inventor of chiropractic.

The chiropractic subluxation is the heart of the split between "straight" and "mixer" chiropractors. Straight chiropractors continue to follow Palmer's vitalistic tradition, claiming that subluxation has considerable health effects and also adding a visceral component to the definition, while mixers, as exemplified by the United Kingdom's General Chiropractic Council, consider it a historical concept with no evidence identifying it as the cause of disease.

Within the chiropractic tradition, a vertebral subluxation complex is believed to be a dysfunctional biomechanical spinal segment which actively alters neurological function, which in turn, is believed to lead to neuromusculoskeletal and visceral disorders. The WHO acknowledges this difference between the medical and chiropractic definitions of a subluxation: medical doctors only refer to "significant structural displacements" as subluxations, whereas chiropractors suggest that a dysfunctional segment, whether displaced significantly or not, should be referred to as a subluxation. This difference has been noted in the proceedings of the chiropractic profession's *Mercy Center Consensus Conference*: "The chiropractic profession refers to this concept as a 'subluxation'. This use of the word *subluxation* should not be confused with the term's precise anatomic usage, which considers only the anatomical relationships."

The chiropractic vertebral subluxation complex has been a source of controversy since its inception in 1895 due to the lack of empirical evidence for its existence, its metaphysical origins, and claims of its far reaching effects on health and disease. Although some chiropractic associations and colleges support the concept of subluxation, many in the chiropractic profession reject it and shun the use of this term as a diagnosis. In the United States and in Canada the term *nonallopathic lesion* may be used in place of *subluxation*.

A 2009 review concluded that epidemiologic evidence does not support the chiropractic subluxation, concluding:

> "No supportive evidence is found for the chiropractic subluxation being associated with any disease process or of creating suboptimal health conditions requiring intervention. Regardless of popular appeal, this leaves the subluxation construct in the realm of unsupported speculation. This lack of supportive evidence suggests the subluxation construct has no valid clinical applicability."

In 2015, 8 internationally accredited chiropractic colleges: AECC, WIOC, IFEC-Paris, IFEC-Toulouse, USD-Odense, UZ-Zurich, UJ-Johannesburg and Durban University of Technology made an open statement which included: "The teaching of the vertebral subluxation complex as a vitalistic construct that claims that it is the cause of disease is unsupported by evidence. Its inclusion in a modern chiropractic curriculum in anything other than an historic context is therefore inappropriate and unnecessary".

History

In 1909 B.J. Palmer wrote that:

> "Chiropractors have found in every disease that is supposed to be contagious, *a cause in the spine*. In the spinal column we *will* find a subluxation that corresponds to every type of disease. If we had one hundred cases of small-pox, I can prove to you where, in one, you *will* find a subluxation and you will find the *same conditions* in the other ninety-nine. I adjust one and return his functions to normal... . There is no contagious disease... . There is no infection... . There is a cause internal to man that makes of his body in a certain spot, more or less a breeding ground [for microbes]. It is a place where they can multiply, propagate, and then because they become so many they are classed as a cause." -- B.J. Palmer, *The Philosophy of Chiropractic*, V. Davenport, IA: Palmer School of Chiropractic; 1909

Definitions, Official Status and ICD Coding

Definitions and Status

The WHO definition of the chiropractic vertebral subluxation is:

> "A lesion or dysfunction in a joint or motion segment in which alignment, movement integrity and/or physiological function are altered, although contact between joint surfaces remains intact. It is essentially a functional entity, which may influence biomechanical and neural integrity."

The purported displacement is not necessarily visible on X-rays. This is in contrast to the medical definition of spinal subluxation which, according to the WHO, is a *"significant structural displacement"*, and therefore visible on X-rays.

As of 2014, the National Board of Chiropractic Examiners states:

> "The specific focus of chiropractic practice is known as the chiropractic subluxation or joint dysfunction. A subluxation is a health concern that manifests in the skeletal joints, and, through complex anatomical and physiological relationships, affects the nervous system and may lead to reduced function, disability or illness."

In 1996 an official consensus definition of subluxation was formed. Cooperstein and Gleberzon have described the situation: "... although many in the chiropractic profession reject the concept of "subluxation" and shun the use of this term as a diagnosis, the presidents of at least a dozen chiropractic colleges of the Association of Chiropractic Colleges (ACC) developed a consensus definition of "subluxation" in 1996. It reads:

> "Chiropractic is concerned with the preservation and restoration of health, and focuses particular attention on the subluxation. A subluxation is a complex of functional and/or structural and/or pathological articular changes that compromise neural integrity and may influence organ system function and general health. A subluxation is evaluated, diagnosed, and managed through the use of chiropractic procedures based on the best available rational and empirical evidence."

In 2001 the World Federation of Chiropractic, representing the national chiropractic associations in 77 countries, adopted this consensus statement which reaffirms belief in the vertebral subluxation.

The ACC paradigm has been criticized by chiropractic authors:

> "All in all, the ambiguities that permeate the ACC's statements on subluxation render it inadequate as a guide to clinical research... Whether the ACC's subluxation claims have succeeded as a political statement is beyond our concern here. These assertions were published as a priori truths (what many chiropractors have traditionally referred to as "principle"), and are exemplary of scientifically unjustified assertions made in many corners of the profession. It matters not whether unsubstantiated assertions are offered for clinical, political, scientific, educational, marketing or other purposes; when offered without acknowledgment of their tentative character, they amount to dogmatism. We contend that attempts to foster unity (among the schools or in the wider profession) at the expense of scientific integrity is ultimately self-defeating. To be sure, the profession's lack of cultural authority is based in part upon our characteristic disunity. However, attempts to generate unity by adoption of a common dogma can only bring scorn and continued alienation from the wider health care community and the public we all serve."

In May 2010 the General Chiropractic Council, the statutory regulatory body for chiropractors in the United Kingdom, issued guidance for chiropractors stating that the chiropractic vertebral subluxation complex "is an historical concept" and "is not supported by any clinical research evidence that would allow claims to be made that it is the cause of disease or health concerns."

ICD Coding

The differences between a medical subluxation and a chiropractic "vertebral subluxation" create confusion and difficulties when it comes to following official ICD-9 and ICD-10 coding. In a 2014 article in *Dynamic Chiropractic* by a chiropractor who is a certified professional coder, these difficulties were discussed in detail. He noted that the WHO recognizes the differences between the two types of "subluxations", and also pointed out certain difficulties for chiropractors:

> "...the official definition of 739 codes is "nonallopathic lesions, not elsewhere classified.... In other words, 739 is a code that does not describe a subluxation. It does not even say what the patient has; it says that there is no code to describe what the patient has.... [T]he elusive "vertebral subluxation complex" I learned about in school has no place in the ICD-9 code set. All we get is 739, which is a code for conditions that do not have a code."
>
> "ICD-9 has never provided a code that truly describes this and differentiates between the chiropractic subluxation and the allopathic subluxation. Chiropractors have been compelled to try to fit a square peg into a round hole for many years."

At the time of writing (August 2014) it was still uncertain which codes in the newer ICD-10 would be useful for chiropractors and how they would be interpreted.

Components

Traditionally there have been 5 components that form the chiropractic subluxation. The vertebral subluxation complex is differentiated by the fifth component, general systemic disturbances secondary to the spinal misalignment (vertebral subluxation).

1. Spinal Kinesiopathology
2. Neuropathophysiology/Neuropathology
3. Myopathology
4. Histopathology
5. Pathophysiology/Pathology

Examination

Historically, the detection of spinal misalignments (subluxations) by the chiropractic profession has relied on X-ray findings and physical examination. At least 2 of the following 4 physical signs and/or symptoms must be documented to qualify for reimbursement:

- Pain and tenderness
- Asymmetry/misalignment
- Range of motion abnormality
- Tissue/tone changes

Background

It has been proposed that a vertebral subluxation can negatively affect general health by altering the neurological communication between the brain, spinal cord and peripheral nervous system.

Although individuals may not always be symptomatic, straight chiropractors believe that the presence of vertebral subluxation is in itself justification for correction via spinal adjustment.

Chiropractic treatment of vertebral subluxation focuses on delivering a chiropractic adjustment which is a high velocity low amplitude (HVLA) thrust to the dysfunctional spinal segments to help correct the chiropractic subluxation complex. Spinal adjustment is the primary procedure used by chiropractors in the adjustment. Adjustment/manipulation has been shown to help with low back pain, neck pain and tension type headaches, but further studies are inconclusive on the use of spinal manipulation outside the treatment of neuromusculoskeletal disorders.

Rationale and Disagreements

In 1910, D.D. Palmer, the founder of chiropractic, wrote:

> "Physiologists divide nerve-fibers, which form the nerves, into two classes, afferent and efferent. Impressions are made on the peripheral afferent fiber-endings; these create sensations which are transmitted to the center of the nervous system. Efferent nerve-fibers carry impulses out from the center to their endings. Most of these go to muscles and are therefore called motor impulses; some are secretory and enter glands; a portion are inhibitory their function being to restrain secretion. Thus, nerves carry impulses outward and sensations inward. The activity of these nerves, or rather their fibers, may become excited or allayed by impingement, the result being a modification of functionating — too much or not enough action — which is dis-ease."

Chiropractors use and have used various terms to express this concept: subluxation, vertebral subluxation (VS), vertebral subluxation complex (VSC), "killer subluxations," and the "silent killer."

They, along with some physical therapists and osteopathic physicians, have also used another term, BOOP, meaning "bone out of place."

Some chiropractors have described the disagreements within the profession about the concept, and have written skeptically about BOOP as an antiquated idea. In 1992 one wrote:

> "The main problem we often run into is the bone out of place (BOOP) concept. It seems we somehow step on toes when we describe the spine as a functioning entity instead of a stack of bones that can be shifted back and forth into the ideal configuration. The BOOP concept will eventually fade, and we are grateful for its contribution to chiropractic. For many decades, it offered a model to work from. This model has been updated by the rest of the healing profession, but chiropractors have been hesitant to let this antiquated model go. Some within our profession hold onto this model with a religious fervor. The chiropractic profession has moved into a new age. The BOOP concept has been updated and science is ever upon us in the 90s. Let's start asking questions again and drive the chiropractic profession kicking and screaming into the 21st century."

One wrote in 1994 about the "brutal civil war":

> "According to various gossip columnists in chiropractic, our profession appears to be currently enmeshed in a brutal civil war between BOOP (bone-out-of-place) practitioners and low back pain practitioners. It should be known that the BOOPers incorrectly call them-

> selves subluxation-based practitioners. My experience has demonstrated that the BOOPers do not know enough about subluxation to call themselves subluxation-based chiropractors. We would all do well to not be subluxation-based in the BOOP sense. It should also be known that this so-called war is really an over-dramatized skirmish between vocal BOOPers and a theoretical group of anti-chiropractic DCs. I have yet to meet any of these anti-chiropractic DCs. Unfortunately, the BOOPers seem to think that those who do not embrace the totality of BOOP philosophy are merely non-BOOPers who are still very pro-chiropractic and appreciate the philosophy of chiropractic from a contemporary and nondogmatic perspective."

Ten years later (in 2004) he openly disparaged the idea still propounded by "modern-day advocates of this concept":

> "... it is essentially impossible to have nerve interference. To summarize, nerve interference is described, by modern-day advocates of this concept, as a reduction of neural or mental impulses, which occurs in response to a bone-out-of-place (BOOP) subluxation... Clearly, the BOOP subluxation model fails miserably when considered in the light of basic neuroscience facts... BOOP subluxationists become angry and defensive when the BOOP model of subluxation is criticized... The reactionary nature of certain BOOP subluxationists is to accuse those who don't buy into the BOOP model of being anti-chiropractic – an astonishing leap of ignorance, to say the least. Furthermore, anyone who does not buy into the model is trying to "medicalize chiropractic" - another example of low-IQ thinking. And if tears do not well up in your eyes when you hear the phrase, "The power that made the body, heals the body," you are accused of having no passion for chiropractic – still another example of depressed, frontal-lobe activity. Even worse, if you don't buy into every bizarre, New Age, tree-hugging notion that comes down the pike and is circularly attached to subluxation, you will be accused of being an atheist – an excellent example of the need for psychiatrists and the drugs they prescribe."

Functional Hypotheses

V. Strang, D.C., describes several hypotheses on how a misaligned vertebra may cause interference to the nervous system in his book, *Essential Principles of Chiropractic*:

- Nerve compression hypothesis: suggests that when the vertebrae are out of alignment, the nerve roots and/or spinal cord can become pinched or irritated. While the most commonly referenced hypothesis, and easiest for a patient to understand, it may be the least likely to occur.
- Proprioceptive insult hypothesis: focuses on articular alterations causing hyperactivity of the sensory nerve fibers.
- Somatosympathetic reflex hypothesis: all the visceral organ functions can be reflexly affected by cutaneous or muscular stimulation.
- Somatosomatic reflex hypothesis: afferent impulses from one part of the body can result in reflex activity in other parts of the body.

- Viscerosomatic reflex hypothesis: visceral afferent fibers cause reflex somatic problems.
- Somatopsychic hypothesis: the effects of a subluxation on the ascending paths of the reticular activating system.
- Neurodystrophic hypothesis: focuses on lowered tissue resistance that results from abnormal innervation.
- Dentate ligament-cord distortion hypothesis: upper cervical misalignments can cause the dentate ligaments to put a stress on the spinal cord.
- Psychogenic hypothesis: emotions, such as stress, causing contraction in skeletal muscles.

The vertebral subluxation has been described as a syndrome with signs and symptoms which include: altered alignment; aberrant motion; palpable soft tissue changes; localized/referred pain; muscle contraction or imbalance; altered physiological function; reversible with adjustment/manipulation; focal tenderness.

Scientific Investigation

Investigation by chiropractors attempting to confirm the existence of vertebral subluxations has been ongoing since it was first postulated in 1895. The early practitioners used palpation and the anatomy of the nervous system as a guide (meric system). In their efforts to be more specific, they seized the newly discovered X-ray technology and introduced the neurocalometer (a heat sensing device). It was during those early years that the medical establishment first criticized the chiropractic profession, saying that the conditions that those early chiropractors were treating were only psychophysiologic disorders. To prove that chiropractic patients had real conditions, BJ Palmer opened a research clinic as a part of the Palmer College of Chiropractic. When a patient entered the clinic, they were first examined by medical doctors and a diagnosis was formulated. They were then sent to the chiropractic part of the clinic, treated, and sent back to the medical doctors for evaluation. Since then, chiropractors have sought a greater understanding of the mechanisms and effects of the vertebral subluxation. Today we see motion x-rays, surface EMG, and digital thermography though none of these methods have been proven to be reliable or valid in the detection of vertebral subluxations.

A 2004 research team at the National University of Health Sciences evaluated changes of the lumbar vertebral column following fixation (immobility) by surgically fusing spinal joints in experimental rats. The fixated joints showed significant degeneration compared to the mobile joints, confirming that surgical fixation results in time-dependent degenerative changes of the zygapophysial joints.

Believers within the chiropractic tradition assert that spinal health and function are directly related to general health and well-being. David Seaman reviewed the work of several researchers concerning autonomic nervous system relationship to the somatic tissues of the spine. He noted that Feinstein *et al.* were the first to clearly describe some symptoms associated with noxious irritation of spinal tissues. They injected hypertonic saline into interspinous tissues and paraspinal muscles of normal volunteers for the purpose of characterizing local and referred pain patterns that might develop. His observations included:

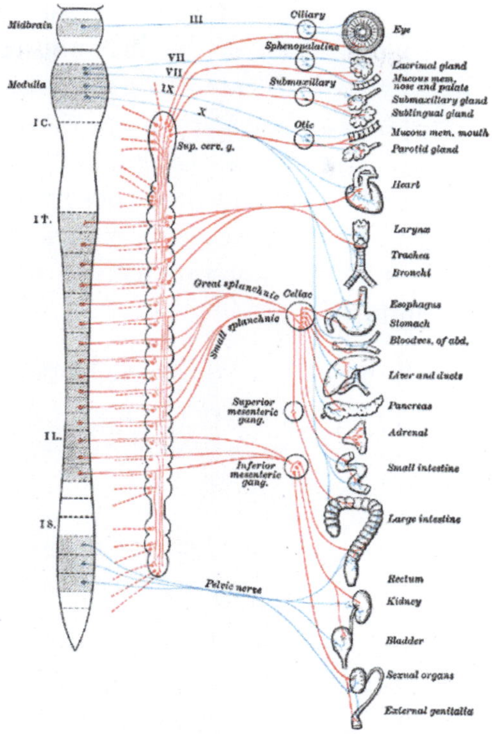

Autonomic nervous system
Blue = parasympathetic
Red = sympathetic

> "The pain elicited from muscles was accompanied by a characteristic group of phenomena which indicated involvement of other than segmental somatic mechanisms ... The manifestations were pallor, sweating bradycardia, fall in blood pressure, subjective faintness, and nausea, but vomiting was not observed. Syncope occurred in two early procedures in the series of paravertebral injections and was subsequently avoided by quickly depressing the subject's head or by having him lie down at the first sign of faintness. These features were not proportional to the severity of or to the extent of radiation; on the contrary, they seemed to dominate the experience of subjects who complained of little pain, but who were overwhelmed by this distressing complex of symptoms."

Feinstein referred to these symptoms as autonomic concomitants. It is likely that these autonomic concomitants were caused by nociceptive stimulation of autonomic centers in the brainstem, particularly the medulla. Feinstein indicated that "this is an example of the ability of deep noxious stimulation to activate generalized autonomic responses independently of the relay of pain to conscious levels." In other words, pain may not be the symptomatic outcome of nociceptive stimulation of spinal structures. Such a conclusion has profound implications for the chiropractic profession. Clearly, patients do not need to be in pain to be candidates for spinal adjustments.

The efficacy and validity of spinal manipulation to address visceral disorders systems remains a source of controversy within the chiropractic profession. Although research is ongoing on this topic, conclusions that support the usefulness of spinal manipulation for organic disorders remains to be seen. Additionally, to complicate matters, chiropractic professors and researchers, Nansel and Szlazak, found that:

> "the proper differential diagnosis of somatic (musculoskeletal) vs. visceral (organ) dysfunction represents a challenge for both the medical and chiropractic physician. The afferent convergence mechanisms, which can create signs and symptoms that are virtually indistinguishable with respect to their somatic vs. visceral etiologies, suggest it is not unreasonable that this somatic visceral-disease mimicry could very well account for the "cures" of presumed organ disease that have been observed over the years in response to various somatic therapies (e.g., spinal manipulation, acupuncture, Rolfing, Qi Gong, etc.) and may represent a common phenomenon that has led to "holistic" health care claims on the part of such clinical disciplines."

Considering this phenomenon, Seaman suggests that the chiropractic concept of joint complex (somatic) dysfunction should be incorporated into the differential diagnosis of pain and visceral symptoms because these dysfunctions often generate symptoms similar to those produced by true visceral disease and notes that this mimicry leads to unnecessary surgical procedures and medications.

Other chiropractic researchers have also questioned some of the claimed effects of vertebral subluxation:

> "The literature supports the existence of somatovisceral and viscerosomatic reflexes, but there is little or no evidence to support the notion that the spinal derangements (often referred to as subluxations by chiropractors) can cause prolonged aberrant discharge of these reflexes. Equally unsupported in the literature is the notion that the prolonged activation of these reflexes will manifest into pathological state of tissues, and most relevantly, that the application of spinal manipulative therapy can alter the prolonged reflex discharge or be associated with a reversal of the pathological degeneration of the affected reflexes or tissues. The evidence that has been amassed is largely anecdotal or case report based and it has attracted much intra disciplinary debate because of its frequent association with certain approaches to management (largely described as being traditional or "philosophical" in nature)."

Still other chiropractic researchers state quite directly:

> "... early chiropractic philosophy ... considered disease the result of spinal nerve dysfunction caused by misplaced (subluxated) vertebrae. Although rejected by medical science, this concept is still [2000] accepted by a minority of chiropractors... Indeed, many progressive chiropractors have rejected the historical concept of the chiropractic subluxation in favor of ones that more accurately describe the nature of the complex joint disfunctions they treat."

Researchers at the RMIT University-Japan, Tokyo studied reflex effects of vertebral subluxation with regards to the autonomic nervous system. They found that "recent neuroscience research supports a neurophysiologic rationale for the concept that aberrant stimulation of spinal or paraspinal structures may lead to segmentally organized reflex responses of the autonomic nervous system, which in turn may alter visceral function."

Professor Philip S. Bolton of the School of Biomedical Sciences at University of Newcastle, Australia writes in Journal of Manipulative and Physiological Therapeutics, "The traditional chiropractic vertebral subluxation hypothesis proposes that vertebral misalignment cause illness, disease, or both. This hypothesis remains controversial." His objective was, "To briefly review and update experimental evidence concerning reflex effects of vertebral subluxations, particularly concerning peripheral nervous system responses to vertebral subluxations. Data source: Information was obtained from chiropractic or, scientific peer-reviewed literature concerning human or animal studies of neural responses to vertebral subluxation, vertebral displacement or movement, or both." He concluded, "Animal models suggest that vertebral displacements and putative vertebral subluxations may modulate activity in group I to IV afferent nerves. However, it is not clear whether these afferent nerves are modulated during normal day-to-day activities of living and, if so, what segmental or whole-body reflex effects they may have."

Conclusions: Monitoring mixed-nerve root discharges in response to spinal manipulative thrusts *in vivo* in human subjects undergoing lumbar surgery is feasible. Neurophysiologic responses appeared sensitive to the contact point and applied force vector of the spinal manipulative thrust. Further study of the neurophysiologic mechanisms of spinal manipulation in humans and animals is needed to more precisely identify the mechanisms and neural pathways involved.

Researchers at the Department of Physiology, University College London studied the effects of compression upon conduction in myelinated axons. Using pneumatic pressure of varying degrees on the sciatic nerves of frog specimens, the study supported the idea of nerve conduction failure as a result of compression.

Critiques

Edzard Ernst has stated that the "core concepts of chiropractic, subluxation and spinal manipulation, are not based on sound science."

An area of debate among chiropractors is whether "vertebral subluxation" is a metaphysical concept (as posited in B. J. Palmer's philosophy of chiropractic) or a real phenomenon.

In an article on vertebral subluxation, the chiropractic authors wrote:

> "Subluxation syndrome is a legitimate, potentially testable, theoretical construct for which there is little experimental evidence. Acceptable as hypothesis, the widespread assertion of the clinical meaningfulness of this notion brings ridicule from the scientific and health care communities and confusion within the chiropractic profession. We believe that an evidence-orientation among chiropractors requires that we distinguish between subluxation dogma vs. subluxation as the potential focus of clinical research. We lament efforts to generate unity within the profession through consensus statements concerning subluxation dogma, and believe that cultural authority will continue to elude us so long as we assert dogma as though it were validated clinical theory."

Since its inception, the concept of *vertebral subluxation* has been a source of definitional debate. Tedd Koren, DC offers this explanation as a possible cause of the confusion:

The vertebral subluxation cannot be precisely defined because it is an abstraction, an intellectual construct used by chiropractors, chiropractic researchers, educators and others to explain the success of the chiropractic adjustment.

This is not a unique state of affairs, abstract entities populate many branches of science...

Subluxations, genes, gravity, the ego and life are all heuristic devices, "useful fictions" that are used to explain phenomenon that are far larger than our understanding. We use them as long as they work for us and discard or limit their application when they become unwieldy or unable to account for new observations...

Critics of chiropractic have incorrectly assumed that chiropractic is based on the theory or principle that vertebral subluxations cause "pinched" nerves that cause disease. They have it backwards. Chiropractic is based on the success of the spinal adjustment. The theory attempting to explain the success of the adjustment (nerve impingement, disease, subluxations) followed its clinical discovery.

Examples of such erroneous criticisms based on this straw man argument abound in the medical literature. Some examples: "The teachers, research workers and practitioners of medicine reject the so-called principle on which chiropractic is based and correctly and bluntly label it a fraud and hoax on the human race." "The basis of chiropractic is completely unscientific." The theory on which chiropractic is based [is false], namely that a "subluxation" of a spinal vertebra presses on a nerve interfering with the passage of energy down that nerve causing disease to organs supplied by that nerve, and that chiropractic "adjustments" can alleviate the pressure thereby treating or preventing such disease. There is no scientific evidence for the validity of this theory."

To be fair, statements by some chiropractors have tended to perpetuate this misunderstanding: "Pressure on nerves causes irritation and tension with deranged functions as a result."

When chiropractors declare that "pinched nerves" "nerve impingement" "spinal fixations" or others mechanisms of action explain how subluxations affect the person and how chiropractic works they are making the same mistake medical critics make – assuming chiropractic is based on theory. Mechanisms and theories are useful tools, but their limitations should always be kept in mind.

Other chiropractors have declared its unproven status as an area that needs reform:

> "Some may suggest that chiropractors should promote themselves as the experts in "correcting vertebral subluxation." However, the scientific literature has failed to demonstrate the very existence of the subluxation. Until and unless sound research published in credible journals demonstrates the existence and reliable identification of vertebral subluxation, and vertebral subluxation is found to be an important public health problem, society at large will not care about its correction. Thus, "subluxation correction" alone is not a viable option for chiropractic's future."

A Beth Israel Deaconess Medical Center article describes the mainstream understanding of vertebral subluxation theory:

Since its origin, chiropractic theory has based itself on "subluxations," or vertebrae that have shifted position in the spine. These subluxations are said to impede nerve outflow and cause disease in various organs. A chiropractic treatment is supposed to "put back in" these "popped out" vertebrae. For this reason, it is called an "adjustment."

However, no real evidence has ever been presented showing that a given chiropractic treatment alters the position of any vertebrae. In addition, there is as yet no real evidence that impairment of nerve outflow is a major contributor to common illnesses, or that spinal manipulation changes nerve outflow in such a way as to affect organ function.

In 2009, four scholarly chiropractors concluded that epidemiologic evidence does not support chiropractic's most fundamental theory. Since its inception, the vast majority of chiropractors have postulated that "subluxations" (misalignments) are the cause or underlying cause of ill health and can be corrected with spinal "adjustments." After searching the scientific literature, the chiropractic authors concluded:

> "No supportive evidence is found for the chiropractic subluxation being associated with any disease process or of creating suboptimal health conditions requiring intervention. Regardless of popular appeal, this leaves the subluxation construct in the realm of unsupported speculation. This lack of supportive evidence suggests the subluxation construct has no valid clinical applicability."

References

- World Health Organization (2005). "WHO guidelines on basic training and safety in chiropractic" (PDF). ISBN 92-4-159371-7. Retrieved 2008-02-29.
- David Chapman-Smith (2000). "Principles and Goals of Chiropractic Care". The Chiropractic Profession: Its Education, Practice, Research and Future Directions. NCMIC Group. p. 160. ISBN 1-892734-02-8.
- Chapman-Smith D (2000). "Current status of the profession". The Chiropractic Profession: Its Education, Practice, Research and Future Directions. West Des Moines, IA: NCMIC. ISBN 1-892734-02-8.
- Singh S, Ernst E (2008). "The truth about chiropractic therapy". Trick or Treatment: The Undeniable Facts about Alternative Medicine. W.W. Norton. pp. 145–90. ISBN 978-0-393-06661-6.
- Anderson M. D. Robert Anderson M. D.; Robert Anderson (October 2009). The Back Door to Medicine: An Embedded Anthropologist Tells All. iUniverse. pp. 59–. ISBN 978-1-4401-7289-2.
- Jonas, Wayne B. (1999). "Foreword – Chiropractic: the return of philosophy to medicine?". In Ian D. Coulter. Chiropractic: a philosophy for alternative health care. Elsevier Health Sciences. pp. ix–xii. ISBN 978-0-7506-4006-0.
- David Chapman-Smith (2000). The Chiropractic Profession: Its Education, Practice, Research and Future Directions. NCMIC Group. p. 160. ISBN 1-892734-02-8.
- WHO guidelines on basic training and safety in chiropractic, World Health Organization, Geneva, 2005. ISBN 92-4-159371-7. available online
- Keating JC Jr (2005). "A brief history of the chiropractic profession". In Haldeman S; Dagenais S; Budgell B; et al. Principles and Practice of Chiropractic (3rd ed.). McGraw-Hill. pp. 23–64. ISBN 0-07-137534-1.
- Robert Cooperstein, Brian J. Gleberzon. Technique systems in chiropractic. Elsevier Health Sciences, 2004, ISBN 0-443-07413-5, ISBN 978-0-443-07413-4.

Evolution of Alternative Medicine

The evolution of alternative medicine focuses on the history of alternative medicine and the progress it has made in the last few decades. The users of alternative medicine believe it has healing effects, but these claims have not been proved scientifically. The following chapter carefully analysis the evolution of alternative medicine and provides an extensive understanding of the subject.

History of Alternative Medicine

The history of alternative medicine refers to the history of a group of diverse medical practices that were collectively promoted as "alternative medicine" beginning in the 1970s, to the collection of individual histories of members of that group, or to the history of western medical practices that were labeled "irregular practices" by the western medical establishment. It includes the histories of complementary medicine and of integrative medicine. "Alternative medicine" is a loosely defined and very diverse set of products, practices, and theories that are perceived by its users to have the healing effects of medicine, but do not originate from evidence gathered using the scientific method, are not part of biomedicine, or are contradicted by scientific evidence or established science. "Biomedicine" is that part of medical science that applies principles of anatomy, physics, chemistry, biology, physiology, and other natural sciences to clinical practice, using scientific methods to establish the effectiveness of that practice.

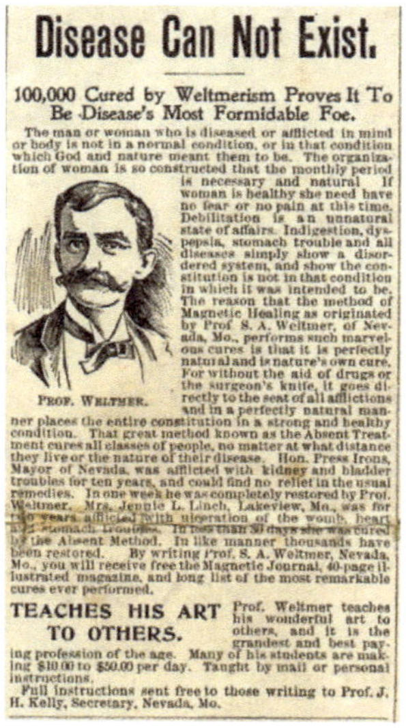

"Disease Can Not Exist", October 1899 advertisement in the *People's Home Journal* for Weltmerism, a form of "magnetic healing"

Much of what is now categorized as alternative medicine was developed as independent, complete medical systems, was developed long before biomedicine and use of scientific methods, and was developed in relatively isolated regions of the world where there was little or no medical contact with pre-scientific western medicine, or with each other's systems. Examples are Traditional Chinese medicine and the Ayurvedic medicine of India. Other alternative medicine practices, such as homeopathy, were developed in western Europe and in opposition to western medicine, at a time when western medicine was based on unscientific theories that were dogmatically imposed by western religious authorities. Homeopathy was developed prior to discovery of the basic principles of chemistry, which proved homeopathic remedies contained nothing but water. But homeopathy, with its remedies made of water, was harmless compared to the unscientific and dangerous orthodox western medicine practiced at that time, which included use of toxins and draining of blood, often resulting in permanent disfigurement or death. Other alternative practices such as chiropractic and osteopathic manipulative medicine, were developed in the United States at a time that western medicine was beginning to incorporate scientific methods and theories, but the biomedical model was not yet totally dominant. Practices such as chiropractic and osteopathic, each considered to be irregular by the medical establishment, also opposed each other, both rhetorically and politically with licensing legislation. Osteopathic practitioners added the courses and training of biomedicine to their licensing, and licensed Doctor of Osteopathic Medicine holders began diminishing use of the unscientific origins of the field, and without the original practices and theories, is now considered the same as biomedicine.

Until the 1970s, western practitioners that were not part of the medical establishment were referred to "irregular practitioners", and were dismissed by the medical establishment as unscientific or quackery. Irregular practice became increasingly marginalized as quackery and fraud, as western medicine increasingly incorporated scientific methods and discoveries, and had a corresponding increase in success of its treatments. In the 1970s, irregular practices were grouped with traditional practices of nonwestern cultures and with other unproven or disproven practices that were not part of biomedicine, with the group promoted as being "alternative medicine". Following the counterculture movement of the 1960s, misleading marketing campaigns promoting "alternative medicine" as being an effective "alternative" to biomedicine, and with changing social attitudes about not using chemicals, challenging the establishment and authority of any kind, sensitivity to giving equal measure to values and beliefs of other cultures and their practices through cultural relativism, adding postmodernism and deconstructivism to ways of thinking about science and its deficiencies, and with growing frustration and desperation by patients about limitations and side effects of science-based medicine, use of alternative medicine in the west began to rise, then had explosive growth beginning in the 1990s, when senior level political figures began promoting alternative medicine, and began diverting government medical research funds into research of alternative, complementary, and integrative medicine.

Alternative Medicine

The concept of alternative medicine is problematic as it cannot exist autonomously as an object of study in its own right but must always be defined in relation to a non-static and transient medical orthodoxy. It also divides medicine into two realms, a medical mainstream and fringe, which, in privileging orthodoxy, presents difficulties in constructing an historical analysis independent of the often biased and polemical views of regular medical practitioners. The description of non-conventional medicine as alternative reinforces both its marginality and the centrality of official medicine. Although more neutral than either pejorative or promotional designations such as "quackery" or "natural medicine", cognate terms like "unconventional", "heterodox", "unofficial", "irregular", "folk", "popular", "marginal", "complementary", "integrative" or "unorthodox" define their object against the standard of conventional biomedicine, entail particular perspectives and judgements, often carry moral overtones, and can be inaccurate. Conventional medical practitioners in the West have, since the nineteenth century, used some of these and similar terms as a means of defining the boundary of "legitimate" medicine, marking the division between that which is scientific and that which is not. The definition of mainstream medicine, generally understood to refer to a system of licensed medicine which enjoys state and legal protection in a jurisdiction, is also highly specific to time and place. In countries such as India and China traditional systems of medicine, in conjunction with Western biomedical science, may be considered conventional and mainstream. The shifting nature of these terms is underlined by recent efforts to demarcate between alternative treatments on the basis of efficacy and safety and to amalgamate those therapies with scientifically adjudged value into complementary medicine as a pluralistic adjunct to conventional practice. This would introduce a new line of division based upon medical validity.

Before The "Fringe"

"Marriage à la Mode, Plate 3, (The Scene with the Quack)" by William Hogarth, 1745

Prior to the nineteenth century European medical training and practice was ostensibly self-regulated through a variety of antique corporations, guilds or colleges. Among regular practitioners, university trained physicians formed a medical elite while provincial surgeons and apothecaries, who learnt their art through apprenticeship, made up the lesser ranks. In Old Regime France, licenses for medical practitioners were granted by the medical faculties of the major universities, such as the Paris Faculty of Medicine. Access was restricted and successful candidates, amongst other requirements, had to pass examinations and pay regular fees. In the Austrian Empire medical licences were granted by the Universities of Prague and Vienna. Amongst the German states the top physicians were academically qualified and typically attached to medical colleges associated with the royal court. The theories and practices included the science of anatomy and that the blood circulated by a pumping heart, and contained some empirically gained information on progression of disease and about surgery, but were otherwise unscientific, and were almost entirely ineffective and dangerous.

Outside of these formal medical structures there were myriad other medical practitioners, often termed irregulars, plying a range of services and goods. The eighteenth-century medical marketplace, a period often referred to as the "Golden Age of quackery", was a highly pluralistic one that lacked a well-defined and policed division between "conventional" and "unconventional" medical practitioners. In much of continental Europe legal remedies served to control at least the most egregious forms of "irregular" medical practice but the medical market in both Britain and American was less restrained through regulation. Quackery in the period prior to modern medical professionalisation should not be considered equivalent to alternative medicine as those commonly deemed quacks were not peripheral figures by default nor did they necessarily promote oppositional and alternative medical systems. Indeed, the charge of 'quackery', which might allege medical incompetence, avarice or fraud, was levelled quite indiscriminately across the varied classes of medical practitioners be they regular medics, such as the hierarchical, corporate classes of physicians, surgeons and apothecaries in England, or irregulars such as nostrum mongers, bonesetters and local wise-women. Commonly, however, quackery was associated with a growing medical entrepreneurship amongst both regular and irregular practitioners in the provision of goods and services along with associated techniques of advertisement and self-promotion in the medical marketplace. The constituent features of the medical marketplace during the eighteenth century were the development of medical consumerism and a high degree of patient power and choice in the selection of treatments, the limited efficacy of available medical therapies, and the absence of both medical professionalisation and enforced regulation of the market.

Medical Professionalisation

In the late eighteenth and nineteenth centuries regular and irregular medical practitioners became more clearly differentiated throughout much of Europe. In part, this was achieved through processes of state-sanctioned medical regulation. The different types of regulatory medical markets created across nineteenth-century Europe and America reflected differing historical patterns of state formation. Where states had traditionally enjoyed strong, centralised power, such as in the German states, government more easily assumed control of the medical regulation. In states that had exercised weaker central power and adopted a free-market model, such as in Britain, government gradually assumed greater control over medical regulation as part of increasing state focus on issues of public health. This process was significantly complicated in Britain by the enduring existence of the historical medical colleges. A similar process is observable in America from the 1870s but this was facilitated by the absence of medical corporations. Throughout the nineteenth century, however, most Western states converged in the creation of legally delimited and semi-protected medical markets. It is at this point that an "official" medicine, created in cooperation with the state and employing a scientific rhetoric of legitimacy, emerges as a recognisable entity and that the concept of alternative medicine as a historical category becomes tenable.

France provides perhaps one of the earliest examples of the emergence of a state-sanctioned medical orthodoxy – and hence also of the conditions for the development of forms of alternative medicine – the beginnings of which can be traced to the late eighteenth century. In addition to the traditional French medical faculties and the complex hierarchies of practitioners over which they presided, the state increasingly supported new institutions, such as the Société Royale de Médecine (*Royal Society of Medicine*) which received its royal charter in 1778, that played a role in policing medical practice and the sale of medical nostrums. This system was radically transformed during the early phases of the French Revolution when both the traditional faculties and the new institutions under royal sponsorship were removed and an entirely unregulated medical market was created. This anarchic situation was reformed under the exigencies of war when in 1793 the state established national control over medical education; under Napoleon in 1803 state-control was extended over the licensing of medical practitioners. This latter reform introduced a new hierarchical division between practitioners in the creation of a medical élite of graduate physicians and surgeons, who were at liberty to practice throughout the state, and the lowly *officiers de santé* who received less training, could only offer their services to the poor, and were restricted in where they could practice. This national system of medical regulation under state-control, exported to regions of Napoleonic conquest such as Italy, the Rhineland and the Netherlands, became paradigmatic in the West and in countries adopting western medical systems. While offering state protection to licensed doctors and establishing a medical monopoly in principal it did not, however, remove competition from irregular practitioners.

Nineteenth-century Non-conventional Medicine

From the late eighteenth century and more robustly from the mid-nineteenth century a number of non-conventional medical systems developed in the West which proposed oppositional medical systems, criticised orthodox medical practitioners, emphasised patient-centredness, and offered substitutes for the treatments offered by the medical mainstream. While neither the medical marketplace nor irregular practitioners disappeared during the nineteenth century, the proponents of alternative medical systems largely differed from the entrepreneurial quacks of the previous century in eschewing showy self-promotion and instead adopting a more sober and serious self-presentation. The relationship between medical orthodoxy and heterodoxy was complex, both categories contained considerably variety, were subject to substantial change throughout the period, and the divisions between the two were frequently blurred. The variety of alternative medical systems which developed during this period can be approximately categorised according to the form of treatment advocated. These were: those employing spiritual or psychological therapies, such as hypnosis (mesmerism); nutritional therapies based upon special diets, such as medical botanism; drug and biological therapies such as homeopathy and hydrotherapy; and, manipulative physical therapies such as osteopathy and chiropractic massage. Non-conventional medicine might define health in terms of concepts of balance and harmony or espouse vitalistic doctrines of the body. Illness could be understood as due to the accretion of bodily toxins and impurities, to result from magical, spiritual, or supernatural causes, or as arising from energy blockages in the body such that healing actions might constitute energy transfer from practitioner to patient.

Mesmerism

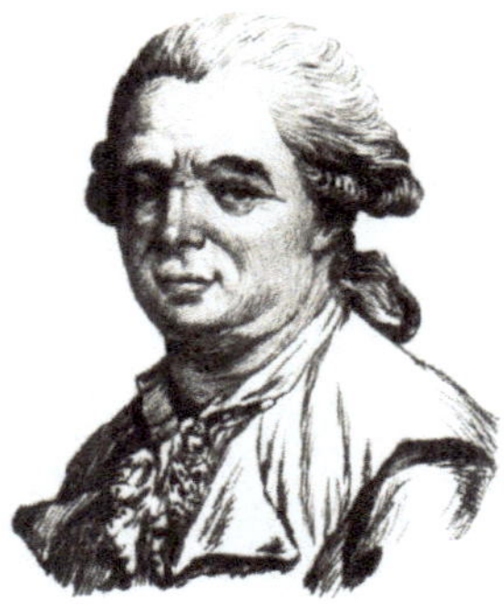

Franz Anton Mesmer (1734–1815)

Mesmerism is the medical system proposed in the late eighteenth century by the Viennese-trained physician, Franz Anton Mesmer (1734-1815), for whom it is named. The basis of this doctrine was Mesmer's claimed discovery of a new aetherial fluid, animal magnetism, which, he contended, permeated the universe and the bodies of all animate beings and whose proper balance was fundamental to health and disease. Animal magnetism was but one of series of postulated subtle fluids and substances, such as caloric, phlogiston, magnetism, and electricity, which then suffused the scientific literature. It also reflected Mesmer's doctoral thesis, *De Planatarum Influxu* ("On the Influence of the Planets"), which had investigated the impact of the gravitational effect of planetary movements on fluid-filled bodily tissues. His focus on magnetism and the therapeutic potential of magnets was derived from his reading of Paracelsus, Athanasius Kircher and Johannes Baptista van Helmont. The immediate impetus for his medical speculation, however, derived from his treatment of a patient, Franzisca Oesterlin, who suffered from episodic seizures and convulsions which induced vomiting, fainting, temporary blindness and paralysis. His cure consisted of placing magnets upon her body which consistently produced convulsive episodes and a subsequent diminution of symptoms. According to Mesmer, the logic of this cure suggested that health was dependent upon the uninterrupted flow of a putative magnetic fluid and that ill health was consequent to its blockage. His treatment methods claimed to resolve this by either directly transferring his own superabundant and naturally occurring animal magnetism to his patients by touch or through the transmission of these energies from magnetic objects.

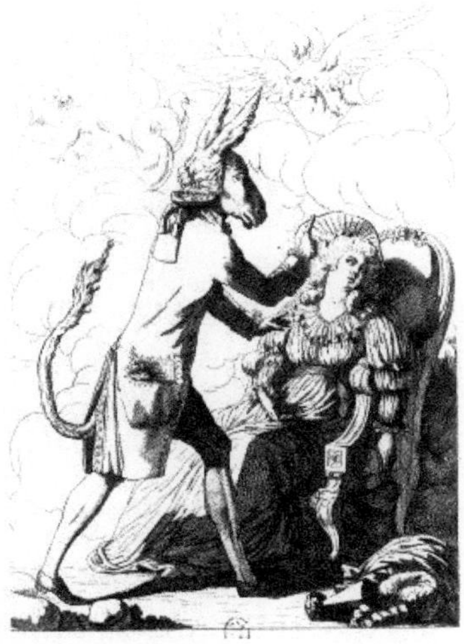

Caricature of a practitioner of animal magnetism treating a patient, *c.* 1780

By 1775 Mesmer's Austrian practice was prospering and he published the text *Schrieben über die Magnetkur an einen auswärtigen Arzt* which first outlined his thesis of animal magnetism. In 1778, however, he became embroiled in a scandal resulting from his treatment of a young, blind patient who was connected to the Viennese court and relocated to Paris where he established a medical salon, "The Society of Harmony", for the treatment of patients. Recruiting from a client-base drawn predominantly from society women of the middle- and upper-classes, Mesmer held group *séances* at his salubrious salon-clinic which was physically dominated by a large, lidded, wooden tank, known as the *baquet*, containing iron, glass and other material that Mesmer had magnetized and which was filled with "magnetized water". At these sessions patients were enjoined to take hold of the metal rods emanating from the tub which acted as a reservoir for the animal magnetism derived from Mesmer and his clients. Mesmer, through the apparent force of his will – not infrequently assisted by an intense gaze or the administration of his wand – would then direct these energies into the afflicted bodies of his patients seeking to provoke either a "crisis" or a trance-like state; outcomes which he believed essential for healing to occur. Patient proclamations of cure ensured that Mesmer enjoyed considerable and fashionable success in late-eighteenth-century Paris where he occasioned something of a sensation and a scandal.

Popular caricature of mesmerism emphasised the eroticised nature of the treatment as spectacle: "Here the physician in a coat of lilac or purple, on which the most brilliant flowers have been painted in needlework, speaks most consolingly to his patients: his arms softly enfolding her sustain her in her spasms, and his tender burning eye expresses his desire to comfort her". Responding chiefly to the hint of sexual impropriety and political radicalism imbuing these *séances*, in 1784 mesmerism was subject to a commission of inquiry by a royal-appointed scientific panel of the prestigious French Académie de Médicine. Its findings were that animal magnetism had no basis in fact and that Mesmer's cures had been achieved through the power of suggestion. The commission's report, if damaging to the personal status of Mesmer and to the professional ambitions of those faculty physicians who had adopted mesmeric practices, did little to hinder the diffusion of the doctrine of animal magnetism.

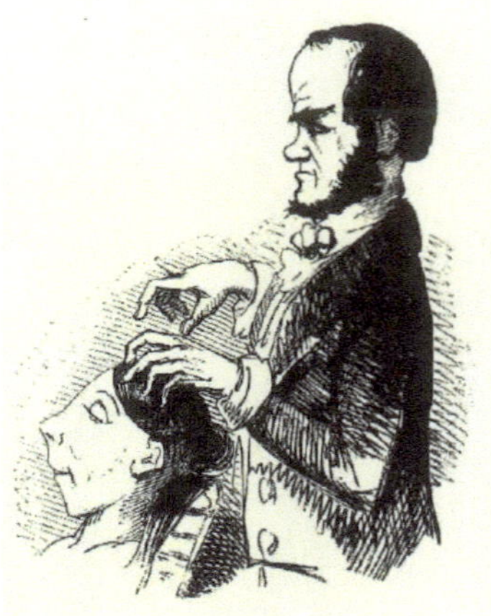

1843 *Punch* magazine caricature depicting John Elliotson "playing the brain" of a working-class, mesmerised woman

In England mesmerism was championed by John Elliotson, Professor of Practical Medicine at University College London and the founder and president of the London Phrenological Society. A prominent and progressive orthodox physician, he was President of the Medico-Chirugical Society of London and an early adopter of the stethoscope in English medical practice. He had been introduced to mesmerism in the summer of 1837 by the French physician and former student of Mesmer, Dupotet, who is credited as the most significant cross-channel influence on the development of mesmerism in England. Elliotson believed that animal magnetism provided the basis for a consideration of the mind and will in material terms thus allowing for their study as medical objects. Initially supported by the *Lancet*, a reformist medical journal, he contrived to demonstrate the scientific properties of animal magnetism as a physiological process on the predominantly female charity patients under his care in the University College Hospital. Working-class patients were preferred as experimental subjects to exhibit the physical properties of mesmerism on the nervous system as, being purportedly more animalistic and machine-like than their social superiors, their personal characteristics were deemed less likely to interfere with the experimental process. He sought to reduce his subjects to the status of mechanical automata claiming that he could, through the properties of animal magnetism and the pacifying altered states of consciousness which it induced, "play" their brains as if they were musical instruments.

Two Irish-born charity patients, the adolescent O'Key sisters, emerged as particularly important to Elliotson's increasingly popular and public demonstrations of mesmeric treatment. Initially, his magnetising practices were used to treat the sisters' shared diagnosis of hysteria and epilepsy in controlling or curtailing their convulsive episodes. By the autumn of 1837 Elliotson had ceased to treat the O'Keys merely as suitable objects for cure and instead sought to mobilise them as diagnostic instruments. When in states of mesmeric entrancement the O'Key sisters, due to the apparent increased sensitization of their nervous system and sensory apparatus, behaved as if they had the ability to see through solid objects, including the human body, and thus aid in medical diagnosis. As their fame rivalled that of Elliotson, however, the O'Keys behaved less like human diagnostic machines and became increasingly intransigent to medical authority and appropriated to themselves the power to examine, diagnose, prescribe treatment and provide a prognosis. The emergence of this threat to medical mastery in the form of a pair of working-class, teenage girls without medical training aroused general disquiet amongst the medical establishment and cost Elliotson one of his early and influential supporters, the leading proponent of medical reform, Thomas Wakley. Wakley, the editor of the *Lancet*, had initially hoped that Elliotson's scientific experiments with animal magnetism might further the agenda of medical reform in bolstering the authority of the profession through the production of scientific truth and, equally importantly in a period when the power-relations between doctors and patients were being redefined, quiescent patient bodies. Perturbed by the O'Key's provocative displays, Wakely convinced Elliotson to submit his mesmeric practice to a trial in August 1838 before a jury of ten gentlemen during which he accused the sisters of fraud and his colleague of gullibility. Following a series of complaints issued to the Medical Committee of University College Hospital they elected to discharge the O'Keys along with other mesmeric subjects in the hospital and Elliotson resigned his post in protest.

This set-back, while excluding Elliotson from the medical establishment, ended neither his mesmeric career nor the career of mesmerism in England. From 1842 he became an advocate of phreno-mesmerism – an approach that amalgamated the tenets of phrenology with animal magnetism and that led to a split in the Phrenological Society. The following year he founded, together with the physician and then President of the Phrenological Society, William Collins Engledue, the principal journal on animal magnetism entitled the *The Zoist: A Journal of Cerebral Physiology and Mesmerism and their Application to Human Welfare*, a quarterly publication which remained in print until its fifty-second issue in January 1856. Mesmeric societies, frequently patronised by those among the scientific and social elite were established in many major population centres in Britain from the 1840s onwards. Some sufficiently endowed societies, such as those in London, Bristol and Dublin, Ireland, supported mesmeric infirmaries with permanent mesmeric practitioners in their employ. Due to the competing rise of spiritualism and psychic research by the mid-1860s these mesmeric infirmaries had closed.

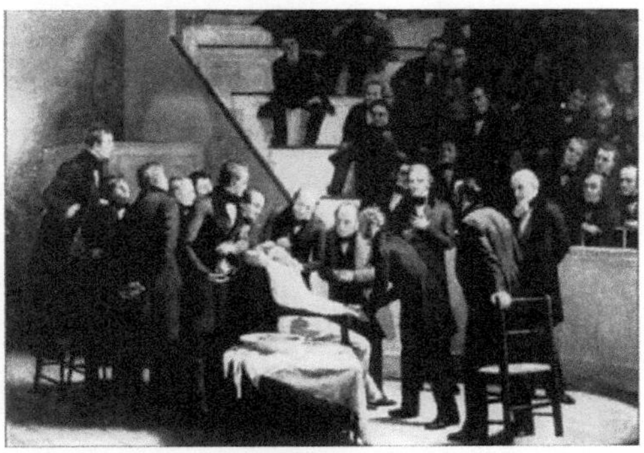

The First Operation under Ether, painted by Robert Hinckley 1881-96. This operation on the jaw of a female patient took place in Boston on 19 October 1846. William Morton acted as the anaesthetist and John Morrow was the surgeon

The 1840s in Britain also witnessed a deluge of travelling magnetisers who put on public shows for paying audiences to demonstrate their craft. These mesmeric theatres, intended in part as a means of soliciting profitable private clientele, functioned as public fora for debate between skeptics and believers as to whether the performances were genuine or constituted fraud. In order to establish that the loss of sensation under mesmeric trance was real, these itinerant mesmerists indulged in often quite violent methods – including discharging firearms close to the ears of mesmerised subjects, pricking them with needles, putting acid on their skin and knives beneath their fingernails.

Such displays of the anaesthetic qualities of mesmerism inspired some medical practitioners to attempt surgery on subjects under the spell of magnetism. In France, the first major operation of this kind had been trialled, apparently successfully, as early as 1828 during a mastectomy procedure. In Britain the first significant surgical procedure undertaken on a patient while mesmerised occurred in 1842 when James Wombell, a labourer from Nottingham, had his leg amputated. Having been mesmerised for several days prior to the operation by a barrister named William Topham, Wombell exhibited no signs of pain during the operation and reported afterwards that the surgery had been painless. This account was disputed by many in the medical establishment who held that Wombell had fraudulently concealed the pain of the amputation both during and after the procedure. Undeterred, in 1843 Elliotson continued to advocate for the use of animal magnetism in surgery publishing *Numerous Cases of Surgical Operation without Pain in the Mesmeric State*. This marked the beginning of a campaign by London mesmerists to gain a foothold for the practice within British hospitals by convincing both doctors and the general public of the value of surgical mesmerism. Mesmeric surgery enjoyed considerable success in the years from 1842 to 1846 and colonial India emerged as a particular stronghold of the practice; word of its success was propagated in Britain through the *Zoist* and the publication in 1846 of *Mesmerism in India and its Practical Application in Surgery and Medicine* by James Esdaile, a Scottish surgeon with the East India Company and the chief proponent of animal magnetism in the subcontinent.

Although a few surgeons and dentists had undertaken fitful experiments with anaesthetic substances in the preceding years, it was only in 1846 that use of ether in surgery was popularised amongst orthodox medical practitioners. This was despite the fact that the desensitising effects of widely available chemicals like ether and nitrous oxide were commonly known and had formed part of public and scientific displays over the previous half-century.

A feature of the dissemination of magnetism in the New World was its increasing association with spiritualism. By the 1830s mesmerism was making headway in the United States amongst figures like the intellectual progenitor of the New Thought movement, Phineas Parkhurst Quimby, whose treatment combined verbal suggestion with touch. Quimby's most celebrated "disciple", Mary Baker Eddy, would go on to found the "medico-religious hybrid", Christian Science, in the latter half of the nineteenth century. In the 1840s the American spiritualist Andrew Jackson Davis sought to combine animal magnetism with spiritual beliefs and postulated that bodily health was dependent upon the unobstructed movement of the "spirit", conceived as a fluid substance, throughout the body. As with Quimby, Davis's healing practice involved the use of touch.

Osteopathy and Chiropractic Manipulation

Deriving from the tradition of 'bone-setting' and a belief in the flow of supernatural energies in the body (vitalism), both osteopathy and chiropractic developed in the USA in the late 19th century. The British School of Osteopathy was established in 1917 but it was the 1960s before the first chiropractic college was established in the UK. Chiropractic theories and methods (which are concerned with subluxations or small displacements of the spine and other joints) do not accord with orthodox medicine's current knowledge of the biomechanics of the spine. in addition to teaching osteopathic manipulative medicine (OMM) and theory, osteopathic colleges in the US gradually came to have the same courses and requirements as biomedical schools, whereby osteopathic doctors (ODs) who did practice OMM were considered to be practicing conventional biomedicine in the USA. The passing of the Osteopaths Act (1993) and the Chiropractors Act (1994), however, created for the first time autonomous statutory regulation for two CAM therapies in the UK.

History of Chiropractic

Chiropractic began in the United States in 1895. when Daniel David Palmer performed the first chiropractic adjustment on a partially deaf janitor, who then claimed he could hear better as a result of the manipulation. Palmer opened a school of chiropractic two years later. Chiropractic's early philosophy was rooted in vitalism, naturalism, magnetism, spiritualism and other unscientific constructs. Palmer claimed to merge science and metaphysics. Palmer's first descriptions and underlying philosophy of chiropractic described the body as a "machine" whose parts could be manipulated to produce a drugless cure, that spinal manipulation could improve health, and that the effects of chiropractic spinal manipulation as being mediated primarily by the nervous system.

Despite their similarities, osteopathic practitioners sought to differentiate themselves by seeking regulation of the practices. In a 1907 test of the new law, a Wisconsin based chiropractor was charged with practicing osteopathic medicine without a license. Practicing medicine without a license led to many chiropractors, including D.D. Palmer, being jailed. Chiropractors won their first test case, but prosecutions instigated by state medical boards became increasingly common and successful. Chiropractors responded with political campaigns for separate licensing statutes, from osteopaths, eventually succeeding in all fifty states, from Kansas in 1913 through Louisiana in 1974.

Divisions developed within the chiropractic profession, with "mixers" combining spinal adjustments with other treatments, and "straights" relying solely on spinal adjustments. A conference sponsored by the National Institutes of Health in 1975 spurred the development of chiropractic research. In 1987, the American Medical Association called chiropractic an "unscientific cult" and boycotted it until losing a 1987 antitrust case.

Histories of Individual Traditional Medical Systems

Ayurvedic Medicine

Ayurveda or ayurvedic medicine has more than 5,000 years of history, now re-emerging as texts become increasingly accessible in modern English translations. These texts attempt to translate the Sanskrit versions that have remained hidden in India since British occupation from 1755-1947. As modern archaeological evidence from Harappa and Mohenja-daro is distributed, Ayurveda has now been accepted as the world's oldest concept of health and disease discovered by man and the oldest continuously practiced system of medicine. Ayurveda is a world view that advocates man's allegiance and surrender to the forces of Nature that are increasingly revealed in modern physics, chemistry and biology. It is based on an interpretation of disease and health that parallels the forces of nature, observing the sun's fire and making analogies to the fires of the body; observing the flows in Nature and describing flows in the body, terming the principle as Vata; observing the transformations in Nature and describing transformations in the body, terming the principle as

Pitta; and observing the stability in Nature and describing stability in the body, terming the principle as Kapha.

Ayurveda can be defined as the system of medicine described in the great medical encyclopedias associated with the names Caraka, Suśruta, and Bhe□a, compiled and re-edited over several centuries from about 200 BCE to about 500 CE and written in Sanskrit. These discursive writings were gathered and systematized in about 600 CE by Vāgbha□a, to produce the *A□□ā□gah□dayasa□hitā* ('Heart of Medicine Compendium') that became the most popular and widely used textbook of ayurvedic medicine in history. Vāgbha□a›s work was translated into many other languages and became influential throughout Asia.

Its prehistory goes back to Vedic culture and its proliferation in written form flourished in Buddhist times. Although the hymns of the Atharvaveda and the □gveda mention some herbal medicines, protective amulets, and healing prayers that recur in the ciphered slokas of later ayurvedic treatises, the earliest historical mention of the main structural and theoretical categories of ayurvedic medicine occurs in the Buddhist Pāli Tripi□aka, or Canon.

Ayurveda originally derived from the Vedas, as the name suggests, and was first organized and captured in Sanskrit in ciphered form by physicians teaching their students judicious practice of healing. These ciphers are termed slokas and are purposefully designed to include several meanings, to be interpreted appropriately, known as 'tantra yukti' by the knowledgeable practitioner. Ayu means longevity or healthy life, and veda means human-interpreted and observable truths and provable science. The principles of Ayurveda include systematic means for allowing evidence, including truth by observation and experimentation, pratyaksha; attention to teachers with sufficient experience, aptoupadesha; analogy to things seen in Nature, anumana; and logical argument, yukti.

It was founded on several principles, including yama (time) and niyama (self-regulation) and placed emphasis on routines and adherence to cycles, as seen in Nature. For example, it directs that habits should be regulated to coincide with the demands of the body rather than the whimsical mind or evolving and changing nature of human intelligence. Thus, for the follower of ayurvedic medicine, food should only be taken when they are instinctively hungry rather than at an arbitrarily set meal-time. Ayurveda also teaches that when a person is tired, it is not wise to eat food or drink, but to rest, as the body's fire is low and must gather energy in order to alight the enzymes that are required to digest food. The same principles of regulated living, called Dinacharya, direct that work is the justification for rest and in order to get sufficient sleep, one should subject the body to rigorous exercise. Periodic fasting, or abstaining from all food and drink for short durations of one or two days helps regulate the elimination process and prevents illness. It is only in later years that practitioners of this system saw that people were not paying for their services, and in order to get their clients to pay, they introduced herbal remedies to begin with and later even started using metals and inorganic chemical compositions in the form of pills or potions to deal with symptoms.

Emigration from the Indian sub-continent in the 1850s brought practitioners of Ayurveda ('Science of Life'). a medical system dating back over 2,500 years, its adoption outside the Asian communities was limited by its lack of specific exportable skills and English-language reference books until adapted and modernised forms, New Age Ayurveda and Maharishi Ayurveda, came under the umbrella of CAM in the 1970s to Europe. In Britain, Unani practitioners are known as hakims and

Ayurvedic practitioners are known as vaidyas. Having its origins in the Ayurveda, Indian Naturopathy incorporates a variety of holistic practices and natural remedies and became increasingly popular after the arrival of the post-Second World War wave of Indian immigrants. The Persian work for Greek,Unani medicines uses some similar materials as Ayurveda but are based on philosophy closer to Greek and Arab sources than to Ayurveda. Exiles fleeing the war between Yemen and Aden in the 1960s settled nearby the ports of Cardiff and Liverpool and today practitioners of this Middle Eastern medicine are known as vaids..

In the USA, Ayurveda has increased popularity since the 1990s, as Indian-Americans move into the mainstream media, and celebrities visit India more frequently. In addition, many Americans go to India for medical tourism to avail of reputed Ayurvedic medical centers that are licensed and credentialed by the Indian government and widely legitimate as a medical option for chronic medical conditions. AAPNA, the Association of Ayurvedic Professionals of North America, www.aapna.org, has over 600 medical professional members, including trained vaidyas from accredited schools in India credentialed by the Indian government, who are now working as health counselors and holistic practitioners in the USA. There are over 40 schools of Ayurveda throughout the USA, providing registered post-secondary education and operating mostly as private ventures outside the legitimized medical system, as there is no approval system yet in the US Dept of Education. Practitioners graduating from these schools and arriving with credentials from India practice legally through the Health Freedom Act, legalized in 13 states. Credentialing and a uniform standard of education is being developed by the international CAC, Council of Ayurvedic Credentialing, www.cayurvedac.com, in consideration of the licensed programs in Ayurveda operated under the Government of India's Ministry of Health and Family Welfare, Dept of AYUSH. In India, there are over 600,000 practicing physicians of Ayurveda. Ayurveda is a legal and legitimate medical system in many countries of South Asia.

Chinese Culture

Traditional Chinese medicine has more than 4,000 years of history as a system of medicine that is based on a philosophical concept of balance (yin and yang, Qi, Blood, Jing, Bodily fluids, the Five Elements, the emotions, and the spirit) approach to health that is rooted in Taoist philosophy and Chinese culture. As such, the concept of it as an alternative form of therapeutic practise is only found in the Western world.

The arrival into Britain of thousands of Chinese in the 1970s introduced Traditional Chinese Medicine – a system dating back to the Bronze Age or earlier that used acupuncture, herbs, diet and exercise. Today there are more than 2,000 registered practitioners in the UK.

Since The 1970S

Until the 1970s, western practitioners that were not part of the medical establishment were referred to "irregular practitioners", and were dismissed by the medical establishment as unscientific or quackery. Irregular practice became increasingly marginalized as quackery and fraud, as western medicine increasingly incorporated scientific methods and discoveries, and had a corresponding increase in success of its treatments. In the 1970s, irregular practices were grouped with traditional practices of nonwestern cultures, and with other unproven or disproven practices that were not part of biomedicine, and the entire group began to be marketed and promoted as "alternative medicine". Following the counterculture movement of the 1960s, misleading marketing campaigns promoting "alternative medicine" as an effective "alternative" to biomedicine, and with changing social attitudes about not using chemicals, challenging the establishment and authority of any kind, sensitivity to giving equal measure to values and beliefs of other cultures and their practices through cultural relativism, adding postmodernism and deconstructivism to ways of thinking about science and its deficiencies, and with growing frustration and desperation by patients about limitations and side effects of science-based medicine, use of alternative medicine in the west began to rise, then had explosive growth beginning in the 1990s, when senior level political figures began promoting alternative medicine, and began diverting government medical research funds into research of alternative, complementary, and integrative medicine.

1970S Through 1980S

1990S to Present

In 1991, after United States Senator Thomas Harkin became convinced his allergies were cured by taking bee pollen pills, he used $2 million of his discretionary funds to create the Office of Alternative Medicine (OAM), to test the efficacy of alternative medicine and alert the public as the results of testing its efficacy. The OAM mission statement was that it was "dedicated to exploring complementary and alternative healing practices in the context of rigorous science; training complementary and alternative medicine researchers; and disseminating authoritative information to the public and professionals." Joseph M. Jacobs was appointed the first director of the OAM in 1992. Jacobs' insistence on rigorous scientific methodology caused friction with Senator Harkin. Harkin criticized the "unbendable rules of randomized clinical trials" and, citing his use of bee pollen to treat his allergies, stated: "It is not necessary for the scientific community to understand the process before the American public can benefit from these therapies." Increasing political resistance to the use of scientific methodology was publicly criticized by Dr. Jacobs and another OAM board member complained that "nonsense has trickled down to every aspect of this office". In 1994, Senator Harkin responded by appearing on television with cancer patients who blamed Dr. Jacobs for blocking their access to untested cancer treatment, leading Jacobs to resign in frustration. The OAM drew increasing criticism from eminent members of the scientific community, from a Nobel laureate criticizing the degrading parts of the NIH to the level a cover for quackery, and the president of the American Physical Society criticizing spending on testing practices that "violate basic laws of physics and more clearly resemble witchcraft". In 1998, the President of the North Carolina Medical Association publicly called for shutting down the OAM. The NIH Director placed the OAM under more strict scientific NIH control.

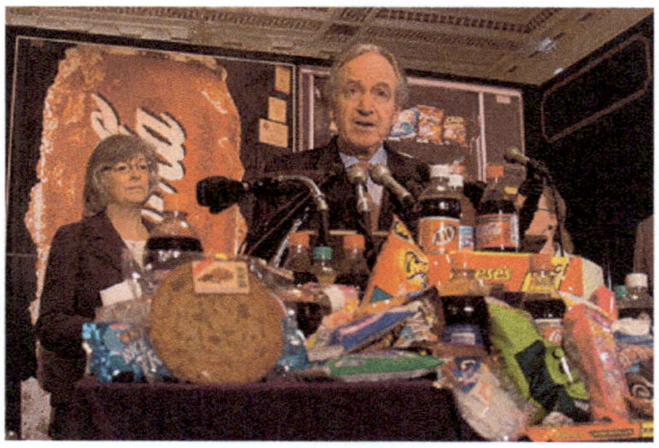

Sen. Tom Harkin at a press conference.

In 1998, Sen. Harkin responded to the criticism and stricter scientific controls by the NIH, by raising the OAM to the level of an independent center, increasing its budget to $90 million annually, and renaming it to be the National Center for Complementary and Alternative Medicine (NCCAM). The United States Congress approved the appropriations without dissent. NCCAM had a mandate to promote a more rigorous and scientific approach to the study of alternative medicine, research training and career development, outreach, and integration. In 2014 the agency was renamed to the National Center for Complementary and Integrative Health (NCCIH). The NCCIH charter requires that 12 of the 18 council members shall be selected with a preference to selecting leading representatives of complementary and alternative medicine, 9 of the members must be licensed practitioners of alternative medicine, 6 members must be general public leaders in the fields of public policy, law, health policy, economics, and management, and 3 members must represent the interests of individual consumers of complementary and alternative medicine.

By 2009, the NCCIH budget had grown from annual spending of about $2 million at its inception, to $123 million annually. In 2009, after a history of 17 years of government testing produced almost no clearly proven efficacy of alternative therapies, Senator Harkin complained, "One of the purposes of this center was to investigate and validate alternative approaches. Quite frankly, I must say publicly that it has fallen short. It think quite frankly that in this center and in the office previously before it, most of its focus has been on disproving things rather than seeking out and approving." Members of the scientific and biomedical communities complained that after a history of 17 years of being tested, at a cost of over $2.5 Billion on testing scientifically and biologically implausible practices, almost no alternative therapy showed clear efficacy.

From 1990 to 1997, use of alternative medicine in the US increased by 25%, with a corresponding 50% increase in expenditures. By 2013, 50% of Americans were using alternative medicine, and annual spending on CAM in the US was $34 Billion.

Other Periods

The terms 'alternative' and 'complementary' tend to be used interchangeably to describe a wide diversity of therapies that attempt to use the self-healing powers of the body by amplifying natural recuperative processes to restore health. In ancient Greece the Hippocratic movement, commonly regarded as the fathers of medicine, actually gave rise to modern naturopathy and indeed much of today's CAM. They placed great emphasis on a good diet and healthy lifestyle to restore equilibrium; drugs were used more to support healing than to cure disease.

Complementary medicines have evolved through history and become formalised from primitive practices; although many were developed during the 19th century as alternatives to the sometimes harmful practices of the time, such as blood-lettings and purgation. In the UK, the medical divide between CAM and conventional medicine has been characterised by conflict, intolerance and prejudice on both sides and during the early 20th century CAM was virtually outlawed in Britain: healers were seen as freaks and hypnotherapists were subject to repeated attempts at legal restriction. The alternative health movement is now accepted as part of modern life, having progressed from a grass-roots revival in the 1960s reacting against environmental degradation, unhealthy diets and rampant consumerism.

Until the arrival of the Romans in AD43, medical practices were limited to a basic use of plant materials, prayers and incantations. Having assimilated the corpus of Hippocrates, the Romans brought with them a vast reparatory of herbal treatments and introduced the concept of the hospital as a centralised treatment centre. In Britain, hydrotherapy (the use of water either internally or externally to maintain health and prevent disease) can be traced back to Roman spas. This was augmented by practices from the Far East and China introduced by traders using the Silk Road.

During the Catholic and Protestant witch-hunts from the 14th to the 17th centuries, the activities of traditional folk-healers were severely curtailed and knowledge was often lost as it existed only as an oral tradition. The widespread emigration from Europe to North America in the 18th and 19th centuries included both the knowledge of herbalism and some of the plants themselves. This was combined with Native American medicine and then re-imported to the UK where it re-integrated with the surviving herbal traditions to evolve as today's medical herbalism movement.

The natural law of similia similibus curantur, or 'like is cured by like', was recognised by Hippocrates but was only developed as a practical healing system in the early 19th century by a German, Dr Samuel Hahnemann. Homeopathy was brought to the UK in the 1830s by a Dr Quinn who introduced it to the British aristocracy, whose patronage continues to this day. Despite arousing controversy in conventional medical circles, homeopathy is available under the National Health Service, and in Scotland approximately 25% of GPs hold qualifications in homeopathy or have undergone some homeopathic training.

The impact on CAM of mass immigration into the UK is continuing into the 21st century. Originating in Japan, cryotherapy has been developed by Polish researchers into a system that claims to produce lasting relief from a variety of conditions such as rheumatism, psoriasis and muscle pain. Patients spend a few minutes in a chamber cooled to −110 °C, during which skin temperature drops some 12 °C.

The use of CAM is widespread and increasing across the developed world. The British are presented with a wide choice of treatments from the traditional to the innovative and technological. Section 60 of the Health Act 1999 allows for new health professions to be created by Order rather than primary legislation. This raises issues of public health policy which balance regulation, training, research, evidence-base and funding against freedom of choice in a culturally diverse societyThe term alternative medicine refers to systems of medical thought and practice which function as alternatives to or subsist outside of conventional, mainstream medicine. Alternative medicine cannot exist absent an established, authoritative and stable medical orthodoxy to which it can function as an alternative. Such orthodoxy was only established in the West during the nineteenth century through processes of regulation, association, institution building and systematised medical education.

Permissions

All chapters in this book are published with permission under the Creative Commons Attribution Share Alike License or equivalent. Every chapter published in this book has been scrutinized by our experts. Their significance has been extensively debated. The topics covered herein carry significant information for a comprehensive understanding. They may even be implemented as practical applications or may be referred to as a beginning point for further studies.

We would like to thank the editorial team for lending their expertise to make the book truly unique. They have played a crucial role in the development of this book. Without their invaluable contributions this book wouldn't have been possible. They have made vital efforts to compile up to date information on the varied aspects of this subject to make this book a valuable addition to the collection of many professionals and students.

This book was conceptualized with the vision of imparting up-to-date and integrated information in this field. To ensure the same, a matchless editorial board was set up. Every individual on the board went through rigorous rounds of assessment to prove their worth. After which they invested a large part of their time researching and compiling the most relevant data for our readers.

The editorial board has been involved in producing this book since its inception. They have spent rigorous hours researching and exploring the diverse topics which have resulted in the successful publishing of this book. They have passed on their knowledge of decades through this book. To expedite this challenging task, the publisher supported the team at every step. A small team of assistant editors was also appointed to further simplify the editing procedure and attain best results for the readers.

Apart from the editorial board, the designing team has also invested a significant amount of their time in understanding the subject and creating the most relevant covers. They scrutinized every image to scout for the most suitable representation of the subject and create an appropriate cover for the book.

The publishing team has been an ardent support to the editorial, designing and production team. Their endless efforts to recruit the best for this project, has resulted in the accomplishment of this book. They are a veteran in the field of academics and their pool of knowledge is as vast as their experience in printing. Their expertise and guidance has proved useful at every step. Their uncompromising quality standards have made this book an exceptional effort. Their encouragement from time to time has been an inspiration for everyone.

The publisher and the editorial board hope that this book will prove to be a valuable piece of knowledge for students, practitioners and scholars across the globe.

Index